# Tenth Edition

## An Outline of
# PSYCHIATRY
● ● ● ● ● ● ● ●

**Clarence J. Rowe, M.D.**
Clinical Professor of Psychiatry Emeritus
University of Minnesota Medical School
Minneapolis, Minnesota

Chief, Medical Staff
The Wilson Center
Faribault, Minnesota

**Walter D. Mink, Ph.D.**
Professor of Psychology
Macalester College
Saint Paul, Minnesota

**WCB Brown & Benchmark**
P U B L I S H E R S

Madison, Wisconsin•Dubuque, Iowa•Indianapolis, Indiana
Melbourne, Australia•Oxford, England

## Book Team

Editor *Michael Lange*
Developmental Editor *Sheralee Connors*
Production Editor *Audrey A. Reiter*

A Division of Wm. C. Brown Communications, Inc.

Vice President and General Manager *Thomas E. Doran*
Editor in Chief *Edgar J. Laube*
Executive Editor *Ed Bartell*
Executive Editor *Stan Stoga*
National Sales Manager *Eric Ziegler*
Director of Course Resource *Kathy Law Laube*
Director of Course Systems *Chris Rogers*
Director of Marketing *Sue Simons*
Director of Production *Vickie Putman Caughron*
Marketing Manager *Carla J. Aspelmeier*
Advertising Manager *Jodi Rymer*
Imaging Group Manager *Chuck Carpenter*
Manager of Visuals and Design *Faye M. Schilling*
Permissions/Records Manager *Connie Allendorf*

## Wm. C. Brown Communications, Inc.

Chairman Emeritus *Wm. C. Brown*
Chairman and Chief Executive Officer *Mark C. Falb*
President and Chief Operating Officer *G. Franklin Lewis*
Corporate Vice President, President of WCB Manufacturing *Roger Meyer*

Cover design by Kay D. Fulton

Copyedited by Joan Torkildson

Library of Congress Catalog Card Number: 91–077551

ISBN 0–697–10490–7

Printed in the United States of America by Wm. C. Brown Communications, Inc.,
2460 Kerper Boulevard, Dubuque, IA 52001

10  9  8  7  6  5  4  3  2  1

# Contents

# Preface to the Tenth Edition

This tenth edition of the *Outline* marks nearly four decades that it has been in print. It was originally intended for courses in entry-level psychiatry, which the senior author had taught to students of nursing, occupational therapy, physical therapy, and some other ancillary medical sciences. In an era when understandable psychiatric texts were scarce, it was an attempt to render, in outline form, a basic knowledge of dynamic and descriptive psychiatry. It was never intended to take the place of a textbook.

Subsequent editions seemed to meet the needs of other groups including medical students, social workers, psychologists, and pastoral counselors.

Beginning with the fourth edition, Walter D. Mink, Ph.D., and his wife, the late Shirley Holt Mink, Ph.D., became collaborators. This continued an association that began when all three of us were colleagues in the Department of Psychiatry at the University of Minnesota and continued into a subsequent private practice relationship.

When the early editions were published, the *Diagnostic and Statistical Manual of Mental Disorders* (*DSM*-I) (1952) was a first attempt by the American Psychiatric Association to develop a uniform classification of mental disorder. *DSM*-II appeared in 1968, followed by *DSM*-III in 1980, which proposed clear descriptions of diagnostic categories. Generally, with some exceptions, it attempted to describe *what* was wrong in mental disorders rather than *how* the disturbances came about.

*DSM*-III-R, a revision, appeared in 1987 and serves as a guide for the present edition (*DSM*-IV is expected in 1993).

Psychiatry has changed significantly in the approximately forty years that have elapsed since the first edition was introduced. We have tried to reflect these changes as we developed subsequent editions—based on our clinical experience in teaching, consulting, and practice. A major change over the years was in the focus of psychiatry from a psychodynamic to an increasingly more biological perspective. However, our continued interest in the field, including our periodic revision of the Outline, still leaves us with a comfortable belief in the validity and usefulness of maintaining a psychodynamic perspective in a more inclusive biopsychosocial approach to our field.

We want to express our gratitude to Ms. Mary Sandra Tarman and her staff at the Boeckman Medical Library, St. Paul, for unending assistance in furnishing us with library materials. To Mrs. Patricia Huiras for seemingly limitless assistance in shepherding the manuscript through all of its phases, to Ms. Ann Shaffer, Audrey Reiter, and other members of the Brown & Benchmark staff for patience and direction and to Jean Jagger-Rowe for researching many of the quotations.

We also wish to thank the following individuals for contributing their insights as reviewers of the Tenth Edition: James Colson, Western New Mexico University; Priscilla Kehoe, Trinity College; Kevin Krycka, Seattle University; William Martin, Lander College; Linda Marks, University of Texas; Marc Oster, Alfred Adler Institute; Ralph Pifer, Sauk Valley College; Laurie Rotando, Westchester Community College; Maureen Travis, St. Joseph College; and Karen Wolford, SUNY-Oswego.

A special acknowledgement to Burtrum C. Schiele, M.D. who served as a critical support in the senior author's embryonic writing efforts!

Clarence J. Rowe
Walter D. Mink

# 1 History

Nor deem the irrevocable past as wholly wasted, wholly vain.
If rising, on its neck at last to something nobler we attain.

Henry Wadsworth Longfellow, *The Ladder of St. Augustine* (1858)

I. **Themes and trends**
  A. The history of psychiatry is in part a history of what mental disorders are called.
    1. In early human history, popular views of madness attributed it to magical influence by another human, to possession by evil spirits, or to divine intervention.
    2. Later in human history, scientific (naturalistic) and professional interpretations emerged, which characterized madness as an illness, a form of disordered behavior, or an expression of social deviance.
  B. Theories of causation have developed in relation to the definition of madness.
    1. Prevailing religious views provided the basis for magical or supernatural influences.
    2. Naturalistic explanations emphasized either physiological influences (somatogenesis) or experiential influences (psychogenesis).
  C. Treatment procedures generally have developed in relation to the view of causation.
    1. Countermagic and exorcism, practiced by shamans or priestly specialists, were used to influence supernatural forces.
    2. Physical treatments were developed to correct the presumed physiological conditions causing the disorder (somatotherapy).
    3. Verbally communicated educational procedures were developed to treat experientially influenced disorders (psychotherapy).
  D. The perspective of a social group toward madness was reflected in popular attitudes and public policies.

1

1. The range of dominant popular attitudes has included indifference and neglect, punishment and exclusion, and humane concern.
2. Similarly, public policies have ranged from exiling people from the community to institutionalization to community-based care.

## II. Eras in Western history

A. Prehistory and the ancients
   1. Stone Age skulls have been found with surgical openings (trephining) in them, suggesting that there was some conception of disorder caused by spirits in the head, which the hole allowed to escape.
   2. Biblical descriptions indicate that many forms of mental disorder were prevalent at that time (e.g., King Saul's depression).
   3. Biblical accounts of the cause of madness emphasized possession by evil spirits, an interpretation that came to dominate Western thought for many centuries.

B. The classical era
   1. Forerunners of most modern views can be found in the variety of views expressed during the classical era.
   2. Mythology and literature of the period provide many descriptions of recognizable mental disorders.
   3. Popular concepts emphasized the supernatural origin of mental disorders.
   4. The temples of Aesculapius, the Greek god of healing, became centers for the treatment of many disorders through a regime of rest, diet, and dream interpretation.
   5. The early Greek philosophers took the understanding of the human mind to be a major quest and claimed rationality was the characteristic of a healthy mind.
      a) Plato (429–347 B.C.) wrote about conflict between higher processes (reason) and lower processes (emotion) and advocated humane treatment for mentally handicapped persons who broke the law, but also believed in the supernatural origin of most mental disorders.
      b) In his many writings about the human mind, Aristotle (384–322 B.C.) gave considerable attention to mental disorders.
   6. A full expression of a naturalistic interpretation of mental disorders is found in the work of Hippocrates (460–377 B.C.)
      a) He denied supernatural intervention as the source of mental disorders, claiming instead that brain pathology was the cause.

    b) He classified mental disorders into three groups: mania, melancholia, and phrenitis (brain fever).

    c) He developed a theory of four basic body fluids (blood, black bile, yellow bile, and phlegm), which he believed to be unbalanced in mental illness (e.g., an excess of black bile caused melancholia).

    d) In treatment he followed the programs of the priests of Aesculapius and also attempted to restore balance of body fluids through bleeding and the use of purgatives and emetics.

7. Galen (A.D. 130–200), the great codifier of the work of Hippocrates, developed a system that became the undisputed Western medical authority for the next fifteen hundred years.

    a) He promoted the theory of the four body fluids and was a strong supporter of the Hippocratic tradition.

    b) Like Plato, he distinguished between mental (rational) and bodily (emotional) processes and also recognized a spiritual organizing influence, which he related to a divine Creator (which no doubt contributed to the favorable assessment of his views during the early centuries of Christianity).

    c) His descriptions of anatomy were very accurate for the times, though he maintained that animal anatomy and human anatomy were identical.

    d) The unquestioning acceptance of his views, largely because of their compatibility with theological views, restricted further empirical investigation of mental disorders.

C. The Middle Ages

1. During the one thousand years of this period (A.D. 500–1500), little scientific inquiry was made into the nature of mental illness, and except for some sanctuaries and retreats maintained by religious groups, little progress was made in humane treatment for disturbed individuals.

2. In the early Middle Ages, demonic possession was the generally accepted popular view of the cause of mental disorders, and exorcism by clergy was the method of treatment.

3. In the late Middle Ages, during a period of famine, epidemic disease, and political disorder, outbursts of mass madness occurred with manifestations of fear and eccentric behavior.

4. In the latter part of the era, as threats to the religious orthodoxy of the time arose, concerns about heresy led to a

preoccupation with witchcraft and to extensive witch-hunts in some parts of Europe.

    5. While it was formerly assumed that many of the victims of witch-hunts were mentally ill, it now appears that during this period, there may have actually been a decline in the belief that the mentally ill were possessed.

D. The Renaissance, the Enlightenment, and the rise of science

    1. While the sixteenth century witnessed in Europe the most extreme expressions of the preoccupation with witchcraft, it was also the time when such thinkers of the time as Francis Bacon, Erasmus, and Thomas More reinvigorated inquiry into human nature and particularly into the nature of the human mind.

    2. Loosening of restrictions on the study of the human body led to the return of empirical inquiry as the basis for the development of medical knowledge.

    3. Naturalistic interpretations were sought to account for occurrences that had been routinely attributed to supernatural causes.

    4. Johann Weyer (1515–1588), a physician, wrote a treatise critical of the demonological interpretation of mental illness and became one of the first physicians to specialize in mental disorders.

## III. Humanitarian reform

A. The trend to naturalistic interpretations of mental illness was accompanied by the development of institutions to care for the mentally ill.

B. While institutional care could be considered an improvement over the punishment, exile, or exorcism that preceded it, the asylums were little more than prisons in which the mentally ill were caged, chained, and put on display to the public.

C. An exception was the shrine at Gheel in Belgium, established in honor of St. Dymphna, which specialized in the care of the mentally disturbed and involved the people of the town in taking them into their homes during pilgrimages to the shrine.

D. Conditions in asylums finally led to much-needed social reform, which transformed the institutional care of the mentally ill during the nineteenth century.

    1. Philippe Pinel (1745–1826), the chief physician at the Bicêtre asylum in Paris, took the significant step of freeing inmates from their chains and allowing them to move freely out of their cells.

    2. In England, the prominent Quaker William Tuke (1732–1822) established the York Retreat, which in its quiet

countryside setting became the model for many other institutions.

3. In the United States, Benjamin Rush (1745–1813), one of the signers of the Declaration of Independence, introduced the principles of moral management, which were based on the assumption that the mentally ill had lost their reason and needed to be helped to regain it.

4. Dorothea Dix (1802–1887) appealed directly to state legislatures in the United States and was directly responsible for action that established or improved hospitals in twenty states.

5. Despite the action of these and other reformers, the benefits of the early reforms were diminished as institutions grew larger and more impersonal and the emphasis of hospitalization shifted to the custodial management of patients, most of whom were slow to recover, if at all.

## IV. Theories of causation in the nineteenth century

A. The somatogenic hypothesis directs the search for causes toward conditions of the body and biological factors that affect them.

1. In the nineteenth century, scientific inquiry into the functions of the human body had established the scientific foundations of medical training and practice.

2. Most physicians interested in mental disorders believed that diagnosis should attempt to establish a physiological cause.

3. Emil Kraepelin (1856–1926) in 1883 published a classification system to help establish the organic basis for mental disorders.

   a) He noted that mental illness, like other medical disorders, displayed symptoms that tended to group together as syndromes.

   b) He viewed mental illness, like other medical disorders, as having typical courses and outcomes.

   c) He proposed two major groups of serious mental disorder: manic-depressive psychosis and dementia praecox (which Eugen Bleuler later renamed schizophrenia).

   d) While Kraepelin could only speculate about causation, he assumed that chemical imbalances or metabolic disorders were the causes of the major mental disorders.

   e) Kraepelin's classificatory scheme and its logic based on other medical diseases established the rationale for the view that mental disorders can be understood as disorders of organic origin.

B. The discovery of organic factors in general paresis provided the first major support for the somatogenic hypothesis.

1. General paresis was first described in 1825 as a specific disorder by the French physician A. L. J. Bayle, on the basis of common features of delusional thinking, increasing paralysis, and a deteriorating course that resulted in death.
2. The clinical observation that many paretic patients also had had syphilis led to a dramatic experiment by Richard von Krafft-Ebing in 1897, which established a clear relationship between paresis and syphilis.
3. The discovery of the syphilitic spirochete in 1905 led later to the verification through postmortem examination that the brains of paretics had been invaded by spirochetes.
4. With the development of the Wassermann blood test in 1906 and treatment procedures by Paul Ehrlich and Julius von Wagner-Jauregg, the pattern of diagnosis and treatment based on a known underlying pathology was complete.

C. The psychogenic hypothesis directs the search for causes toward events in the life of the individual, particularly those that influence the development of personality and styles of adjustment to environmental demands.
   1. While the medical approach to mental disorders focused attention on the brain and conditions that affected its function, other thinking about the nature of mind directed attention to issues of consciousness and unusual phenomena of consciousness.
   2. Franz Mesmer (1734–1815) intrigued the salons of Vienna and Paris with his demonstrations of the use of animal magnetism (what we recognize today as hypnosis) in the relief of physical symptoms of his patients.
   3. While Mesmer and his ideas were viewed as quackery by most other physicians, some were intrigued by the mental effects of his techniques and began the serious study of hypnosis.
   4. The establishment of the first laboratory in experimental psychology by Wilhelm Wundt in 1879 formalized the study of factors that affect such normal mental processes as sensation and perception.
   5. As psychology developed as a discipline, study shifted to the processes that establish and maintain learning, particularly the conditions of learning known as classical conditioning established by Ivan Pavlov (1848–1936).

D. The study of hypnosis and its application to the treatment of hysteria led to the first formulation of the psychogenic hypothesis.
   1. Hysteria (what is today referred to as conversion disorder) is a condition in which patients show physical symptoms that seem to suggest neurological disorder (e.g., paralysis,

sensory loss) but for which no neural pathology can be found.
2. The patients whom Mesmer "cured" were probably mostly hysterics.
3. The French neurologist Jean Charcot (1825–1893) was persuaded by his students to investigate the use of hypnosis in instigating and relieving symptoms in his hysteric patients.
4. In 1885 Sigmund Freud (1856–1939), a young specialist in neurology, studied with Charcot and became acquainted with the work of other French physicians who were investigating hypnosis.
5. Freud, on returning to Vienna, joined practice with Josef Breuer (1842–1925), who had developed a technique of having patients talk about their problems under hypnosis (the cathartic method).
6. Breuer and Freud published their *Studies in Hysteria* (1895), which described the role of emotional experiences and unconscious mental processes in hysteria.
7. Breuer and Freud's treatise showed that psychological processes could also be causative in some forms of mental disorder, a position that Freud was to elaborate later in his theory of psychoanalysis.

V. **Twentieth-century developments (to 1965)**
   A. While the somatogenic point of view was adhered to by many psychiatrists, its successes were limited to the early part of the century.
   1. Nothing followed comparable to the explanation of general paresis.
   2. Schizophrenia, the most challenging of the severe mental disorders, was the target of intensive research into its possible pathology, with no success.
   3. A number of somatic treatments were developed involving the induction of coma or seizures or surgical intervention in the brain, but results were, with a few exceptions, not striking and there were no clear explanations of the effects.
   4. The situation was radically changed, however, in the 1950s when the first effective antipsychotic and antidepressant drugs were introduced, leading the way to the "pharmacological revolution," which has reestablished the somatogenic perspective as the dominant viewpoint in contemporary psychiatry.
   5. The rapid pace of discovery in molecular genetics, brain function, and neural mechanisms that began in the middle of the century began to provide a substantial base of supporting information for the somatogenic hypothesis.

B. While the somatogenic point of view languished in the early part of the century, the psychogenic perspective flourished.
   1. The development of psychoanalysis provided both a psychological theory of causation and a psychological treatment based on the theory.
      a) Freud's theory of personality focused attention on unconscious determinants of behavior, emotional conflict, early childhood experiences, and the central role of anxiety and defenses against anxiety in neurotic symptoms.
      b) His method of treatment involved the use of free association, dreams, memories of childhood experiences, and interactions with the therapist, which were interpreted to find meaning in terms of unconscious motives, conflicts, and developmental distortions.
      c) Freud's "talking cure," in which patient and therapist use focused conversation to achieve therapeutic goals, became the model for the large number of psychotherapeutic practices that emerged in succeeding years.
   2. Freud became the center of a group of psychoanalytic practitioners, but soon differences of opinion about the nature of the unconscious, the primary causes of mental disorders, and the effective procedures in psychotherapy led to other variants of the psychodynamic approach (see chapter 2).
      a) Early associates Alfred Adler (1870–1937) and Carl Jung (1875–1961) were the first to develop theories that departed significantly from those of Freud.
      b) Others, while retaining many of Freud's ideas, introduced a greater role for cultural factors, found greater significance in adult styles of coping, and liberalized psychoanalytic practice.
      c) Karen Horney (1885–1952) and Harry Stack Sullivan (1892–1949) in particular placed great emphasis on the role of experiences in the family and society as determining influences in personality, and directed their therapy toward the resolution of disturbed interpersonal relationships.
   3. A major influence on American psychiatry was Adolf Meyer (1866–1950).
      a) Meyer viewed mental illness as evidence of an individual's maladaptive interaction with the environment.
      b) His emphasis on objective observation of patient behavior and on habit as the mechanism in maladaptive behavior was compatible with the psychology of learning that was being elaborated by American psychologists.

    c) His views anticipated the biopsychosocial model that is currently held by many psychiatrists.
  4. Advances in the psychology of learning led to the application of learning principles to problems of child behavior and later to adult behavior.
    a) John Watson (1878–1958), the founder of behaviorism, demonstrated how fears could be conditioned in children and advocated the use of conditioning principles in the raising of children.
    b) B. F. Skinner (1904–1990) developed principles of operant conditioning, which were later used by psychologists as the basis for behavior modification.
    c) In 1950 John Dollard and Neal Miller published *Personality and Psychotherapy,* which attempted to reinterpret psychoanalytic theory in terms of classical and operant conditioning.
    d) The elaboration of learning-based approaches to behavioral problems developed into a major alternative to psychodynamic therapeutic approaches.
C. Provision for the mentally ill became much more of a governmental concern first at the state and county level and later at the national level.
  1. The reform zeal of Dorothea Dix was continued into the twentieth century with the development of the mental hygiene movement.
    a) Clifford Beers described his own recovery from mental illness in his book, published in 1908, *A Mind That Found Itself.*
    b) He, with the support of psychologist William James and psychiatrist Adolf Meyer, undertook a national campaign to educate the public about the problem of mental illness.
    c) He formed the National Committee for Mental Hygiene, which set as its goal reform of state institutions, public education, and early intervention through the establishment of child and family clinics (now called the National Association for Mental Health).
  2. In the early part of the century, state institutions remained pretty much as they had in the previous century, housing an increasing number of chronically disabled patients whose unrelieved disorders made them unacceptable in their communities.
  3. Some institutions, however, also became centers for research into the characteristics of psychotic disorders.

4. The advent of drugs that effectively relieved some of the symptoms of chronic disorders changed the role of state hospitals from custodial caretaking to treatment centers and allowed many patients to be discharged to less restrictive settings.
5. At the same time, many community hospitals introduced psychiatric services to support psychiatric treatment with the new drugs.
6. The deinstitutionalization movement in the 1960s resulted in greater legal protection for the rights of mentally ill patients and further shifted the emphasis from long-term hospitalization in public hospitals to treatment in the patient's community.
7. The Community Mental Health Centers Act was passed by Congress in 1963 to provide comprehensive mental health care clinics in the community and to support educational and preventive measures.
8. The deinstitutionalization movement, together with the establishment of community clinics, appears to have fulfilled the goals of the mental hygiene movement, but other problems have emerged from deinstitutionalization that continue to challenge the development of effective public policy.

## References

Alexander, F. G., and S. T. Selesnick. *The History of Psychiatry*. New York: Harper & Row, 1966.

Carson, R. C., J. N. Butcher, and J. C. Coleman. *Abnormal Psychology and Modern Life*. 8th ed. Glenview, Ill.: Scott, Foresman, 1988.

Zegans, L. S., and B. S. Victor. "Conceptual Issues in the History of Psychiatry." In *Review of General Psychiatry*. 2d ed., edited by H. H. Goldman. Norwalk, Conn.: Appleton & Lange, 1988.

# 2 Psychodynamic Foundations

There is occasions and causes why and wherefore in all things.

**Shakespeare, *King Henry V***

## I. Introduction
  A. *Psychodynamics* is one set of factors that is important to the understanding of the formation of personality and the development of mental disorders.
  B. Just as the human organism undergoes a process of physical development from the moment of conception (fusion of sperm and ovum) until it reaches physical maturity, so, too, a person undergoes a process of psychological development (maturation). Both are influenced by genetic determinants and experiential forces (environmental influences). Included in the latter are parental relationships, peer relationships, and cultural and social experiences.

## II. Personality development
  A. Personality
    1. Personality has been defined in various ways. Simply stated, personality is the sum total of the individual's internal and external patterns of adjustment to life.
    2. Personality is, in part, determined by one's genetically transmitted organic endowment and in part by one's life experiences.
    3. As individuals develop, their behavior also changes. Thus, a newborn reacts differently to a given environmental stimulus than an adolescent or adult.
    4. For the various stages of personality development, see chapter 5.
  B. In this chapter, we will discuss various psychosocial conceptions of human behavior as well as the psychosocial forces operant in mental disorders.

## III. Psychodynamic concepts
  A. Definition

1. *Psychodynamics* is the study, explanation, or interpretation of behavior or mental states in terms of mental or emotional forces or processes. It recognizes the role of *unconscious* motivation and assumes that one's behavior is determined by past experience, genetic endowment, and current reality. It is the science of mental forces in action (see Campbell, *Psychiatric Dictionary,* 5th ed., and the APA *Psychiatric Glossary,* 6th ed.).
2. Psychoanalytic theory is the foundation of psychodynamic (dynamic) psychiatry, which chiefly explains mental disorder as the consequences of the conflict from unconscious drives.

B. History

Much of the material covered in this chapter might have been included in the chapter on history, but it seemed more appropriate to consider all of those who have contributed to psychodynamic foundations in one section.

1. As noted in the previous chapter on history, Sigmund Freud became the center of a group of psychoanalytic practitioners including Alfred Adler, Carl Jung, Karen Horney, and Harry Stack Sullivan (all of whom will be discussed later in this chapter).
2. Sigmund Freud

   Most of the current psychiatric conceptions of behavioral development and psychopathology originated with the work of Sigmund Freud, who created psychoanalysis. Psychoanalysis is

   a) A theory of how the mind works: including attempts to comprehend and explain both normal and abnormal functioning at all ages.
   b) An investigative or research method: basically using the free association technique to gain access to the patient's conscious and unconscious thoughts.
   c) A specific form of therapy using free association to obtain data in the form of thoughts, feelings, memories, fantasies, and dreams. It also involves "working through" and the development of insight (for additional information see chapter 9).
3. Origins

   Psychoanalysis developed out of the teachings and opinions that prevailed at the time of Freud's work. Its basic elements (including dynamics of psychic processes, the classification of these processes into primary [psychological expressions of the underlying basic drives] and secondary processes [the reasonable and acceptable ways in which underlying basic drives are controlled and permitted expression according to the demands of the outside world] and into the unconscious and conscious [topography], and their economy [pleasure/displeasure]) were prefigured in Herbart, Fechner, Helmholtz, and Meynert.

4. Among the early theorists were the following:

   a) Gottfried Wilhelm Liebniz (1646–1716), the German philosopher and mathematician, believed that perception of elements occurred unconsciously. He presented the first systematic statement of degrees of consciousness.

   b) Johann Fredrick Herbart (1776–1841) developed the dynamic theory of unconscious mental processes some seventy years before Freud. Herbart's central thesis was that it must eventually be possible to describe mental processes in terms of scientific laws. And he dreamed of the "mathematical psychology."

   c) Gustav Theodor Fechner (1801–1887) referred to "negative sensations" that occurred below the threshold of consciousness. He employed not only a concept of inhibition but also repression. He also worked toward a "mathematical psychology."

   d) Hermann Helmholtz (1821–1894), a nineteenth-century scientist who made contributions to physiology and other scientific fields, coined the term "unconscious inference" and explained the associations of perception to past experience.

   e) Theodore Meynert (1833–1892) was a German neurologist and psychiatrist who advocated the localization theory (mental and emotional life is dependent on the brain). Like Freud, he accorded a position of central importance to associations.

   f) Josef Breuer, a Viennese neurologist, published with Freud the classic *Studien Uber Hysterie* (*Studies in Hysteria*) (1895), which Freud said were the "products of Breuer's mind."

   g) Eduard von Hartman (Karl Robert) (1842–1906) was a metaphysical philosopher who was called "the philosopher of the unconscious." He authored a book entitled *Philosophy of the Unconscious,* published in Berlin in 1869. He based his philosophical system on the premise that the unconscious permeates both will and reason.

   h) Perhaps one could also include the great philosopher Immanuel Kant (1724–1804), who stated,

      "Innumerable are the sensations and perceptions where of we are not conscious. . . . The clear ideas indeed are but an infinitely small fraction of the same exposed to consciousness."

5. Psychoanalysis derived from two great antithetical traditions: the deterministic and materialistic framework of nineteenth-century science, which was strongly oriented toward physics and evolutionary biology (from the rationalism of the Enlightenment); and the vision of the romantic poets and philosophers of the nineteenth century, a cultural movement that rejected and undermined the dominant ideas of the Enlightenment and explored the "night side of life." For example, Samuel Taylor Coleridge referred to the "unconscious" and "twilight realms of consciousness." Schopenhauer's concept of "unconscious will" was roughly equivalent to the "id" as seen by psychoanalysts. For Freud the importance of psychoanalysis lay in its contribution to knowledge and not in its therapeutic benefits (Rolo 1963).

Although Freud was dependent on other contributions, he remains the first cartographer of the unconscious.

C. A comprehensive resume of psychoanalytic theories is beyond the scope of this outline. However, a few of the basic psychoanalytic concepts that have been found useful in general psychiatry will be listed.

## IV. Sigmund Freud (1856–1939)

A. Thinking

Freud viewed thinking as composed of primary and secondary processes. This differentiation is viewed by many of his followers as his greatest accomplishment.

1. Primary processes

These are the psychological expressions of the underlying basic drives. They are assumed to be largely unconscious and present at birth, and thus can be considered innate. They are the more primitive modes of thinking. They are manifested in dreams but are also present during waking life. Thinking at this level follows the *pleasure principle*— the seeking of pleasure and the avoidance of pain.

2. Secondary processes

These are the reasonable and acceptable ways in which the underlying basic drives are controlled and permitted expression according to the demands of the outside world. They are characteristic modes of preconscious and conscious thinking and follow the *reality principle.*

B. Drives

There are certain significant desires and drives that are repressed. These constitute the *dynamic unconscious,* and they resist conscious expression because of their basic unacceptability.

C. Resistance

An individual resists attempts to make these repressed forces conscious through the use of defenses. This constitutes what Freud called *resistance*.

D. Transference

*Transference* is the displacement of feelings for significant people in one's earlier life onto the physician or therapist.

E. Mind

To help explain all of these phenomena, Freud postulated a mind composed of the conscious, the preconscious (foreconscious), and the unconscious.

1. *The conscious* is composed of ideas, feelings, drives, and urges of which the person is aware. It is the scene of purposeful behavior.

2. *The preconscious,* which is midway between the conscious and the unconscious, comprises feelings, ideas, drives, and urges that are out of the individual's continuous awareness but that can be readily recalled. For example, you may not think about what you ate for supper last night, but you could easily recall the menu if asked.

3. *The unconscious* is made up of drives, feelings, ideas, and urges that are outside of the individual's awareness. One does not acknowledge or label them.

F. Divisions of personality

Structurally, Freud divided personality into three parts. This tripartite division included the id, ego, and superego.

1. Id

The *id* is the unconscious reservoir of primitive drives (instincts). The id is dominated by the primary process manner of thinking and the pleasure principle. It exists in all humans and in modified forms in all other animal life. Components of the id are:

a) *Eros,* the name Freud gave to the creative forces, the life instinct. (Eros was the Greek god of love and originally represented the primeval power that created order and cohesion out of chaos.)

b) *Thanatos,* Freud's term for the aggressive, destructive, or death forces. (Thanatos was the Greek god who personified death and was the twin brother of Hypnos, or sleep.)

c) *Homeostasis,* the individual's tendency to maintain a relatively stable psychological condition with respect to contending drives, motivations, and other psychodynamic forces. Freud felt that psychological growth depended on a proper balance between the creative and aggressive forces, with somewhat of a preponderance of the former.

d) *Libido,* Freud's term for the emotional energy broadly derived from these underlying instincts (psychosexual energy) and presumably present at birth. The id serves as a reservoir for the libido, which has two general forms.

   (1) *Ego libido* is libido concentrated on the self, or narcissism. *Primary narcissism* is the original state of the newborn. (Narcissus was a Greek youth who fell in love with his own reflection in the water.)

   (2) *Object libido* is libido that is directed outward toward another person or thing.

e) *Cathexis,* the name Freud gave to the process by which the unconscious primitive drives are vested with psychic energy (i.e., attachment of feeling and significance to object, idea, or person).

2. Ego

The *ego* is the part of the personality that meets and interacts with the outside world; it is the "integrator" or "mediator" of the personality.

a) The ego functions to help the individual deal with the world and yet to satisfy the underlying needs of the id through coping and problem solving.

b) It functions at all three levels of consciousness (conscious, preconscious, and unconscious).

c) The adaptive functions of the ego are the defenses against anxiety.

d) The opposition of ego energy to id energy is called *countercathexis.*

e) The ego is the executive function of the personality.

f) The part of the ego devoted to the development of parental substitutes (parental imagoes) is called the *ego ideal.* This is a part of a developing ego that is set aside, so to speak, to contain the mental images of the parents—for identification.

3. Superego

The *superego* is the censoring force of the personality. It is composed of the morals, mores, values, and ethics of the individual and is largely derived from one's parents.

a) The conscious part of the superego is called *conscience,* but it operates at all three levels of consciousness.

b) Most of us are conscious of our moral and ethical beliefs but remember only a portion of the training and experience that contributed to the formation of those beliefs.

     c) If the ego contemplates violation of the superego's code, anxiety results; if the person carries out the contemplated violation despite the anxiety, guilt feelings ensue.

     d) The infant's superego is primitive and undeveloped. It begins to develop in the second year and takes definite form at the age of four or five.

     e) The punitive aspect of superego concerns itself with prohibitions, self-criticism, and guilt feelings (bad conscience).

     f) The nonpunitive, positive aspect of the superego is sometimes separately designated as the *ego ideal*.

     g) An overly strict superego usually leads to the development of a rigid, compulsive, unhappy person. A weak, defective superego permits a person to express hostile and antisocial strivings without anxiety or guilt.

G. Libido development (stages of psychosexual development)

Freud believed that the major development of adult personality takes place in infancy and early childhood.

  1. The oral phase

     a) The first twelve to eighteen months of life are characterized chiefly by preoccupation with feeding. Pleasure is derived mainly through the mouth. This period is called the *oral phase*.

     b) The early part of the oral phase, the *sucking stage*, is passive.

     c) The later oral phase, or *biting stage*, is aggressive (oral-sadistic).

  2. The anal phase

     a) From the eighteenth month until the end of the third year, the infant's attention is centered on excretory functions. This is the *anal phase*.

     b) This is the first time the infant must adjust his or her behavior to the demands of others.

     c) This stage is also the foundation for the development of the superego.

     d) *Expulsive and retentive phases* are part of the anal phase, just as passive and aggressive ones are part of the oral phase.

  3. The narcissistic or pregenital phase

The oral and anal phases considered together are called the *narcissistic or pregenital phase* because the child's libido is satisfied within his or her own body.

  4. The phallic phase

The *phallic phase* extends from the end of the third year to the seventh year. The child becomes aware of his or her genitalia. During this stage, for the first time, the child's libido is directed outward and requires others for its satisfaction. It is characterized, psychosexually, by:

a) *Castration anxiety,* which results from the boy's fear of damage to or loss of his genitals. It includes the childhood fantasy that female genitals result from the loss of the penis.

b) *Penis envy,* which is the girl's desire to possess a penis and, thus, to become masculine.

c) *The Oedipus complex,* which is the attachment of the child to the parent of the opposite sex, accompanied by envious and aggressive feelings toward the parent of the same sex.

    (1) This complex of aggressive feelings in the girl is called the *Electra complex.*

    (2) The resolution of this complex is usually accomplished by subsequent identification with the parent of the same sex.

5. Latency

*Latency* is the stage between the Oedipal period and the adolescent years. In general, during this period, the person learns to recognize and cope with reality.

6. The genital phase

The *genital phase* is the final stage of psychosexual development.

a) It begins with puberty, with the physiological capacity for orgasms as well as the capacity for object love and mature heterosexuality.

b) The early adolescent stage is narcissistic in that selfish interests predominate.

c) Following this, there is a temporary homosexual phase in which adolescents prefer to meet in gatherings of the same sex.

d) As adolescence progresses, attraction to the opposite sex begins to assert itself more strongly and the capacity for object love and mature heterosexuality emerges.

H. Adult character structure

1. Adult character includes the ego's usual mode of dealing with the id, the superego, and the external world. It is patterned on an individual's experiences during the previous stages.

2. Character types

According to Freudian theory, adults could be certain character types, based on fixations (from unresolved conflicts) at any of the stages.

a) Oral character. This person has a passive-receptive orientation toward life and has oral preoccupations (eating, drinking, smoking, etc.).

b) Anal character. This frugal, orderly, obstinate person needs to feel in control of himself or herself in the environment.

c) Phallic character. In the male, overcompensatory behavior is a reaction against underlying castration fears and grows out of a need to demonstrate his masculinity. In the female, the reaction to penis envy would be to assume "masculine" roles.

d) Genital character. This concept is "an ideal." Such a person has successfully passed through all the developmental stages and is able to maturely participate in meaningful relationships with members of the opposite sex.

  I. Few psychiatrists or psychoanalysts accept all of the previously described Freudian concepts. However, it is necessary to know them in order to understand the influence Freud had on other investigators and how his work contributed to other theoretical formulations.

## V. Alfred Adler (1870–1937)

A. Individual psychology

Adler founded the school of *individual psychology*—each person has his or her own special goals and unique manner of achieving them.

B. Organ inferiority (he later expanded the concept to human inferiority).

Adler placed more emphasis on the ego than on sexuality.

1. He regarded organ inferiority as the most important etiological factor.

2. He believed that the individual's development was determined by the adaptive push for superiority, or the drive to power. (The specific type of superiority depends upon the individual's biological background and early environment.)

3. In this quest for power, a particular *life-style*—the individual's stepwise, active, unique adaptation to the social milieu—evolves.

C. Personality

Adler regarded personality as developing out of the individual's attitudes toward herself or himself, toward other people (especially family), and toward society.

D. Inferiority complex

1. Adler coined the term *inferiority complex* to describe the conflict, partly conscious and partly unconscious, that impels the individual to attempt to overcome the distress

accompanying feelings of inferiority (which are derived from the helplessness of the infant).

2. He believed that a neurotic disposition is caused by over-protection, neglect, or both, during childhood.

3. The person with strong feelings of inferiority may, however, compensate by trying to become superior in some special area.

4. The struggle for superiority may be successful, if modified by the demands of reality.

5. Thus, in the Adlerian formulation, neurosis represents the various maladaptive psychological processes by which the individual seeks to cope with his or her inferiority.

E. Masculine protest

1. *Masculine protest* is Adler's term for the individual's (male/female) attempt to escape from the feminine submissive role. Women become tomboys or tyrannical wives or mothers. Men become Don Juans. This concept can be regarded as the main motive force in neurotic disorder. It is tied in with self-esteem: the neurotic purpose is the enhancement of self-esteem, the simplest form of which can be recognized in the exaggerated masculine protest.

2. Masculine protest may derive from the subject's own uncertainty of his or her role.

VI. **Carl G. Jung (1875–1961)**

A. Analytic psychology

Jung's modification of psychoanalysis was called *analytic psychology.*

B. Introversion and extroversion

Jung stressed life goals and the role of introversion and extroversion in personality development.

1. He defined *introversion* as inwardly directed libido, reflected in the tendency to be preoccupied with oneself.

2. *Extroversion* was his term for outwardly directed libido.

C. The libido

1. Like Adler, Jung minimized the role of sexuality in personality dynamics.

2. He believed that the libido was broadly derived from all life energy (not just from sex).

D. The unconscious

1. In addition to the *personal* unconscious, Jung postulated a *collective* unconscious (racial or archaic unconscious), believing that there was an inheritance of primitive racial ideas and impulses.

2. He believed the personal unconscious to be superficial and hence more accessible than the collective unconscious.

3. The collective unconscious was later called the *objective psyche*. It included both
   a) *Autochthonous ideas*, ideas originating within the psyche without external stimuli.
   b) *Primordial images*, a phylogenetic memory heavily laden with mythological reference.
E. The shadow
   This is the term Jung gave to the objective counterpart of the underlying personal unconscious and collective unconscious. Coming to terms with it requires maturity and perspective (which usually emerge during the second half of life).
F. The persona and anima
   1. The *persona* is the social facade assumed by an individual (so named from the mask worn by actors in ancient Greek drama, which characterized the mood portrayed). The individual behaves in conformity with what is expected of him or her.
   2. The *anima* is the true inner self, or soul. In addition,
      a) The *animus* is the masculine component of the female personality.
      b) The *anima* is the female component of the male personality.
G. Self
   According to Jungian psychology, the self does not really come into awareness until the individual has dealt with his shadow and anima or animus.
H. Basic psychological functions
   1. Jung described four basic psychological functions: feelings, thinking, sensation, and intuition. (The first two are usually conscious; the second two are usually unconscious.)
   2. In addition, he saw people as having two general attitudes: extroversion and introversion.
   3. Thus, there were eight possible combinations.
I. Therapy
   Jung believed that psychiatric treatment should deal with current problems and plans for the future as well as attempts to uncover past causal experiences.

**VII. Otto Rank (1884–1939)**
A. The birth trauma
   Rank proffered the theory that the *birth trauma* was central to the individual's experience.
   1. The process of birth produces primal anxiety in response to feelings of helplessness.

2. Separation from the mother is the original trauma, a sudden, violent change from the security of intrauterine existence to the uncertainties of the outer world.
3. Subsequent separations of any type are also traumatic.
4. Every pleasure is a seeking of the reestablishment of intrauterine primal pleasure.

B. Conflict and therapy
1. As the child becomes conscious of himself as separate from his mother, he develops conflict.
2. The desire for separation leads to guilt feelings.
3. According to Rank, a person has difficulty asserting his or her will.
4. In adulthood, a person possesses a "good" portion (approved by his parents and society) and a "bad" portion, called *counterwill* (which is disapproved).
5. Relieving guilt feelings is the central focus of treatment.

C. Personality
Rank described three character types:
1. The normal or average person (who accepts the will of the group)
2. The creative person (who sets his or her own ideals and governs himself or herself accordingly)
3. The neurotic person (who is not free to express his or her own will, but cannot conform to the group)

D. As the only nonmedical member of Freud's inner circle, he brought a world view to the psychoanalytic movement. His psychology and therapeutic method were precursors of the *third force,* or *humanistic psychology.*

VIII. **Karen Horney (1885–1952)**
A. The social and emotional environment
Unlike Freud and Jung, Horney felt that conflict is an outgrowth of social conditions and not part of human nature. She focused on the dynamics of social and environmental factors in personality development.

B. Sexuality
1. Horney did not accept the Freudian theory of the libido and his emphasis on infantile sexuality.
2. She discounted the theory of penis envy.

C. Anxiety
Horney stressed the principle of basic anxiety.
1. The child's apprehension and insecurity result from relationships with parents who are overindulgent, dominating, erratic, or indifferent.
2. As a consequence, the child is left without a feeling of belonging.

3. Hostility and conflict derive from this basic anxiety.

D. Personality
   1. She delineated three main directions a child could take in coping with the environment:
      a) *Moving toward people* (i.e., accepting one's helplessness and attempting to win the affection of others);
      b) *Moving against people* (fighting the surrounding hostility); or
      c) *Moving away from people* (remaining apart and neither belonging nor fighting).
   2. Three types of persons would typify these three basic attitudes.
      a) Compliant
      b) Aggressive
      c) Detached

E. Self
   Central to Horney's theory is the concept of *self*, which could be viewed in three ways.
   1. The *actual self* (the sum total of an individual's experiences)
   2. The *real self* (the unique total force and sense of integration found in each person)
   3. The *idealized self* (a glorified self-image, closely related to the current concept of narcissism, and a sign of neurosis)

F. Therapy
   In therapy, she emphasized the self and the environment, concentrating on:
   1. Self-realization
   2. Self-actualization
   3. Dealing with the here and now

G. Although the influence of culture and the importance of the here and now are commonly accepted today, they were unacceptable to the larger psychoanalytic community in Horney's time. A very important contribution to our present-day understanding of women was her belief that much of female behavior was the result of cultural reinforcement.

H. Both Horney and Harry Stack Sullivan emphasized the environmental and social aspects of personality and disease.

I. They emphasized the importance of security, trust, and warmth in avoiding and resolving conflicts.

IX. **Harry Stack Sullivan (1892–1949)**
A. Interpersonal theory of psychiatry
   1. Harry Stack Sullivan espoused an *interpersonal theory of personality;* that is, interpersonal relationships provide the

experiences that are crucial in personality formation, both normal and abnormal.

2. Interpersonal relations mediate the basic human needs, which Sullivan believed are tenderness, security, intimacy, and peers.
3. Social psychiatry has developed from Sullivan's principles.

B. Anxiety
1. Sullivan emphasized the need for security, which he felt could be satisfied only through interpersonal relationships.
2. He conceived of anxiety in the infant as stemming from a disturbance in the relationship between the child and the mothering one.
3. He regarded anxiety as the major factor in personality development as well as in the development of all emotional illnesses and psychopathology.

C. Parataxic distortions
This was a term coined and used by Sullivan to describe attitudes toward other persons that are based on distorted evaluations of them or on an identification of such persons with figures from one's past life. As a consequence, one develops certain manners of coping with the significant people in his or her life and uses these in later interpersonal relationships.

D. Personality
1. Sullivan believed that personality evolves from the action of personal and social forces in the individual from the time of birth onward.
2. He believed that the *power motive* underlies all other impulses and operates from birth onward to overcome an inner sense of helplessness.
3. He regarded intrapsychic conflicts (from within the personality) as being derived from interpersonal conflicts—that is, they are internalized interpersonal conflicts.

E. Therapy
Sullivan believed that treatment must include management of the patient in his or her milieu (environment).

F. Both Sullivan and Horney were greatly influenced by concepts of learning theory (simply stated: behavior is modified as a function of learning).

X. **Melanie Klein (1882–1960)**
A. Klein was a controversial but inspiring British child psychiatrist who originally described *object relations theory* (experiences of the external world are internalized).
B. She described the psychodynamic process by which the child handles conflict with the parents by introjecting the relationship

and dealing with it at an intrapsychic level (intrapsychic introjects).

   C. Others who subscribed to object relations theory were Ronald Fairbairn (1889–1964) and Donald Winnicott (1897–1971), a pediatrician who became a psychoanalyst and who described the emergence of what he called "transitional objects "(objects that assume special value for infants when under stress, particularly when going to sleep).

## XI. Erik Erikson (1902–    )

   A. Theory

Erikson's psychosocial theory of personality extends beyond the nuclear Freudian model to the social world. He views development as extending beyond the infantile sexuality of Freud. (Thus, he rejects the notion that the childhood experiences are the sole determinants of development.) He introduced the term *epigenesis* to refer to the stages of ego and social development.

   B. Identity

     1. Erikson emphasizes the concepts of *identity* (an inner sense of sameness that perseveres, despite external changes), *identity crisis,* and *identity confusion.*

     2. His contributions are built upon basic Freudian tenets (in this regard he differs from Jung, Adler, and Horney, who rejected Freud's theories and substituted their own).

     3. Like Adler, he minimizes the role of sexuality in personality dynamics.

   C. Psychosocial stages

Erikson identifies eight *psychosocial stages* in personal development (the human life cycle or ego development).

     1. Sensory-oral

The *sensory-oral stage* is characterized by trust versus mistrust (corresponds to Freud's oral stage and usually extends through the first year of life).

     2. Muscular-anal

The *muscular-anal stage* is characterized by autonomy versus doubt (corresponds to the anal stage; spans the second and third years of life).

     3. Genital

The *genital stage* takes place during ages four and five; this is the play age.

     4. Latency

*Latency* involves industry versus inferiority (ages six to eleven; this is the school age).

     5. Puberty and adolescence

a) *Puberty and adolescence* involve ego identity versus role confusion (roughly, ages twelve to eighteen, when the adolescent is developing a personal identity).

b) *Identity crisis* is a term used by Erikson to describe the inability of the adolescent to accept a role he or she believes to be expected by society.

6. Young adulthood

*Young adulthood* is characterized by intimacy versus isolation (roughly, the period of courtship and early family, extending from late adolescence until middle age).

7. Adulthood

*Adulthood* is characterized by generativity versus stagnation or self-absorption (middle age).

8. Maturity

*Maturity* is characterized by ego integrity versus despair (the individual's major efforts are nearing completion, and there is time for reflection and the enjoyment of any grandchildren).

D. At each stage of development, basic psychosocial crises must be resolved. How each of these crises is resolved impacts on subsequent development stages.

## XII. Ego psychologists

A. Heinz Hartmann, Ernst Kris, Rudolph Lowenstein

B. *Ego psychology* shifted the emphasis from depth psychology to increased emphasis on autonomous or independent functions of the ego (reality testing, control of movement, perception, thinking, etc.).

C. Ego psychology involved the part of the personality that is most attuned to the outer world and which has the task of maintaining a relationship through reality. This new interest in the ego included but was not limited to those aspects of the ego functioning that are more or less conscious or preconscious.

D. Ego psychology described an undifferentiated phase from which both the id and the ego are gradually formed.

E. Contemporary ego psychology really began with Anna Freud (*Ego and the Mechanisms of Defense*) (1936). Ego psychology complemented but did not replace the id psychology of Sigmund Freud.

## XIII. Heinz Kohut (1913–1981)

A. Kohut is considered the founder of modern self-psychology.

B. Kohut focused attention on "holistic" matters, dealing with the problems of the whole person. His ultimate concern was the future of humans as complete beings and the primacy of "self-transmission" throughout succeeding generations—the "Odysseus complex" (through focusing on the disorders of self-experiences).

C. He viewed people as composed of a confluence of psychic forces (versus Freud's perceptual bias, envisioning people as being made up of isolated mental fragments).

D. Only through persistent empathy and comprehension of the narcissistic superstructure of the modern world was it possible to assess these "tragic" humans and aid them through the trials and tribulations of their mechanized jungle (insane society).

E. Kohut defined empathy as "vicarious introspection"—the mode of cognition attuned to the affective and cognitive states of another.

F. Kohutian psychotherapy (self-psychological psychotherapy) is identical to classical psychoanalysis and its basic tenets: free association and transference analysis. However, it involves the analysis of the whole personality as opposed to drive derivatives and formulates this interpretation with that bias.

## XIV. Margaret Mahler (1897– )

A. Mahler described the separation-individuation process—the child's sense of separateness from the world about him or her.

B. This process begins in the fourth or fifth month of life and is completed by age three.

C. She described four phases.

1. Differentiation—the ability to distinguish between self and others

2. Practicing period—the infant's discovering the ability to separate by crawling and climbing, and later by upright ambulation (from seven to ten months until fifteen to sixteen months)

3. Rapprochement—the need and desire for the mother to share the infant's newly found experiences and skills (sixteen months to twenty-five months of age)

4. Consolidation—achievement of individuality and attainment of a certain degree of object constancy (twenty-five to thirty-six months of age)[1]

## XV. Existential psychoanalysis

A. Existential psychoanalysis is based on the findings of modern philosophy, especially of the works of Sartre and Kierkegaard.

B. This theoretical approach stresses the here and now rather than the past in the evaluation of personality disorder.

1. It primarily focuses on three themes:

a) The person and himself or herself;

b) The person and other persons; and

c) The person and the world he or she lives in.

---

1. H. I. Kaplan and B. J. Sadock, *Modern Synopsis of Comprehensive Textbook of Psychiatry/III,* 3d ed. (Baltimore: Williams & Wilkins, 1981), pp. 19, 20.

2. Anxiety is seen as resulting from the fear of not being—the fear of death.
3. Therapy emphasizes the use of the therapist's own inner feelings as a therapeutic tool. Emphasis is on expression of feelings by both the patient and the therapist and on the uniqueness of each individual and his or her "way-of-being-in-the-world." In contrast to behavior therapy, existential therapy calls for the therapist to share his or her feelings, values, and existence. The therapeutic process is highly subjective.
4. Like psychodynamic psychotherapy, existential therapy is not for everyone, but rather is directed primarily toward the intelligent and verbal individual who appears to be having an existential crisis.
5. Among its contributors have been Karl Jaspers, Ludwig Binswanger (1888–1966), Medard Boss, and R. D. Laing.
6. *Logo therapy* is an existential psychoanalytic method used by Viktor Frankl. It is a type of psychotherapy based on a system of spiritual values. It stresses the search for the meaning of human existence.
7. This theoretical approach has had little influence on present-day psychiatry.

C. Rollo May (1909–      )

Rollo May's special contributions to self-theory come from the European influence of existentialism.

XVI. **Humanistic perspectives on personality**

The ascendance of humanistic psychology as a "third force" in psychology (in addition to psychoanalysis and behaviorism) is attributed particularly to the influence of Abraham Maslow and Carl Rogers.

A. General characteristics of humanistic psychology
1. It is defined as the study of the experiencing person.
2. It is concerned primarily with choice, creativity, and self-realization.
3. Personally and socially significant problems are taken as a special focus of interest.
4. The goal of study is the enhancement of the lives and dignity of human beings.

B. Maslow's motivational theory
1. A distinction is made between higher needs and lower needs, in which higher needs emerge later in evolutionary and individual development, are less directly related to survival, and have more environmental preconditions to their satisfaction.
2. Needs form a hierarchy (from lowest to highest levels)

a) Physiological needs (e.g., food, water, sex, sleep)
b) Safety (e.g., structure, security, predictability)
c) Belongingness and love
d) Esteem (e.g., recognition, acceptance, confidence)
e) Self-actualization (e.g., full knowledge, acceptance of one's personal trend toward integrity, and expression of human potential)

3. Relative satisfaction of needs more basic in the hierarchy is necessary for the next level of needs to emerge.
4. Self-actualization is a level of need that is reached by few people, according to Maslow. (The concept of self-actualization was first expounded by Kurt Goldstein in 1939.)
5. Maslow objected to personality theories developed from the study of abnormal people and developed his approach to personality from the study of healthy, creative people. He informally collected information about a group he considered to be self-actualized. Among these people were historical figures such as Abraham Lincoln, Henry David Thoreau, Eleanor Roosevelt, Albert Einstein, and some of Maslow's friends.

C. Rogers's phenomenological theory
1. The major motivating influence in personality development is the *actualizing tendency,* the striving to maintain and enhance the experiencing person.
2. The actualizing tendency motivates the person toward greater complexity, greater independence, and greater social responsibility.
3. It is *phenomenological reality,* the subjective, personal interpretation of experience rather than physical reality, that determines behavior.
4. The best conditions for development are those that encourage a positive self-regard and feeling of worth.
5. Distortions of self-regard may occur when a person is confronted with an *incongruency* between perceived experience and self-concept.
6. Under conditions of incongruency, a person is vulnerable to anxiety and may respond with defensive denial or distortion to such a degree that psychotherapy is required to reduce the incongruency.

D. Humanistic therapy
1. Humanistic therapy is oriented toward releasing the individual's potential by encouraging self-acceptance "as is" with both strengths and weaknesses.
2. The therapy is viewed as an "authentic" encounter between two individuals, and the client plays a major role in

directing the course of treatment. The assumption is that people have within themselves the resources to understand and alter their view of the self and direct their own behavior.

3. The role of the therapist is largely a demonstration of empathetic understanding and unconditional positive regard.

## XVII. Adolf Meyer (1866–1950)

A. Psychobiology

1. Adolf Meyer founded *psychobiology* ("Psychobiology studies not only the person as a whole, as a unit, but also the whole man").

2. His therapy theory was characterized as distributive analysis and synthesis.

   a) Patients, under the guidance of the therapist, critically evaluate the situations with which they are confronted and their responses to them.

   b) Through discussion and reasoning, the patients try to formulate a way of dealing with their problems more constructively.

3. Meyer's was a comprehensive or pluralistic approach to the understanding of mental illness. Thus, he emphasized the need to consider all pertinent information about the life of an individual as a biological, psychological, and social organism.

4. This is sometimes called *holism*, or the holistic approach (the understanding of the individual personality is based on the interplay of inherited structure, uniqueness, and the cultural pattern in which the individual lives).

5. Despite Meyer's holistic approach, he did not focus at all on the family.

6. American psychiatry has been greatly influenced by Meyerian thinking.

7. His approach has relevance to the community mental health movement.

B. Ego development

1. Meyer did not systematize his thinking and never outlined developmental stages and their critical tasks.

2. He spoke of reactions rather than diseases.

C. Therapy

1. He introduced the concept of *commonsense* psychiatry, which refers to understanding the patient in the simplest terms possible.

2. He believed that treatment began with the first patient contact, and that one of the first steps in the evaluation of the patient was an assessment of the patient's assets and liabilities.

3. The essential goal of therapy was to help the patient modify unhealthy adaptations ("habit training"). The emphasis was always on the current life situation.
D. He really anticipated the biopsychosocial model—an attempt to integrate three perspectives into one overall comprehensive view.

**XVIII. Deficit Model of Disorder**
A. In addition to the conflict model of disorder (as espoused by most of the previously mentioned theorists) present-day psychodynamic psychiatry includes the *deficit model* of disorder.
B. This model views an absence or weakening of sound psychic structures as causal in the production of mental disorder.
C. Examples
1. Alexithymic deficit milieu of psychosomatic symptoms (emotions are defined only in terms of somatic sensations as, for example, the somatoform disorders (either because of some innate ego defect or as resulting from hidden primitive ego defenses).
2. The *negative* symptoms of schizophrenia (restricted affect, poverty of thought, apathy, and anhedonia) with apparent genetic linkage could be explained by an "absence of function."

**XIX. Psychodynamic Psychiatry**
A. Psychodynamic psychiatry is heavily indebted to psychoanalytic theory as discussed in this chapter (especially is indebted to Freud).
B. Most of the early psychodynamic formulations were based on a *conflict model*.
C. Recently the deficit model has been considered a part of psychodynamics.
D. To summarize, the critical ingredients of psychodynamic psychiatry represent an approach to diagnosis and treatment of mental disorders based on unconscious conflict, internal object relations, and deficit and distortions of psychic structures.

# References

Blum, G. S. *Psychodynamics: The Science of Unconscious Mental Forces.* Belmont, Calif.: Brooks/Cole, 1966.

Bromberg, W. *The Mind of Man.* New York: Harper & Brothers, 1959.

Ewalt, J. R., and D. L. Farnsworth. *Textbook of Psychiatry.* New York: McGraw-Hill, 1963.

Freinhar, J. P. "Oedipus or Odysseus: Developmental Lines of Narcissism." *Psychiatric Annals* 16 (August 1986): 476–85.

Gabberd, G. O. *Psychodynamic Psychiatry and Clinical Practice.* Washington,

D.C.: American Psychiatric Press, 1990.

Goldman, H. H., ed. *Review of General Psychiatry.* Los Altos, Calif.: Lange Medical Publications, 1988.

Kaplan, H. I., and B. J. Sadock. *Modern Synopsis of Comprehensive Textbook of Psychiatry/V.* 5th ed. Baltimore: Williams & Wilkins, 1989.

Kolb, L. C., and H. K. H. Brodie. *Modern Clinical Psychiatry.* 10th ed. Philadelphia: Saunders, 1982.

Millon, T. *Theories of Psychopathology.* Philadelphia: Saunders, 1967.

Nicholi, A. M., Jr., ed. *The New Harvard
Guide of Modern Psychiatry.*
Cambridge: Belknap Press of
Harvard University, 1988.
Rolo, C. *Psychiatry and American Life.*
New York: Delta (Dell Publishing),
1963.
Wyss, D. *Psychoanalytic Schools, From
the Beginning to the Present.* New
York: Jason Aronson, 1973.

# 3 Behavioral and Cognitive Foundations

The ideas of goblins and sprights have really no more to do with darkness than light; yet but a foolish maid inculcate these often on the mind of a child . . . possibly he shall never be able to separate them again so long as he lives but darkness shall forever afterward bring with it those frightful ideas. . . . Many children imputing the pain they endured at school to their books . . . so join those ideas together that a book becomes their aversion . . . and thus reading becomes a torment to them, which otherwise possibly they might have made the greatest pleasure of their lives.

**John Locke**

I. **Introduction**
A. The psychogenic perspective on mental disorders implies that the effect that experiences have on the shaping of personality is through mechanisms of learning.
B. The experimental psychology of learning and behavior change has been the source of many concepts and techniques that have been applied in the explanation and treatment of psychiatric disorders.
C. In the first half of the century, the dominant view in psychology emphasized the control of behavior by environmental stimuli and the alteration of behavior by the manipulation of environmental stimuli.
D. In the second half of the century, there has been a shift in interpretative emphasis to a view of behavior as the outcome of the processing of environmental information in relation to the accumulated knowledge of the individual.
E. While the behavioristic emphasis on explaining the acquisition and performance of responses remains very much a part of contemporary psychology, considerable attention is given to the cognitive processes that are involved in the acquisition and use of knowledge, including knowledge about oneself and other persons.

## II. Assumptions

A. Those who usually rely on principles of learning in their explanations of psychiatric disorders interpret the symptoms of the disorders as the outcome of experiences in which inappropriate or maladaptive learning, particularly emotional learning, has occurred.

B. It is generally assumed that the same principles of learning that account for the development of disordered behavior can be applied in its correction.

C. Cognitive approaches to psychiatric disorders stress distortions that may occur in the ways people perceive themselves and their circumstances, the beliefs they hold, and the expectations and judgments they express in their behavior.

D. Cognitively based corrective approaches are directed toward altering false or unwarranted beliefs and judgments.

## III. Learning

A. Classical (Pavlovian) conditioning

1. Modern experiments in learning began in Russia with Ivan Pavlov, the Nobel Prize–winning physiologist who discovered classical conditioning during his studies of digestion.

2. Pavlov showed that a reflexive response can, with proper training, be linked to a stimulus that does not normally produce it.

    a) His famous experiments demonstrated that salivation, which occurs reflexively when food is put in the mouth, can also be caused to occur predictably in the presence of a neutral stimulus such as a bell's sound or a light.

    b) His training procedure involved the presentation of a neutral stimulus (e.g., a bell) slightly before putting food, which causes a dog to salivate, into a dog's mouth.

    c) Repeated pairings of the bell and the food eventually resulted in salivation when the bell alone was presented.

    d) In the standard terminology of classical conditioning, a conditioned stimulus (CS), such as a bell, is repeatedly presented slightly before an unconditioned stimulus (US), such as a piece of food, elicits salivation, an unconditioned reflex or response (UR); the CS will eventually elicit the response, which is then referred to as a conditioned reflex or response (CR).

    e) Schematically:

    US → UR
    (food) (salivation)
    CS → CR
    (bell) (salivation)

3. Other phenomena in the conditioning of reflexes include:

a) Extinction, which refers to the decrease and eventual disappearance of a CR when the CS is repeatedly presented without the US
b) Generalization, which refers to the tendency of the CR to occur to stimuli that resemble the CS used in training (e.g., a bell tone of a frequency different from the one used in training)
c) Discrimination, which refers to the result of training to respond to a CS but not to respond, during the same training, to another stimulus that is similar to the CS

4. Classical conditioning may occur particularly in learned reactions that are mediated by the autonomic nervous system, as is the case with emotional reactions.
5. Some food aversions reflect the powerful one-trial conditioning of food characteristics, such as taste or odor, to experiences of nausea and disgust.
6. The rapid conditioning of some responses such as fears and aversions suggests that there may be a kind of biological preparedness or predisposition to acquire certain classes of conditioned responses.

B. Behaviorism
1. In the United States, psychologist John Watson formulated a methodological position in psychology that he called behaviorism.
a) Watson believed that psychology should be the study of observable behavior and should avoid references to unobservable mental functions such as consciousness.
b) He insisted that the experimental study of animal behavior could contribute to the understanding of human behavior and used Pavlov's principles of conditioning to explain the acquisition and alteration of human habits.
2. In 1920 Watson and Rosalie Raynor demonstrated that fears could be induced by classical conditioning.
a) An eleven-month-old boy named Albert became fearful (CR) of a white rat (CS), which had not frightened him previously, when a loud noise (US) made by striking an iron bar behind him frightened him (UR) while he was playing with the rat.
b) After a few trials, Albert became fearful of any rat without the noise, and his fear generalized to other furry animals and objects.
c) Later, Mary Jones replicated Watson's findings and also demonstrated that the conditioned fear response could be eliminated by the conditioning procedures that produced extinction.

3. Watson was a vigorous champion of his position and influenced developing American psychology to emphasize the study of learning in accordance with the methodological tenets of behaviorism (stimulus-response or S-R psychology).

C. Operant (instrumental) conditioning

1. While Pavlov and Watson emphasized the conditions of the elicitation of responses by stimuli, Edward Thorndike (1874–1949), an American psychologist, investigated the effects of the consequences of behavior.

a) Studying what was viewed as trial-and-error behavior, such as a cat learning to unlatch a box in which it was enclosed, Thorndike decided that the acquisition of the correct problem-solving response was the outcome of the instrumental stimulus-response connection being strengthened by the consequences of the successful response.

b) Thorndike referred to this principle of instrumental learning as the law of effect.

2. B. F. Skinner, an American psychologist, working in the tradition of Watson's behavioristic methodology, which he called the experimental analysis of behavior, reformulated Thorndike's law of effect as a principle of reinforcement and explored the conditions of acquisition and maintenance of operant responses (responses that "operate" on the environment).

a) The experimental investigation of operant conditioning involves making available to a subject a response (such as a lever that can be pressed), which will produce a consequence (such as providing a pellet of food if the subject is hungry) and observing the changes in the frequency with which the response is made in relation to its success in producing the outcome.

(1) There are several notable features of operant conditioning.

(a) The temporal relation of an act to an outcome, such as food or escape from an annoying situation, influences the likelihood that the act will be repeated; the occurrence together in time of a response and a consequence is called a contingency.

(b) In the terminology of operant conditioning, the consequence of a response is called reinforcement (e.g., if pressing a lever results in the delivery of a food pellet, the food serves to reinforce the response tendency to press the lever).

    (i) Positive reinforcement is the presentation of a rewarding stimulus.

    (ii) Negative reinforcement is the removal of a noxious or aversive stimulus.

    (iii) In either case, the response that produces the changed situation for the subject is the one that is reinforced.

  (c) Stimulus control of a response can be established by reinforcing a response only in the presence of a particular stimulus (such as a light).

    (i) The controlling stimulus is referred to as a discriminative stimulus.

    (ii) Schematically:

S —————→ R —————→ S

discriminative stimulus     reinforcement
(light)        (lever press)  (food)

(2) Some other phenomena of operant conditioning

  (a) Extinction, in the operant conditioning case, occurs when a response is repeated in the absence of reinforcement.

  (b) Discrimination results when a response to one stimulus, but not to another present at the same time, is reinforced (e.g., reinforced responding to a green light but not to a red light).

  (c) Schedules of reinforcement that involve varying the amount of time between reinforcements (interval schedules) or the required number of responses between reinforcements (ratio schedules). These schedules influence the rate of response and the resistance of the response to extinction.

    (i) Fixed schedules conform to a consistent value of time or number of responses between reinforcements.

    (ii) Variable schedules, as the term indicates, allow time intervals or the number of responses between reinforcements to change from trial to trial according to some patterned or random sequence.

    (iii) Generally variable schedules are more difficult to acquire but are more resistant to extinction.

b) Learning under aversive conditions

(1) Sometimes the consequences of an action that have an effect on learning are unpleasant or painful.

(2) Punishment occurs when an aversive or noxious stimulus follows a response.

(3) The effect of punishment is to suppress a response but not necessarily to extinguish it.

(4) Escape learning occurs when a response is learned that terminates an aversive stimulus or allows withdrawal from its source.

(5) Avoidance learning occurs when the onset of aversive stimulation is signaled by another stimulus or a response is made to the signal that presents the onset of the aversive stimulus.

3. Applications of operant conditioning

a) The principles of operant conditioning have been used to analyze social learning, aggressive behavior, classroom learning, and many other forms of complex behavior.

b) Many students and collaborators of Skinner have interpreted disordered behaviors in operant terms and have developed training procedures for use in hospitals and other institutional settings (behavior modification).

c) Within limits, operant conditioning affects autonomic responses, as in the self-regulation of muscle tension, heart rate, blood pressure, and skin temperature (biofeedback).

## IV. Social Learning

A. Social learning approaches pay particular attention to the ways in which people learn life skills, cultural rules, and values through interactions with others.

B. As they have developed, social learning interpretations of learned behavior have incorporated concepts about such things as expectations, judgments, and self-appraisal, which are also important in current cognitive interpretations of behavior.

C. The conditions of social learning allow for implicit learning and mediated learning in which the performance of responses during acquisition and the contingency of response and reinforcer are more subtle and less obvious than in traditional models of learning.

D. In social learning approaches, reinforcement is often considered as a source of information about behavioral outcomes that may influence future behavior.

E. Julian Rotter (1954) asserts that effective living is guided by people's expectancies about sources of potential reward and punishment in their lives.

1. Expectancies about the probable outcome of an action are functions of the significance of the action and the subjective value (good or bad) of the outcome.
2. People are also guided by generalized assumptions or beliefs about the source of major influences in their lives.
   a) Those who attribute major influences in their lives to factors in the environment or the chance factors have an external locus of control.
   b) Those who feel that the control of the important outcomes of their lives is a function of their own judgments and choices have an internal locus of control.
F. Albert Bandura (1985) has provided detailed elaborations of his position in which he emphasizes the reciprocal interaction of social learning experiences, the cognitive processes involved in understanding these learning experiences and planning reactions to them, and the coping behaviors with which people try to manage their social environment.
   1. Humans have the capability to learn through observation, imitation, and modeling, and most important social learning takes place in this way.
   2. A central role in Bandura's theory is given to the capability for self-regulation.
      a) One's own behavior is selectively observed on dimensions of performance that are relevant to the situation.
      b) Self-observations produce self-reactions that are influenced by both personal standards of performance and comparison to social norms and the performance of others.
      c) Self-evaluations form the basis for incentives for future action and for reinforcing self-reactions.
   3. The capability for self-reflection allows people to gain knowledge from their experience and to develop beliefs and expectations about the future relation between their behavior and the consequences of their behavior.
      a) Outcome expectancies refer to assumptions about what will happen if particular actions are taken.
      b) Efficacy expectancies refer to assumptions about one's capabilities to influence and determine the outcomes of actions.

## V. Cognition

A. The current reformulation of learning in psychology emphasizes behaviors that are mediated by processes traditionally called "mental" but which are themselves inferred from behavior.
B. Cognitive interpretations of behavior emphasize the way in which information about the environment and behavioral inter-

actions with it are received, identified, and incorporated into new or existing systems of knowledge.

C. Behavior in a given situation is considered to be a product of the current perceptual interpretation of the situation and relevant knowledge based on memory of previous experiences and skills.

D. Images, thoughts, memories, and other mental phenomena figure prominently in the theorizing and research of cognitive psychologists in ways that strict behavioral approaches would not utilize.

E. Cognitive activities and processes

   1. Sensation and perception are concerned with the registration and interpretation of the physical and social environment.

   2. Attention refers to the selective processes that control the flow of information and the allocation of cognitive resources.

   3. Memory is concerned with the acquisition and later utilization of knowledge about the world and individual experience in it.

   4. Thinking and problem solving involve the transformations and manipulation of knowledge in order to make decisions and reassess experience.

   5. Language is the system in which most knowledge is encoded, modified, and communicated to others.

F. Cognitive development

   1. The way in which knowledge and strategies for obtaining knowledge are demonstrated in the developing child is of particular interest to cognitive psychologists.

   2. The eminent Swiss psychologist Jean Piaget (1896–1980) viewed the cognitive development of the child as a sequence of stages involving both the assimilation of knowledge into developing mental structures and the accommodation of mental structures to permit the assimilation of new information.

     a) The sensorimotor period extends from birth to about two years and involves the internal (symbolic) representation of initially behavioral (reflexive) representations of the simple cause-effect relations of the world.

     b) The preoperational period extends from the beginnings of language to about seven years and involves the development of thinking and languages from a relatively rigid and egocentric view of relations in the world to a more flexible approach that can incorporate the perspectives of others.

c) The period of concrete operational thought extends from seven years to eleven years and is characterized by a child's ability to deal with situations as if certain general rules or relationships hold for classes of relationships (although the child may not necessarily be able to state or identify the rule).

d) The period of formal operational thought extends from eleven years to adulthood and is expressed in abstract thinking of the kind that is involved in scientific and mathematical concepts and theory.

3. Piaget's ideas and findings have generated considerable research, much of which has contributed to the revision and elaboration of his pioneering work.

4. Current investigations of cognitive development look for the kind of knowledge that young children have about the world, the cognitive skills that they use in acquiring and using their knowledge, and the acquisition and use of language.

5. Infants and children apparently possess more knowledge and more cognitive competencies than was formerly assumed.

G. Social cognition

1. Some social psychologists have concerned themselves with the way people seek answers to their questions about causes (attribution theory).

2. Studies of human reasoning about the explanation of relationships in conditions of uncertainty reveal some consistent errors and biases.

a) A self-serving attributional bias generally influences people to take personal responsibility for successful accomplishments but to attribute failures to external circumstances.

b) Belief in the effective control of one's life results in the belief that one can bring about desired outcome and the failure to do so is the fault of the victim.

c) There is a tendency to underestimate situational influences, to misperceive the base rates of human events, and to assume that familiar examples are also the most representative.

d) People tend to attribute the causes of their own behavior to factors different from the causes of the behavior of others.

e) In the judgment of similarity of oneself to others, there are indications of both false consensus and false similarity.

f) People may display characteristic attributional styles that may in some cases be related to tendencies toward some mental disorders or to the maintenance of mental health.

H. Current developments in cognitive psychology
   1. The study of implicit and automatic processes in cognition has led to a reformulation of unconscious processes in cognitive rather than psychodynamic terms.
   2. A multiprocess approach to the interpretation of memory has contributed to a modular view of information processing in which different components of cognition are carried out in semi-independent, parallel ways.
   3. Interpretations of automatic processing and modular organization have led to new ways of characterizing consciousness.
   4. The related roles of cognition and affect in behavior are receiving increased research attention, particularly in the relationship of emotion and mood to memory.

VI. **Learning, cognition, and psychiatry**
   A. Basic research in learning and cognition has been applied to the interpretation of many psychiatric concepts and symptoms.
      1. Psychodynamic concepts of anxiety, defense, and symptom formation have been interpreted as involving mechanisms of learning.
         a) Anxiety may be interpreted as an autonomic nervous system reaction that occurs in fearsome or threatening situations and becomes conditioned to other aspects of the situation (e.g., Albert's fear of the white rat).
         b) Since situations that produce or rearouse anxiety are aversive, behaviors that escape or avoid the situation may be reinforced.
         c) Symptoms of some mental disorders may be viewed as learned reactions that are the result of the reinforcing effects of such outcomes as avoiding anxiety or receiving support and attention from others.
         d) If symptoms persist in situations, it is because something in the situation is reinforcing them.
         e) Symptoms, like any other learned response, can be altered by changing the conditions of reinforcement.
      2. Studies of the learned control of autonomic responses have provided research basis for biofeedback training.
         a) Laboratory studies have shown that within limits, operant conditioning can affect changes in such responses as heart rate, muscle tension, EEG alpha wave, blood pressure, and skin temperature.

b) If subjects receive information about alterations in autonomic indicators, they can achieve a degree of self-regulation of some of the processes.

c) Biofeedback training procedures directed toward altering autonomic and muscular responses (e.g., relaxation, increasing or decreasing peripheral blood flow) are used in the practice of the new field of behavioral medicine.

3. Martin Seligman and his associates have developed a learned helplessness model of depression based on the behavior of animals who receive inescapable shock.

a) Animals given unpredictable electric shocks in a situation in which they can neither escape nor avoid the shock show a deficit in behavior in later situations where escape or avoidance are possible.

b) When placed in situations where shock can be escaped or avoided by making appropriate responses, the animals given "helplessness" training remain in the location, receive the shock, and make no attempt to deal with the circumstances.

c) Some human subjects show similar tendencies in learning situations that resemble those used in the studies with animals.

d) The learned helplessness syndrome of loss of coping skills, failure to detect opportunities to change situations, and passive capitulation to circumstances has characteristics similar to clinical depression.

e) Studies by Jay Weiss suggest that the helplessness response may be related to a temporary depletion of norepinephrine in the brain.

f) Seligman has developed a reformulation of the learned helplessness model as applied to human depression, which incorporates the cognitive concept of attribution.
   (1) In the revised model, helplessness also depends on the way the person explains failure.
   (2) If failure is attributed to global factors, the effects are likely to be general.
   (3) If failure is attributed to stable factors, the effect is likely to be persistent.
   (4) If failure is attributed to internal factors, the effect is likely to diminish the sense of self-worth.

4. The predictability of outcome and control over outcome has been related to the effects of stress.

a) Animals placed in situations in which shock is delivered on an unpredictable or uncontrollable basis are more likely to develop symptoms of chronic stress (e.g., help-lessness syndrome, gastric ulceration).

b) Animals presented with an anticipatory signal before receiving the shock and animals who can escape the shock after it begins show less effects to stress although they receive the same number of shocks.

c) Predictability of environmental events and information from the environment about the outcome of actions contribute to coping abilities that help prevent or reduce stress and its effects.

B. Behavioral and cognitive concepts have provided the basis and rationale for some applications in the treatment of psychiatric disorders. (Examples will be developed more fully in chapter 9.)

1. Classical conditioning techniques of counterconditioning and desensitization have been applied to the treatment of fears.

2. Operant conditioning principles are applied in a variety of behavior modification procedures.

3. Imitative learning is applied in modeling, role playing, and rehearsal activities in which patients observe and attempt to emulate the successful behavior of others.

4. Cognitive strategies emphasize the modification of beliefs, attitudes, and expectations that influence emotions and behavior.

5. Successful cognitive therapy techniques have been developed, particularly in the treatment of depression.

## References

Abramson, L., ed. *Social Cognition and Clinical Psychology*. New York: Guilford, 1988.

Bandura, A. "Model of Causality in Social Learning Theory." In *Cognition and Psychotherapy*, edited by M. Mahoney and A. Freeman. New York: Plenum, 1985.

Bloom, F., and A. Lazerson. *Brain, Mind, and Behavior*. New York: Freeman, 1988.

Davison, G., and J. Neale. *Abnormal Psychology*. 5th ed. New York: Wiley, 1990.

Hersen, M., A. Kazdin, and A. Bellak, eds. *The Clinical Psychology Handbook*. New York: Pergamon, 1983.

Kaplan, H. I., and B. J. Sadock, eds. *Comprehensive Textbook of Psychiatry/ V*. Vol. 1, 5th ed. Baltimore: Williams & Wilkins, 1989.

Rotter, J. B. *Social Learning and Clinical Psychology*. Englewood Cliffs, N.J.: Prentice-Hall, 1954.

Tataryn, D., L. Nadel, and W. Jacobs. "Cognitive Therapy and Cognitive Science." In *Comprehensive Handbook of Cognitive Therapy*, edited by A. Freeman, K. Simon, L. Beutler, and H. Arkowitz. New York: Plenum, 1989.

# 4 Neurobiological Foundations

No twisted thought without a twisted molecule.

Ralph Gerard, *Neurophysiology: Brain and Behavior* (1959)

I. **Introduction**
   A. In the United States the period of the 1990s has been officially declared (by act of Congress) the Decade of the Brain.
   B. This proclamation recognizes that in the past thirty years, there have been advances in the understanding of the human brain that could only be dimly envisioned at the start of the century.
   C. These developments have revolutionized psychiatric theory both by providing new techniques for examining brain functions and by offering new ways of thinking about brain dysfunctions in psychiatric disorders.
   D. Any detailed account of brain structure and function is beyond the scope of this outline, but the following sections will present some information to assist those who would like to understand more about the possible relation of mental disorder to brain disorder.

II. **Neuroscience**
   The many disciplines that contribute to the understanding of the brain are referred to collectively as neuroscience. The following list gives some idea of the many contributing areas of research, which extend from studies of the fine structure of the membranes of nerve cells to the nonintrusive observation of brain activity in human participants.
   A. Neuroanatomy
   B. Neurophysiology
   C. Neurochemistry
   D. Neuroendocrinology
   E. Neuroimmunology
   F. Neurogenetics
   G. Neuropharmacology
   H. Behavioral neuroscience
   I. Cognitive neuroscience

**Figure 4.1** *The major brain structures active in sensing and internal regulation, as well as those in the limbic system and brain stem. Source: Floyd Bloom and Arlyne Lazerson,* Brain, Mind, and Behavior *(New York: W. H. Freeman, 1985), fig. 1.7.*

## III. Brain organization

A. Basic structures (see figures 4.1, 4.2 and 4.3)

1. The nervous system consists of two basic divisions.

a) The central nervous system (CNS) lies within the skull (brain) and spinal column (spinal cord) and is a complex collection of centers of neural activity and neural pathways that connect one region with another.

b) The peripheral nervous system (PNS) includes all of the nervous system that lies outside the skull and the spinal column.

(1) The somatic division of the PNS consists of the nerve fibers that carry sensory information from the surface of the body to the CNS and the nerve fibers that carry motor signals from the CNS to the skeletal muscles.

(2) The autonomic nervous system (ANS), together with the enteric nervous system (digestive tract), regulates the internal environment that controls and maintains basic bodily processes.

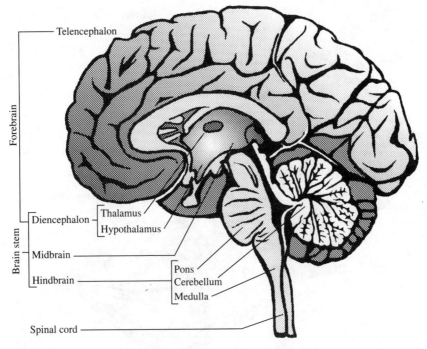

**Figure 4.2** *The major anatomical divisions and subdivisions of the brain. The midbrain is very small relative to the forebrain and hindbrain and has few distinctive features, so it is difficult to illustrate. Source: Floyd Bloom and Arlyne Lazerson,* Brain, Mind, and Behavior *(New York: W. H. Freeman, 1985), fig. 1.4.*

     (a) The parasympathetic division of the ANS controls bodily processes during relaxed states (as in rest and digestion).

     (b) The sympathetic division of the ANS mobilizes body resources for action during times of stress.

2. The brain stem and cerebellum

   a) The brain stem is the transition structure between the spinal cord and the forebrain.

   b) The brain stem is subdivided into the midbrain and the hindbrain.

   c) Attached to the hindbrain is the cerebellum.

3. The forebrain

   a) The major subdivisions of the forebrain are the diencephalon and the telencephalon.

   b) The diencephalon includes the structures of the thalamus and the hypothalamus.

   c) The telencephalon consists of the cerebral hemispheres.

     (1) The cortex, or thin covering of the cerebral hemispheres, is a network of millions of nerve cells.

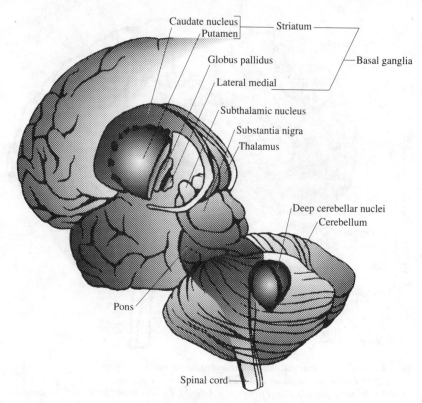

Caudate nucleus
Putamen
Striatum
Globus pallidus
Basal ganglia
Lateral medial
Subthalamic nucleus
Substantia nigra
Thalamus
Deep cerebellar nuclei
Cerebellum
Pons
Spinal cord

**Figure 4.3** *The basal ganglia, an alliance of brain places linked together within the extrapyramidal components of the motor system. The information flowing among the basal ganglia coordinates large muscular movements, initiating and terminating them.*
*Source: Floyd Bloom and Arlyne Lazerson,* Brain, Mind, and Behavior *(New York: W. H. Freeman, 1985), fig. 4.23.*

(2) One set of structures embedded in the cerebrum is loosely organized in what is called the limbic system. (Two of the major structures of the limbic system are the hippocampus and the amygdala.)

(3) Another set of structures deep in the cerebrum is referred to as the basal ganglia (included in this set are the caudate nucleus and the putamen).

B. The anatomic structures of the nervous system are organized into functional systems that integrate the behavioral capabilities and actions of the individual.

1. Much of the nervous system engages in activity that provides sensory information about the world and organizes and directs movement.

a) Some regions of the cerebral cortex are the primary reception areas for sensory experience.

b) The control of muscular activity is hierarchically organized involving the cerebral cortex, the basal ganglia, and the cerebellum.
2. The regulation of bodily processes is centrally influenced by structures of the brain stem and the hypothalamus in association with the pituitary gland.
3. The limbic structures of the brain in association with the cerebral cortex play a role in the regulation of emotion, motivation, and memory.
4. The complex circuitry of the cerebral cortex (particularly frontal and temporal regions) supports the cognitive functions involved in knowing and interpreting the world and solving the problems that it presents (which in humans includes the capacity for and the use of language).
C. The implied relation between brain function and mental state is increasingly supported in psychiatrically significant ways by current brain research (relevant examples will be provided in later sections of the outline).

IV. **Neurotransmission**
A. The neuron
1. Neurons are specialized cells that are the operational units of the nervous system.
2. Neurons vary considerably in shape and to a degree in function, but generally they consist of a cell body (soma), a set of extending processes that convey information to the cell body (dendrites), and an extended process that carries information away from the cell (axon).
3. The membrane that covers the cell and its processes is excitable and capable of transmitting voltage changes from one part of the membrane to another.
4. Part of the information that is conveyed in neurons is in the form of voltage changes.
5. The voltage change that is carried by an axon (the nerve action potential) allows a neuron to influence other neurons that its axon reaches.
B. The synapse
1. Neurons are associated with other neurons by areas of contact, or synapses, that axons make with the cell body or processes of other neurons.
2. The synaptic areas are actually minute spaces that separate parts of the neuron membrane that are specialized to release molecules of chemical substances (presynaptic) and to receive and be activated by those molecules (postsynaptic).
3. Whether or not a neuron transmits a message in its axon is determined by whether the net synaptic action on the cell is

excitatory (facilitates an action potential) or inhibitory (prevents an action potential).

4. It is assumed that the representation of learning in the nervous system involves some modification of synapses in neural networks.

C. Neuroactive substances

   1. Neuroactive substances are molecules that can interact with the membranes of neurons and alter the membrane voltage and/or influence the metabolic processes of the neuron.

     a) The effects of neuroactive substances can be relatively short acting, with a time course of one millisecond to a second or more.

     b) Some neuroactive substances, however, may facilitate or depress activity in neurons for minutes, hours, or even longer.

   2. Neurotransmitters are released from activated axons of neurons (and some dendrites) and act to excite or inhibit or to modify excitability in the postsynaptic cell.

   3. Neuromodulators are substances that tend to amplify or dampen the degree of neurotransmitter action.

   4. Many endocrine substances are also neuroactive (neurohormones).

   5. As naturally occurring neuroactive substances are added to the list, it can be seen that the nervous system is part of a large, as yet incompletely understood, regulatory system that includes the endocrine system and most likely the immune system.

D. The sequence of synaptic transmission

   1. Neurotransmitters are synthesized and stored in neurons.

   2. When an action potential is induced in an axon, on reaching the terminus it causes molecules of neurotransmitters to be released into the synapse.

   3. The neurotransmitter molecules bind to specialized molecules in the postsynaptic membrane (receptors).

   4. The effect of receptor binding is to allow a change in ion flow across the membrane (changing the membrane voltage) and/or to initiate a change in the metabolic processes of the cell (through a "second messenger" system).

   5. The precise effect of a neurotransmitter depends on the particular characteristics of the receptor; there are multiple subtypes of receptors for many neurotransmitters.

   6. Neurotransmitter molecules are released back into the synapse, where they may be inactivated by metabolic processes or taken up back into the releasing cell depending on the nature of the neurotransmitter.

7. The synthesis, release, binding, and inactivation of neuro-transmitters are complex chemical processes that can be influenced by other substances and conditions, including drugs.

E. Neurotransmitters

Neurotransmitters are proteins and are classified according to the complexity of their structure.

  1. Amino acids

    a) The simplest in structure of the neuroactive substances are the amino acids.

    b) The majority of the synapses in the brain are amino acid synapses.

    c) The amino acids that exert excitatory synaptic effects are glutamate and aspartate.

    d) The amino acids that exert inhibitory synaptic effects are gamma-aminobutyric acid (GABA) and glycine.

    e) Some amino acid receptor types are very complex in structure and function.

      (1) One type of GABA receptor also has locations that react to sedatives, anxiolytic drugs, and perhaps alcohol.

      (2) The NMDA (n-methyl-d-aspartate) type of glutamate-aspartate receptor has been identified as playing a possible role in the neuronal changes that accompany learning.

  2. Monoamines (biogenic amines)

    a) The monoamine neurotransmitters were the first to be clearly identified in the brain, and the study of their synthesis and effects provided the experimental basis for modern psychopharmacology.

    b) While a relatively small proportion of synapses in the brain are responsive to these neurotransmitters, the distribution of the synapses in the cortex, limbic system, and basal ganglia exerts strong modulatory effects on the activities of these structures.

    c) Many of the drugs that are used in the treatment of schizophrenia and affective disorders affect the release, receptor binding, and reuptake of some of these neurotransmitters.

    d) Examples of monoamines

      (1) Epinephrine

      (2) Norepinephrine (NE)

      (3) Dopamine (DA)

        (a) These three substances are also referred to collectively as catecholamines.

        (b) In synthesis dopamine is a precursor of norepinephrine, and norepinephrine is a precursor of epinephrine.

        (4) Serotonin (5–HT, 5–hydroxytryptamine)

        (5) Histamine

        (6) Acetylcholine (ACh)

  3. Neuropeptides

    a) Neuropeptides are recent entries in the classification of neuroactive substances, but vigorous research into their identification in the CNS has produced a continually growing list of these large proteins.

    b) Sources of the neuropeptides are found both in the nervous system and in the endocrine system.

    c) In the central nervous system, a neuropeptide and a neurotransmitter may be stored in the same neuron and co-released.

    d) The neuropeptides that have been most extensively studied include somatostatin, vasopressin, cholecystokinin, substance P, and neurotensin.

    e) Of particular significance is the family of neuropeptides that have been shown to have central nervous system effects like those of opiates.

        (1) Collectively they are called endorphins (for endogenous morphine-like).

        (2) The endorphins appear to have many effects, but their involvement in the regulation of pain, anxiety, and memory suggests their significance to the understanding of mental disorders.

## V. Psychopharmacology

  A. The development of psychiatric drugs and progress in the understanding of the neurotransmitter systems of the brain have occurred in complementary fashion in recent years.

  B. Major classes of psychoactive drugs. (Information will be presented in greater detail in chapter 10.)

    1. Antipsychotics

    2. Mood modifiers

      a) Antidepressants

      b) Antimanics

    3. Anxiolytics

    4. Sedative-hypnotics

    5. Stimulants

    6. Analgesics

C. Sites of action of psychoactive drugs
  1. Drugs modify brain systems in relation to the distribution and concentration of the neurotransmitter pathways that are affected.
  2. Since there are subtypes of receptors for each major neurotransmitter, drug effects will be determined by which of the receptor subtypes are affected.
     a) Some drugs affect more than one neurotransmitter system (e.g., many antidepressants affect both catecholamine and serotonin transmission).
     b) Some drugs are considered to be broad spectrum or narrow spectrum depending on the number of receptor subtype synapses that are affected.
  3. In principle a drug could affect any step of the neurotransmission process from synthesis of the neurotransmitter in the neuron to the inactivation of the neurotransmitter in the synapse. However, the more common mechanisms of drug effects are:
     a) Increasing the release of neurotransmitters at synapses
     b) Binding to synaptic receptors and simulating a neurotransmitter effect (agonists)
     c) Preventing the enzymatic breakdown of neurotransmitters in synapses or on reuptake in the presynaptic cell
     d) Blocking the effect of neurotransmitters by competing for receptor sites (antagonists)
     e) Blocking the reuptake of a neurotransmitter in a synapse thereby increasing its relative availability
     f) Binding to a complex receptor and modulating the normal effect of a neurotransmitter
D. Since drugs can affect neurotransmission at sites other than those that are targeted for psychiatric reasons, drugs will have side effects, some of which may produce unpleasant or risky symptoms.
E. The effectiveness of some drugs in psychiatric treatment has led to the development of models of underlying pathology based on those effects (e.g., the dopamine theory of schizophrenia).

VI. **Molecular genetics**
A. The distribution of mental disorders in populations, especially as investigated in family and twin studies, indicates the possible role of genetic factors in many disorders.
B. It is a reasonable assumption that the structural, metabolic, and regulatory proteins that control such activities as the assembly of synaptic receptors and the synthesis of neurotransmitters depend on the expression of specific gene products.

C. Recently developed techniques in molecular genetics are now being utilized to gain new knowledge about the structure and function of neurons.
   1. It is possible to clone gene information and produce usable amounts of purified selected samples.
   2. It is possible to learn the molecular sequencing that determines the complete structure of genes.
   3. Genetic engineering can control gene expression and alter the structure of the products of genes.
D. While neuroscientists have just begun to characterize the genes that are responsible for the development, organization, and functions of the normal brain, many investigators believe that it is only a matter of time until mental disorders will be related to variations and abnormalities in gene expression and regulation.

## VII. Prospects

Recent advances in neuroscience and the prospect of many more to come have persuaded many psychiatrists that the organic perspective, which was largely an article of faith at the beginning of the century, will be the established scientific foundation of the practice of psychiatry in the next century.

## References

Bloom, F. E., and A. Lazerson. *Brain, Mind, and Behavior.* 2d ed. New York: Freeman, 1988.

Grebb, J. A., V. I. Reus, and N. B. Freimer. "Neurobehavioral Chemistry and Physiology." In *Review of General Psychiatry.* 2d ed. edited by H. H. Goldman. Norwalk, Conn.: Appleton & Lange, 1988.

Judd, L. L., and P. M. Groves, eds. *Psychiatry.* Vol. 4, *Psychobiological Foundations of Clinical Psychiatry.* Philadelphia: Lippincott, 1986.

Kaplan, H. I. and B. J. Sadock, eds. *Comprehensive Textbook of Psychiatry/ V,* Vol. 1, 5th ed. Baltimore: Williams & Wilkins, 1989.

# 5 Etiology of Mental Disorders

The mind of men is a mystery; and, like the plant, each one of us naturally appropriates and assimilates that about him which responds to that which is within him.

Joseph Roux, "Prelude," *Meditations of a Parish Priest (1886)*

I. **Introduction**
  A. Definition
      1. Etiology refers to the study or demonstration of causes.
      2. It also refers to the causes themselves that contribute to the expression of a phenomenon, disorder, or illness.
  B. Since the essential causes of most mental disorders are unknown or incompletely understood, it is necessary to consider all the factors that could play a role in the development of a particular disorder.
      1. Some causes are remote in time and are difficult to determine convincingly in the absence of direct evidence (e.g., childhood abusive experiences).
      2. A single cause may have multiple effects and, likewise, a single effect may have multiple causes.
  C. Causes vary in the significance of their contributions to the expression of a disorder.
      1. Some factors are both necessary for the expression of a condition and sufficient to determine the condition (e.g., Huntington's disease is caused by the presence of a single gene).
      2. Some factors are necessary but not in themselves sufficient to produce a disorder (e.g., the ingestion of alcohol is necessary for the expression of alcoholism, but not all people who drink alcohol become alcoholics).
      3. Some factors may contribute to susceptibility or facilitate the conditions in which a mental disorder occurs but are neither necessary nor sufficient to the expression of the disorder (e.g., conditions of poverty or physical handicap).

D. A commonly held view is that mental disorder is the outcome of an interaction of the person (personality) with predisposing, precipitating, and perpetuating factors.
1. Predisposing factors are those that render the personality susceptible or vulnerable and generally are present over a long period of time though they may not be expressed in clinical form (subclinical).
2. Precipitating factors are events that precede and contribute to the clinical onset of a disorder.
3. Perpetuating factors are conditions that maintain, prolong, or exacerbate the symptoms or course of a disorder.
   a) For example, a person who develops a severe anxiety disorder may withdraw from social activities and limit the opportunities for social support.
   b) Sometimes these secondary factors may themselves become the object of therapeutic intervention.
   c) It is particularly important to distinguish between what is intrinsic to a disorder and what develops as a consequence of the disorder.
4. The severity of predisposing factors determines the person's vulnerability or susceptibility to precipitating factors.
5. Precipitating factors of varying severity may produce disorders in mildly predisposed persons.
   a) For example, a loosely organized schizophrenic may be inordinately upset by a mild social rebuff.
   b) Conversely, a well-integrated person may develop an anxiety reaction to a catastrophe such as a flood or a fire.
6. Predisposing factors may endure throughout the life of the individual and tend to be cumulative and connected.
7. Precipitating factors occur intermittently through life though some may be related to special developmental periods of life (e.g., adolescence, retirement).
E. As a general rule, human behavior at any time is determined by the individual's physical and psychological status and his or her capacity, at that moment, to adapt to the requirements of the immediate environment.
F. Historically, two major hypotheses have been advanced to account for the occurrence of mental disorders.
1. Proponents of the *somatogenic hypothesis* regard mental disorder as resulting from the malfunction of the central nervous system and associated regulatory systems, reflecting physical influences or genetically transmitted conditions, in a way that affects cognitive, emotional, and expressive processes.

2. Proponents of the *psychogenic hypothesis* regard mental disorder as the outcome of psychosocial (environmental) factors that influence the development of personality and the adequacy of the individual to manage the satisfaction of personal needs and the requirements of the circumstances of one's life.
3. The somatogenic and psychogenic hypotheses have been viewed as conflicting alternatives, but this view is unnecessarily dualistic.
4. All factors interact whether they are categorized as psychosocial or organic, and it is the interaction of these factors that must be considered in any etiology.

G. The diathesis-stress model views mental disorders as the product of a predisposition toward the development of a particular disorder (diathesis) and conditions operating on a person that require an adjustive response (stress).

## II. Epidemiology

A. Epidemiology is the study of the temporal and geographic distribution of a disorder within a specified population.
B. Epidemiological studies are concerned with the occurrence of a disorder in groups of people rather than in individual cases.
C. Epidemiological studies obtain information about the rates, correlates, and potential etiological factors of a disorder in a given population.
D. Prevalence studies are concerned with the proportion of a population that has or has had the disorder that is being studied.
   1. Point prevalence refers to the rate that is determined on the particular occasion of the study.
   2. Period prevalence refers to rates based on frequencies of a disorder accumulated over a specified period of time.
   3. Lifetime prevalence refers to the proportion of a sample that has experienced a disorder in their lives up to the time of the study.
   4. In cohort studies, a group of people may be followed for a period of time to observe the onset or change in a disorder.
   5. Prevalence studies of various diagnostic groups are particularly useful in the planning of mental health services.
E. Incidence refers to the number of new cases of a disorder that occur in a given period of time (e.g., annual rates of new admissions of various diagnostic groups to the mental health facilities of a region).
F. Risk or vulnerability refers to a condition or circumstance that, if present, increases the probability of a disorder in a population (e.g., a high cholesterol level increases the risk for heart disease).

G. While epidemiological studies alone cannot provide convincing evidence about causal factors in mental disorders, they can indicate relationships that might provide clues for causal studies. For example, the following relationships occur in some disorders:
   1. Differences in prevalence or incidence rates of a disorder for men and women
   2. Different rates of prevalence or incidence associated with socioeconomic level
   3. Different incidence rates associated with age
   4. Differential risk associated with ethnic or national group membership
H. The *Diagnostic and Statistical Manual of Mental Disorders,* third edition, revised (*DSM*-III-R), contains information about prevalence and other epidemiological findings for disorders where there have been adequate studies.

III. **Predisposing factors**
   A. Predisposing factors are those that increase the risk of developing a mental disorder by increasing vulnerability to stressful precipitating factors.
      1. Factors that increase vulnerability may be either biological or psychosocial in nature.
      2. Currently attention in research is being directed toward conditions and characteristics that increase invulnerability as well as to those that contribute to vulnerability.
   B. Genetic influences
      1. Genetic influences control both the characteristic development of members of a species but also are a source of individual differences.
      2. The influence of genes begins at conception and may be expressed at any time throughout life.
      3. Chromosomal aberrations and faulty genes may result in metabolic and biochemical dysfunctions that may predispose individuals to particular disorders.
         a) Variations in chromosomal structure and number are related to such outcomes as *Down's syndrome* (a common form of mental retardation, once called mongolism and caused by an autosomal anomaly) and *Turner's syndrome* (a chromosomal defect in women with a karyotype of XO and with forty-five rather than the usual forty-six chromosomes), but none of the major mental disorders have been linked to chromosomal abnormalities.
         b) Huntington's disease, a degenerative disorder of the basal ganglia and cortex characterized by progressive intellectual loss and motor dysfunction, is related to a

dominant gene, but such simple genetic models have not been found in major mental disorders.

   c) Genetic markers have been reported in some studies of bipolar disorder.

   d) The search for a genetic cause of schizophrenia has produced many studies, but at present no accurate genetic model has been developed and no genetic marker has been discovered.

4. Genetic influences are presumed to operate through mechanisms that affect the development of the nervous system, the organization of critical structures, the metabolism of neurotransmitters, and the regulation of the production and location of receptors.

5. Advances in genetic research holds much promise for unraveling the complicated effects of genetic makeup in personality and mental disorders.

   a) Family risk and pedigree studies, while in themselves are incapable of discriminating the interaction of genetic and environmental influences, can point in directions for other research to follow.

      (1) It is important to note that pathological ways of feeling and thinking may be transmitted within families by parents' pathological behavior and example rather than through genetic transmission.

      (2) In such examples it is appropriate to talk of familial disorders that are not necessarily hereditary.

   b) Adoptive studies, in which frequency and risk for mental disorder can be assessed in both biological and adoptive parents, help separate the relative contributions of genetic and environmental influences.

   c) Twin studies permit the investigation of co-occurrence (concordance) rates for monozygotic (identical) and dizygotic (fraternal) twins.

   d) Linkage studies look for predisposing genes that cluster together with marker genes that have identifiable characteristics and known modes of inheritance.

   e) Techniques of molecular genetics hold great promise for localizing and mapping genes and determining the biochemical processes that they regulate and control. (The analysis of the genetic basis of Huntington's disease provides a remarkable model of the successful application of these techniques.)

C. Constitutional factors

1. Characteristics are considered to be constitutional if they are either innate or acquired so early (as early as in the

prenatal environment) that the effects are similar to those of genetically determined characteristics.

2. Physique and appearance
   a) While earlier hypotheses about the relationship between body type and mental disorder have not been substantiated, tendencies toward particular body configurations or size may be related to a higher probability of certain kinds of social experiences and styles of reaction.
   b) The value placed on physical characteristics by a society (e.g., beauty) can influence experiences of social acceptance and rejection and the attitudes one has toward one's own appearance.

3. Congenital defects
   a) Abnormalities in fetal development or environmental conditions operating before, at, or shortly after birth may produce abnormalities that affect later development and behavior.
   b) Premature birth and low birth weight (which may be the result of a number of influences) have been associated with developmental disturbances though not to specific syndromes of mental disorders.
   c) Nicotine, alcohol, and other chemical use are associated with higher risk for premature birth and low birth weight (e.g., "crack babies"), but the long-term consequences of these factors have not yet been reliably established.
   d) Heavy alcohol consumption during pregnancy can produce the symptoms of fetal alcohol syndrome—physical distortions of the head and face, small stature, and mental retardation.
   e) The effects of environmental pollutants, toxins, and low-level radiation on prenatal and early postnatal development are possible sources of vulnerability.

4. Newborns differ in basic reaction patterns or temperament, and these patterns influence the style of parental interaction between the infant and its care-givers.

D. Group membership
   1. Risk has been associated with a variety of group membership variables but the mechanisms that account for the risk relationships are obscure and undoubtedly quite complex.
   2. Gender
      a) Sex differences occur in the frequency with which some psychiatric diagnoses are made.
         (1) Major affective disorders, generalized anxiety disorder, somatization disorder, and multiple personality

are among the diagnoses made more frequently in women.

   (2) Alcoholism, antisocial personality disorder, and paranoid personality disorder are among the diagnoses made more frequently in men.

b) Since social roles are profound influences on how one develops styles of behavior and self-assessment in relation to the expectations of others, it is difficult to separate factors that are role related from those that are constitutional or dimorphic (chromosomally determined).

c) Current analyses of gender-related differences indicate a number of methodological issues that must be considered in making interpretations of risk associated with gender differences.

   (1) Sex role stereotypes have been shown to operate in the models of mental health and mental illness that many people hold; it is possible that such biases may influence diagnostic judgments.

   (2) Expectations about responsibilities and power may pose particular problems for women who may be perceived as departing from conventional social roles.

   (3) It has been proposed by some investigators that women's risk may be increased by the greater stress, frustration, and dissatisfaction associated with the position they occupy in a society.

3. Age

a) Certain periods of life are considered to be times of special vulnerability, not only because of the occurrence of physical changes but also because of special psychological demands that may be confronted during the period.

b) Adolescence (puberty), middle life (the involutional period), and old age (the senium) are often considered to be periods of special stress.

4. Racial and ethnic group membership

a) Relative frequency differences in some mental disorders have been found in studies of groups within a dominant culture and in cross-cultural studies, but the interpretation of the complex factors that contribute to such findings does not yield any simple conclusions about either genetic factors or cultural differences.

b) Members of groups that are targets of prejudice and discrimination within a larger society may be placed in chronic circumstances of social, political, and economic disadvantage.

c) Coping with the chronic stress of social disadvantage because of one's racial or ethnic identification may sometimes lead to adaptive responses that may be perceived by the larger society as maladaptive (e.g., increased sensitivity to prejudice and discrimination may be interpreted as paranoid suspicion).

5. Economic status

a) Some now-classic studies have shown relationships between socioeconomic standing, frequency with which certain diagnoses are made and the kind of treatment that is received.

b) A correlation between low economic status and the frequency of a number of physical and mental disorders is well established, but the direction of causation is not indicated in such correlational studies.

c) Poverty is a circumstance that increases the level of a number of risk factors (e.g., malnutrition, inadequate prenatal care, disorganized family structures).

E. Early deprivations

1. Chronic malnutrition may retard physical and mental growth and produce lowered resistance to environmental stress.

2. Extreme isolation from human contact during infancy and early childhood can produce chronic deficits in cognitive and social functioning.

3. Retrospective studies suggest that extreme physical and sexual abuse may have both general effects on the capacity for relationships, particularly with children, and may increase the vulnerability to some mental disorders (e.g., multiple personality).

IV. **Precipitating factors**

A. As with predisposing factors, precipitating factors may be either biological or psychosocial.

B. Essentially, precipitating factors arise in the environment and are frequently referred to as environmental factors.

1. The environment includes those physical and biological variables that affect the functioning of the body and the psychosocial variables that influence interpersonal relations and determine the deficiencies and rewards that affect psychological well-being.

2. Environmental variables can be assessed objectively, but it is important also to consider the way that they are perceived and interpreted by a person.

3. Potential precipitating factors are so numerous that no exhaustive account will be attempted here.

C. Psychosocial stressors
   1. The *Diagnostic and Statistical Manual of Mental Disorders* (*DSM*-III-R) recognizes a number of precipitating factors and rates their severity on Axis IV of the multiaxial diagnostic procedure that the manual recommends.
   2. Among the factors mentioned are the following:
      a) Various family events and interactions (e.g., engagement, marriage, separation, death, parenthood)
      b) Other interpersonal relationships (e.g., difficulties with friends, neighbors, or work associates)
      c) Living circumstances (change in residence, immigration)
      d) Financial conditions (loss of wage earner, investment losses, inadequate financial resources)
      e) Legal affairs (being arrested, suing or being sued, custody settlement)
      f) Occupation
         (1) Job-related stresses (conflict with a supervisor, competition for promotion).
         (2) Overwork is usually considered a symptom of a problem rather than as a cause in itself.
         (3) Special occupational hazards.
         (4) Women's occupations in which they have to contend with sexist attitudes (e.g., less pay or benefits, expected stereotypical feminine behavior, insensitivity to child-care issues).

D. Physical illness or physical handicap
   1. Physical illness may pose both practical and emotional problems.
      a) Pain, discomfort, enforced idleness
      b) Financial problems such as cost of hospitalization and treatment and disruption of earning capacity
      c) Emotional side effects such as reactivation of feelings of dependency or inadequacy
      d) Distortions of body image as in such mutilative surgery as mastectomy
      e) Effects of illness or treatment that affect sexual adequacy or arouse concerns about sexual adequacy
   2. Physical handicaps may arouse feelings of inadequacy, helplessness, or resentment or may produce maladaptive overcompensations, but most people with physical handicaps do not manifest enduring emotional problems.
   3. Drugs (both prescribed and self-administered) may be taken in toxic doses that produce organic mental disorders.

4. Environmental and industrial toxins (e.g., insecticides, solvents) may also induce symptoms of organic mental disorders.

5. Some infectious diseases may lead to delirium with accompanying hallucinations and delusions.

6. Some diseases (e.g., syphilis, encephalitis, AIDS) may produce changes in the nervous system that in some cases may produce mental symptoms).

7. Brain trauma may produce reversible or irreversible changes with accompanying personality effects or mental symptoms.

E. Deprivations and deficiencies

1. Starvation or special dietary deficiencies may lead to personality changes and symptoms of mental disorder.

2. Sensory deprivation may in some instances lead to hallucinations and other distortions of perception and judgment such as are experienced by some people who are required to have their eyes bandaged over a period of time or by lone explorers or sailors.

3. Deprivation of sleep may lead to temporary mental and personality changes such as inability to concentrate, restlessness, loss of interest, and occasionally hallucinatory experiences.

4. Even something as simple as reduction of sunlight may trigger depressive reactions in some predisposed persons (as in seasonal affective disorder).

F. Disasters and catastrophes

1. Most people experience at least short-term reactions to being involved in accidents, fires, earthquakes, floods, and events of war.

2. Some people may experience more prolonged reactions or recurring reactions (post-traumatic stress syndrome).

3. Not only the victims but also those who work with the victims and the effects of disasters may experience unexpected emotional reactions as an aftermath of their involvement.

4. Post-traumatic effects may also occur in people who have been raped, assaulted or robbed.

V. **Developmental perspectives**

A. Predisposing and precipitating factors act on and in individuals who have developed the characteristic vulnerabilities and competencies in managing their lives (what we generally refer to as personality).

B. Many personality theories attempt to account for the occurrence of personality and mental disorders in terms of the adequacy of the development of individual personality structures and adaptive mechanisms for meeting the demands and circumstances of adult life.

1. Early development is frequently conceived of as involving certain kinds of situations to be mastered and certain competencies to be acquired and exercised.
   a) Particularly important in early development are the experiences that affect interpersonal relations, socialization, and a sense of self-esteem.
   b) Sometimes early childhood circumstances may introduce deprivation, conflict, or trauma that interferes with normal personality development and may leave the person vulnerable to later experiences or with inadequate ways of dealing with them.
   c) Accordingly, some people may be predisposed to develop adult disorders if circumstances of adult life challenge their vulnerabilities or inadequate responses.

2. Adult development may also be viewed as a continuum of situations and problems to be met and mastered, particularly in areas of personal relationships and achievement.
   a) For convenience of description and discussion, the continuum is often divided into stages that summarize the special cultural expectations and opportunities that are associated with periods of adult life span.
   b) These developmental stages serve as a background against which to consider sources of stress associated with particular developmental tasks and requirements.
   c) These commonly faced challenges and opportunities of adult life may for some people be a source of precipitating factors for the occurrence of a mental disorder.

C. Freud's well-known stages of psychosexual development provide an example of how early experiences can be considered to shape the development of personality in a way that might predispose a person to a personality or mental disorder (see chapter 2 for a description of Freud's stages and other developmental perspectives).

D. Erik Erikson, in a more sociocultural approach, modified the account of Freud's psychosexual stages and extended the stages of development through the adult life span.

1. For Erikson, each stage from infancy to old age is seen as involving a developmental challenge or "crisis" to be managed and, ideally, resolved by the accomplishment of a value; to fail to do so leaves the person less well equipped to deal with later challenges and may result in personality disorders.

2. For example, the early childhood stage that Freud called "anal" for Erikson involves a conflict between autonomy versus shame and doubt and is resolved productively by the accomplishment of a sense of will.
3. Adult stages deal with issues of identity (adolescence), intimacy (young adulthood), generativity (adulthood), and integrity (late adulthood) and are resolved positively by the accomplishment of a sense of fidelity, love, care, and wisdom, respectively.

E. The life span developmental perspective has led to a number of studies of the cycles of adult life in men and women and several descriptive models.
   1. These models usually consider the development of and commitment to an adult organization of one's life that provides a pattern of key choices, goals, and values.
   2. Transitions from one stage to another become the occasions for self-evaluation and the modification of patterns.
   3. Transition periods may also be periods of particular stress for some people depending on the opportunities and pressures for change and the rigidity or flexibility of their life patterns.

## VI. Etiology of mental disorders

A. The etiology of mental disorders should be regarded as a complex interaction of genetic, physical, and psychosocial factors.
   1. Some factors are probably inherent to the individual, some develop or occur so early in life that they become an integral part of the basic personality structure, and others exert their influence later in life.
   2. The major factors to consider can be summarized briefly:
      a) Genetic factors may include presence or absence of mental disorder in the family, metabolic balances affecting nervous system function, innate adaptive tendencies, physical endowment, and the like.
      b) Early environmental influences that influence emotional learning and development such as parental attitudes, family interactions, and sociocultural influences.
      c) The characteristic coping and defensive styles that a person learns to use in handling interpersonal relations and developmental requirements.
      d) Stress, which includes both physical and psychosocial sources of threat or loss.
   3. The etiology of mental disorder, thus, may result from an interaction of predisposing and precipitating organic and psychosocial factors with the personality organization of a person, as in the following schema:

Hereditary factors + early environmental influences (lead to) → defensive and coping strategies + stress (may lead to) → mental disorder.

B. This approach is sometimes referred to as the biopsychosocial model of mental disorder.

C. Some aspects of psychosocial concepts are reviewed in chapters 2, 3, and 6. Organic concepts are reviewed in chapter 4.

## References

Carson, R., J. Butcher, and J. C. Coleman. *Abnormal Psychology and Life*. 8th ed. Glenview, Ill.: Scott, Foresman, 1988.

Costin, F., and J. Dragus. *Abnormal Psychology*. New York: Wiley, 1989.

Gelder, M., D. Gath, and R. Mayou. *Oxford Textbook of Psychiatry*. 2d ed. Oxford: Oxford University Press, 1988.

Gould, R. "Adulthood." In *Comprehensive Textbook of Psychiatry/V*. Vol. 2, 5th ed., edited by H. I. Kaplan and B. J. Sadock. Baltimore: Williams & Wilkins, 1989.

Maxman, J. *Essential Psychopathology*. New York: Norton, 1986.

# 6  Stress and Anxiety

Joy, interrupted now and again by pain and terminated ultimately by death, seems the normal course of life in nature. Anxiety and distress, interrupted occasionally by pleasure, is the normal course of man's existence.

Joseph Wood Krutch, "May," *The Twelve Seasons* (1949)

I. **Introduction**
   A. For much of the twentieth century, anxiety was a key explanatory concept in psychopathology, not only in the psychodynamic theory of neurosis, but in other disorders as well.
   B. During the past twenty-five years, anxiety has come to be viewed much less as a primary theoretical concept but still remains useful as a term to identify both a subjective state and a pattern of response that are common in normal experience as well as in psychiatric practice.
   C. During the same time, *stress* has become a prominent concept in psychiatry and is a common term in popular usage.
   D. While the terms are not exactly synonymous, it is useful to consider them together.

II. **Stress**
   A. Stress is defined and discussed in a variety of ways, but commonly the description of stress includes the following:
      1. The external events or stressors that affect the individual
      2. The individual differences in the interpretation and recognition of stressors and their impact
      3. The effects of stress on the individual
         a) Subjective experiences of stress
         b) Physiological and behavioral effects of stress
         c) Physiological adaptations to persistent stressors
      4. The behavioral coping strategies used by individuals to adapt to stressful situations
   B. Acute stress produces physiological changes during which the body is alerting itself and preparing for vigorous body activity (fight or flight)

1. Certain body processes are stimulated while others are inhibited.
   a) The cardiovascular system is stimulated, the heart beats faster, and blood pressure is maintained or elevated to force more blood to the muscles.
   b) The liver makes more energy available through glucose release.
   c) The adrenal glands secrete epinephrine (adrenalin).
   d) The gastrointestinal system is inhibited, and its secretions and peristaltic activity are reduced.
2. These body adjustments prepare the individual for activity. The blood that is redirected from the gastrointestinal tract is made available to the muscular system.
3. The sympathetic division of the autonomic nervous system regulates these ''emergency'' reactions with norepinephrine serving as the neurotransmitter that influences the peripheral physiological targets of the system.

C. Stress is coming to be understood in terms of the mediation of stress responses by the actions of the hypothalamic-pituitary-adrenal axis.
   1. The stressor through its specific effects excites the sympathetic nervous system and the hypothalamus.
   2. The hypothalamus secretes corticotrophic hormone releasing factor (CRF), which is relayed to the anterior pituitary.
   3. The pituitary discharges adrenocorticotrophic hormone (ACTH) into the bloodstream.
   4. ACTH reaches the adrenal cortex and stimulates the release into the bloodstream of corticoids such as cortisol and corticosterone.
   5. The corticoids mobilize sources of energy for adaptive reactions and facilitate other responses.
   6. The corticoids also feedback to the hypothalamus inhibiting the secretion of ACTH if corticoid levels are high.
   7. There are probably other central nervous system mechanisms involved, particularly those influenced by the norepinephrine pathways of the brain stem.

D. Hans Selye (1976) made a particularly important contribution to the analysis of stress by describing the general adaptation syndrome, a sequence of stages that the body passes through when stress is particularly intense or prolonged.
   1. The alarm reaction is the first response to stress. It functions to increase alertness and sensitivity stimuli (vigilance) and is accompanied by increased emotionality, tension, and sympathetic nervous system activity.

2. The stage of resistance is the adaptation to persisting stress. Coping responses are directed toward maintaining task-oriented activity, which may reduce the excesses of the alarm reaction but may also introduce some potentially maladaptive features.
3. The stage of exhaustion follows prolonged stress in which the adaptation of the stage of resistance leaves the individual vulnerable to and unable to respond appropriately to additional stress (decompensation).
4. Selye's general adaptation syndrome has been applied particularly to the interpretation of stress-related diseases, but it also provides a useful way to think about psychological adaptation and defense.

E. Psychosocial stressors
  1. All situations that require some adjustive response might be considered stressful. Selye distinguishes between two types of stress.
    a) Eustress refers to positive stress situations that require adaptation but are generally viewed favorably (e.g., marriage, a work promotion).
    b) Distress refers to negative stress situations that require adaptation but involve losses or threat (e.g., death of family member, reduction of financial resources).
  2. Stressors are often highly individual, and their effect may depend on:
    a) A person's vulnerability (stress tolerance)
    b) The nature of the stress
    c) A person's psychological resources such as capacity to cope and available defenses
    d) The self-perception of the person's adaptive capabilities
  3. A common feature of negative life events that may add to their stressfulness is the unpredictability and/or uncontrollability of the event and its consequences.
  4. DSM-III-R considers the severity of psychosocial stressors on Axis IV and provides a rating scale for coding severity.
    a) The scale severity ranges from mild to catastrophic.
    b) Stressors are specified as either acute (duration less than six months) or enduring (duration greater than six months).
  5. Types of psychosocial stressors considered in DSM-III-R.
    a) Conjugal (marital and nonmarital) (e.g., discord, separation, or divorce)
    b) Parenting (e.g., illness of a child)
    c) Other interpersonal relations (e.g., disagreement with a neighbor)
    d) Occupational (e.g., job loss, retirement)

e) Living circumstances (e.g., moving to another city)
f) Financial (e.g., bank closure, stock market crash)
g) Legal (e.g., arrest, being sued)
h) Developmental (e.g., turning forty)
i) Physical illness or injury
6. Holmes and his colleagues have developed a scale of impact of life stresses (Social Readjustment Rating Scale).
a) High-rated stressors include such events as death of a spouse, divorce, personal injury, or illness.
b) Low-rated stressors include such events as a change in social activities, a vacation, and minor law violations.
c) When assessed over a period of time, the scale provides a way to consider cumulative stress.
d) Research has indicated that persons who are exposed to a number of life stresses over a period of time have a high risk for an accident and for developing a major illness in the years immediately following the period of exposures.

F. Reactions to stress
1. General responses to stress
a) Responses that maintain an orientation toward solving problems posed by the stress, such as changing the situation or one's behavior (problem-focused responses)
b) Responses that protect the individual from the discomfort or disorganizing effect of the stressor but do not alter the stressor (emotion-focused responses)
2. Decompensation under severe stress
a) Whether stress is "excessive" is a function of predisposing and precipitating events and the tolerance and coping styles of the individual.
b) Excessive stress is signaled by a general lowering of effectiveness with which a person handles other life activities.
c) If severe stressors require mobilization of personal resources to their limit, there may be lowering of resistance to the effects of other stressors.
d) Decompensation may be both psychological and physical (lowered resistance to disease).

## III. Managing stress
A. Since stress is a highly distressing state, individuals usually act to reduce it or be rid of it.
1. Conscious attempts to manage stress are usually called coping strategies.
2. Unconscious ways of handling stress traditionally have been called defenses.

B. Coping strategies can call on cognitive, emotional, and behavioral resources to deal with stress.
   1. Some strategies are directed toward solving the problem directly.
   2. Others may be directed toward managing the emotional effects of a stressor.
   3. Still others may be directed toward changing ways of thinking about a stressful situation or problem, about plans, or even about one's basic orientation to life.
C. The denial or suppression of the emotional and cognitive significance of stressors is a common response and may be effective in acute or short-term stress situations.
D. Horowitz (1988) describes cognitive coping strategies that involve choices about what to think about and do.
   1. Changing what is thought about includes intensively focusing on the situation, avoiding thinking about it by focusing on something else, and "taking the long view."
   2. The modality of thinking may be shifted to utilize or avoid such things as vivid images about the stress-producing circumstances.
E. Coping styles
   1. Research has been directed toward assessing individual differences in the ways people cope with stress.
   2. Some of the general findings of this research are:
      a) Men tend to use direct action a little more and distraction, emotional catharsis, and social support a little less than women.
      b) The way in which a problem is assessed is significantly related to the way people attempt to handle it.
      c) Most people are flexible in their coping styles. While they may have a preferred approach, they combine it with other strategies as the problem requires.

IV. **Anxiety**
A. Comparison of anxiety and stress
   1. Stress, as has been noted, refers, in its negative instances, to conditions that are extremely unpleasant, noxious, or demanding and that produce both the experience of stress and effects on physiological state and behavior.
   2. Anxiety, in traditional psychiatric usage, has been defined as a diffuse unpleasant uneasiness, apprehension, or fearfulness stemming from anticipated danger, the source of which is uncertain or unidentifiable.
   3. The experiential or "state of mind" aspects of stress have much in common with the experience of anxiety.

B. Characteristics of anxiety
   1. Anxiety can be viewed as an alerting or signaling process that warns the individual of impending danger and stimulates preparations to deal with the threat.
   2. It can be a highly distressing state and if sustained may call into play coping or defensive behaviors.
   3. The physiological manifestations of anxiety are products of the action of the sympathetic nervous system as enhanced by the response of the adrenal glands.
      a) Dermatological responses include pallor of the skin, sweating, and erection of skin hairs.
      b) Cardiovascular responses include tachycardia and increase in systolic blood pressure; occasionally the cardiovascular response is one of decreased activity with resulting fainting.
      c) Gastrointestinal responses include anorexia (loss of appetite), nausea, "butterflies in the stomach," diarrhea, and constipation.
      d) Respiratory responses include rapid breathing and hyperventilation.
      e) Genitourinary responses include urinary urgency and frequency, impotence, dysmenorrhea, dyspareunia, and frigidity.
      f) Vasomotor responses include sweating or flushing.
      g) Musculoskeletal responses may appear as trembling, tension headaches, tension in the muscles of the back of the neck, quavering voice, and feelings of discomfort in muscles and joints.
   4. The psychological manifestations of anxiety include both the conscious experience of body responses and a sense of apprehension or dread. Often there is an obsessive preoccupation with worrisome thoughts and concerns about physiological symptoms and what they might mean.
   5. General behavioral reactions include restlessness and general indications of muscular tension.
C. The role of anxiety in psychodynamic theory
   1. The concept of anxiety in the psychodynamic perspective is based on Freud's analysis of the term.
      a) Anxiety is intrapsychic, originating in the personality and the dynamics of personality formation and development.
      b) Anxiety arises from conflict.
      c) Anxiety is a normal response to threat and is an essential warning process.

d) Anxiety is a driving force for many human adjustive responses during development.

e) The mechanisms for coping with anxiety or defending against it form the basis of psychodynamics and psychopathology.

f) The consistent use of certain defenses is involved in the development of personality character traits.

## V. Defense mechanisms

A. Defense mechanisms, in psychodynamic usage, are specific, unconscious, intrapsychic adjustments that represent attempts to resolve emotional conflict and reduce anxiety.

B. They are variously referred to as mental mechanisms, mental dynamisms, ego defense mechanisms, and adjustive techniques.

C. They function to keep people from being anxious or to reduce their anxiety, and to protect the consistency of one's sense of self (ego) though with some distortion in perception and interpretations of reality.

D. In psychodynamic interpretations, they also maintain and bolster repression.

E. In behavioral terms, defense mechanisms function as escape or avoidance reactions that are learned and maintained by the reinforcing effects of reducing or terminating the aversive stimulation of anxiety.

## VI. Specific defenses

A. Repression

*Repression* is the involuntary, automatic banishment of unacceptable ideas, impulses, or feelings into the unconscious (motivated unconscious forgetting).

1. It is best known of all the ego defenses and one of the most commonly employed.

2. It retains the central position in psychodynamic theory that was allotted to it by Freud in relation to ego defenses and symptom formation.

3. It is sometimes used as a generic term for all defense mechanisms. It is a primary defense against anxiety and as such is considered the cornerstone of psychodynamics. If it is unsuccessful in preventing anxiety, it may then be coupled with other defense mechanisms to permit the emergence of repressed material in disguised form. Two such combinations follow.

a) *Repression plus displacement,* also termed *focalization,* produces phobic responses that veil the repressed wish. For example, a thirty-six-year-old mother developed the fear that her two-year-old daughter would contract a serious illness. The phobia was a defense against her repressed hostility toward, and rejection of, the girl.

b) *Repression plus conversion,* also termed *symbolic somatization,* produces a hysterical response. For example, a twenty-year-old soldier developed paralysis of his right hand when firing on the rifle range. His paralysis was a defense against his repressed hostility toward his father, who had abandoned the family.

4. In psychodynamic theory, conflicts that remain repressed are unchanged in quality and intensity. Because they retain their dynamic drive, they constantly seek expression. This is usually called *cathexis.* This requires a constant expenditure of emotional energy, *countercathexis,* to prevent the conflictual material from appearing in awareness. Often such repressed material reemerges in other ways: in our dreams, for example, in slips of the tongue, or in other aspects of everyday behavior. Freud referred to these as *the psychopathology of everyday life.*

5. Not all repressed conflicts cause psychopathology in the individual. Repression is a universally used defense mechanism. For example, we all sometimes forget the name of a well-known person or a frequently called telephone number. Only if abnormal behavior results is repression considered pathological.

B. Suppression

*Suppression* is the voluntary, intentional relegation of unacceptable ideas or impulses to the foreconscious (volitional exclusion, or conscious forgetting).

1. Technically, since suppression is a conscious process, it is not considered a true defense mechanism by many authorities.

2. The conflict can be readily recalled because it remains in the foreconscious.

3. It is a commonly employed coping mechanism of normal personalities and, thus, is considered a mature defense.

4. Conscious control requires a strong ego.

5. Examples of suppression
   a) A person who behaved foolishly under the influence of alcohol the previous evening may consciously try to forget the behavior the following day.
   b) A student who wishes to study for an examination may consciously set aside distracting fantasies.

C. Regression

*Regression* is the unconscious return to an earlier level of emotional adjustment at which gratification was assured (turning back the maturational clock and going back to earlier modes of dealing with the world).

1. The retreat may be partial, total, or symbolic.
2. Many symptoms of emotional disorder have a regressive aspect, since mature modes of adjustment are replaced by behavior that represents a reversion to an earlier level of adjustment. It is not a desirable adaptation because, in the process, some developmental maturity is lost.
3. Regression may occur normally, as in the following examples:
   a) It occurs normally in play and sleep.
   b) A toilet-trained, firstborn child may temporarily lose bladder and bowel control in response to the arrival of a second child in the family.
   c) A person promoted to a more responsible position may experience the rearousal of underlying uncertainty, insecurity, and indecision, and hence ask to be returned to the old job.
   d) A person hospitalized for any kind of illness may experience the rearousal of underlying, unmet dependency, and hence make unnecessary requests and demands for attention and care.
4. Regression may be a symptom of pathology.
   a) Excessive dependence on oral gratification can represent a return to the breast. This is seen, for example, in alcoholics.
   b) It is a primary defense in the production of obsessive-compulsive disorders.
   c) Schizophrenia is profound regression, in the psychological sense. In the more severe forms, regression is seen in many aspects of the individual's personality.

D. Fixation

*Fixation* is the arrest of maturation at an immature level of psychosexual development.

1. Fixation may occur when there is excessive gratification or excessive frustration at a particular developmental level.
2. Examples of fixation
   a) An overly dependent attachment to a parent that remains the same over a long period.
   b) The continued attachment to a nursing bottle beyond infancy.
   c) The infantile behavior sometimes seen in psychosis may be interpreted as fixation or regression.

E. Identification

*Identification* is the unconscious, wishful adoption, or internalization, of the personality characteristics or identity of another individual, generally one possessing attributes that the subject envies or admires.

1. Normal identification
   a) Identification plays a decisive role in normal personality development, especially the development of the superego (including the conscience), and occurs within the family setting. It requires the continuing presence and emotional support of the parenting ones.
   b) Normally, a boy identifies principally with his father, a girl, with her mother.
   c) Children often emulate other important parent figures, for example, teachers, scout leaders, athletes, or television and movie personalities.
   d) A person's adult identification, or adult individuation, evolves from the success of identification with all of these important figures.
   e) Identification is to be distinguished from imitation, which is a conscious mimicking of the behavior of others.
   f) *Empathy* is the capacity for participating in, or vicariously experiencing, another's feelings, volitions, or ideas. This ability to feel with another is a form of identification found in mature, well-integrated personalities.
   g) The transference occurring in the therapist-patient relationship in psychotherapy may be based on identification with important figures in one's early life (see chapter 9).

2. Identification may be distorted.
   a) A person may internalize certain undesirable personality traits of parent or authority figures. This is sometimes called *hostile identification.*
   b) *Identification with the aggressor* is the unconscious internalization of the characteristics of a frustrating or feared person.
   c) A severely pathological kind of identification is seen in the psychotic person who believes he or she is God or some other important personage.
   d) This mechanism operates in induced paranoid disorder, or *folie à deux* (see chapter 26).

F. Incorporation

*Incorporation* is a primitive defense mechanism in which the psychic image of another person is wholly or partially assimilated into an individual's personality. Incorporation is a psychoanalytic term.

1. It is a special type of introjection (see the following).
2. It is the primary mechanism in identification.
3. It is assumed to begin during the oral phase of personality development and to be related to the nursing experience. An example is the infantile fantasy that the mother's breast has been ingested and has become a part of oneself.

G. Introjection

*Introjection* is the symbolic internalization or assimilation (taking into oneself) of a loved or hated person or external object.

1. This mechanism is the converse of projection (see the following).
2. It is sometimes regarded as a form of identification. It is also closely related to incorporation.
3. It plays a fundamental role in the early development of the ego (it antedates identification).
4. It also plays an important role in the development of the superego; that is, the child internalizes parental values and ideals.
5. It operates in the process of mourning as sadness appropriate to a loss.
6. It tends to obliterate the distinction between the loved object and the person.
7. Instead of expressing anger or aggression toward others, people sometimes turn these unacceptable tendencies into self-criticism, self-depreciation, and self-accusation. This is also referred to as turning against the self.
8. In depressive disorders, individuals direct unacceptable aggressive and hostile impulses toward themselves—that is, toward the introjected objects or persons within themselves.

H. Projection

*Projection* is the attributing, to another person or object, the thoughts, feelings, motives, or desires that are really one's own disavowed and unacceptable traits.

1. Normal projection
   a) Mild forms of projection are found in normal, everyday activities. We call them alibiing: the "blind" referee, the unfair supervisor, the scapegoat, and various prejudices and other types of suspiciousness and hypervigilance to external danger.
   b) In mythology, human qualities are often attributed to nonhuman things or events. This is also called anthropomorphism. In the novel *Main Street,* by Sinclair Lewis, Carol Kennicott takes a walk in Gopher Prairie shortly

after her arrival. Looking up the street, "oozing out from every drab wall, she felt a forbidding spirit which she could never conquer."

    c) Many of us are often critical of our own shortcomings in other people and, as a consequence, tend to hold others responsible for our own difficulties.

  2. Projection as a symptom

    a) To some extent, projection, like rationalization (see the following), is a misinterpretation or distortion of reality, and hence is potentially dangerous.

    b) It is associated with immaturity and vulnerability.

    c) It is a form of displacement and closely associated with denial (see the discussion of denial later in this chapter).

    d) In a pathological sense, this is the mechanism operating in paranoid disorders of all types (paranoia, induced paranoid disorder, acute paranoid disorder, and paranoid schizophrenia). If the ego becomes disorganized, it leads to

      (1) Delusions or *projected ideation.* The ego loses the capacity to distinguish inner fantasies from external reality.

      (2) Hallucinations, or projections of perception.

      (3) Ideas of reference, also a projection of ideation.

I. Rationalization

*Rationalization* is the ascribing of acceptable or worthwhile motives to one's own thoughts, feelings, or behavior that really have unrecognized motives. One does something and invents a reason for the action. It can also be thought of as unconscious, retrospective justification (proclaiming logical reasons for actions actually performed for other reasons, usually to avoid stress or self-blame; rationalization is also used to justify avoiding unpleasant duties).

  1. Rationalization, which is an unconscious mechanism, is not to be confused with pretending or lying, both of which are conscious processes because the individual recognizes that the "reasons" for his or her behavior are fictitious.

  2. It is a very common defense. Much of our behavior has multiple determinations; that is, several motives are involved. When we "explain" our behavior by the most acceptable of these motives, we are rationalizing.

  3. It helps one preserve self-respect and avoid accountability and guilt.

  4. It can even be positive in that it enhances self-esteem.

  5. A minor element of truth is often involved.

  6. Although rationalizing is self-protective, it is also self-deceiving and hence potentially dangerous. As J. B. S.

Haldane has written, "Let him beware of him in whom reason has become the greatest and most terrible of passions."
7. Examples of rationalization
   a) Punishing someone else, personally or legally, may be a rationalization.
   b) Imbibing extra cocktails may involve rationalization.
   c) The teenager who does not know how to dance, but really wants to, may say that he prefers to stay home.
   d) The "sour grapes" response is a rationalization. In Aesop's fable, "The Fox and the Grapes," the fox, who was very hungry, strove to obtain some "charming ripe grapes." He failed, then said, "Let him who will take them! . . . They are green and sour."
J. Intellectualization
   *Intellectualization* is the overuse of intellectual concepts and words to avoid affective experience or expressions of feelings.
   1. It is closely related to rationalization.
   2. It is a way of controlling affects and feelings by thinking about them instead of experiencing them.
   3. Examples of intellectualization
      a) The adolescent who wants to avoid acknowledging his or her sexual impulses.
      b) Borderline personalities.
      c) Patients suffering from obsessive-compulsive disorders.
K. Compensation
   *Compensation* is a conscious or unconscious attempt to overcome real or fancied inferiorities.
   1. Status seems to be an important need in all of us; thus, compensatory behavior is universal.
   2. Compensation may be
      a) Socially acceptable—for example, the blind person who becomes proficient in music, the paraplegic who becomes successful in politics
      b) Socially unacceptable—for example, the physically handicapped person who becomes a bully or a boor; the physically small person who becomes aggressive and domineering ("the small man syndrome" or "the banty rooster syndrome")
   3. Compensation may also be
      a) Direct—that is, an attempt to achieve in an area in which one has failed
      b) Indirect—that is, an attempt to achieve in a different field than the field in which one has failed
   4. *Overcompensation* is an exaggerated attempt to overcome inferiorities. (The term was made popular by Alfred Adler.)

5. William Wordsworth (1770–1850), in "Character of the Happy Warrior," describes compensation:

> who, doomed to go in company with pain
> and Fear, and Bloodshed, miserable train!
> Turns his necessity to glorious gain!

L. Reaction formation

*Reaction formation* is the direction of overt behavior or attitudes in precisely the opposite direction of the individual's underlying, unacceptable conscious or unconscious impulses. (A warded-off idea or feeling is replaced by an unconsciously derived but consciously felt emphasis on the opposite.)

1. It is a two-step defense.
   a) An unacceptable desire is repressed.
   b) The repression is followed by the conscious expression of its antithesis (thus, employing countercathexis).
2. The conscious intent of reaction formation is often altruistic.
3. The use of this adaptive pattern often leads to the production of lasting changes in an individual's behavior. For example:
   a) Uriah Heep, the hypocritical clerk in Charles Dickens's *David Copperfield,* insists that he is a very "humble" person, but his underlying nature is detestable, sly, and conniving.
   b) "Don Juans" may be masking underlying doubts about their masculinity.
   c) Excessive politeness or courtesy may disguise underlying hostility.
   d) Overt oversolicitousness and overprotectiveness toward a child may hide a parent's hostile and rejecting feelings.
   e) Submissiveness, excessive amiability, or excessive concern may be reaction formations against underlying hostility or aggressiveness.
   f) Compulsive meticulousness may cover up strong impulses to soil.

M. Sublimation

*Sublimation* is the diversion of unacceptable, instinctual drives into socially sanctioned channels. (It is the process whereby one replaces an unacceptable wish with a course of action that is similar to the wish but does not conflict with one's value system. For example, aggressive wishes may be sublimated into working hard to solve social problems.)

1. This is socialization of emotion.

2. It is a term often reserved for successful defense mechanisms because, while the underlying impulse is gratified and the goal is retained, they are redirected from socially unacceptable to socially acceptable paths.
3. Unlike other defenses, there is no countercathexis. The emotional energy from an unacceptable impulse is transferred to a new goal-directed activity that is decided upon by the ego and approved by the superego.
4. Since sublimation offers some gratification of the underlying instinctual drive, it is usually considered healthy and often regarded as the most desirable of the mental mechanisms.
5. Examples of sublimation
   a) Sports and games may be sublimations of hostile and aggressive impulses.
   b) Various types of creative activity may be sublimations of sexual drives.
   c) Vocational choices may be sublimations of underlying unacceptable impulses.

N. Denial

*Denial* is the unconscious disavowal of a thought, feeling, wish, need, or reality that is consciously unacceptable. One behaves as if the problem does not exist. Denial is to be distinguished from lying, which is a conscious process. It is also known as negation (avoidance of awareness of some painful reality).
1. Dynamically, denial is the simplest form of ego defense, closely related to rationalization.
2. It is a very primitive defense mechanism, much used by young children. The shutting of the infant's eyes, to avoid seeing a threatening situation, is the prototype of this defense.
3. Denial is also sometimes used to defend oneself against catastrophes.
4. It is also much used by deteriorated psychotics, who may replace the rejected reality with a more satisfying fantasy.
5. Examples of denial
   a) The small child who disclaims pain when a finger has been smashed in the door.
   b) The deaf individual who refuses to admit a hearing loss.
   c) The alcoholic who refuses to admit that he or she cannot handle liquor.
   d) The dissatisfied employee who believes that a change in jobs will solve all of his or her vocational problems.
   e) Magical thinking ("pay no attention and it will go away") also plays a powerful role in denial.

6. Some say it is the most frequently encountered defense in general medical practice, and within limits it is a normal process (as, for example, in response to bad news). However, denial can be maladaptive if it interferes with rational action.

O. Substitution

*Substitution* is an unconscious replacement of a highly valued but unattainable or unacceptable emotional goal or object by one that is attainable or acceptable.
1. It is comparable to displacement.
2. To be satisfactory, the substitutive activity must have certain similarities to the original forbidden one. For example, murderous or intensely hostile impulses may be replaced by some impersonal destructive act, such as striking a punching bag or shooting a target rifle.

P. Restitution

*Restitution* is the supplanting of a highly valued object that has been lost through rejection by, or death or departure of, another object.

Q. Displacement

*Displacement* is the redirection of an emotion from the original object to a more acceptable substitute. (The avoided ideas and feelings are transferred to some other person, object, or situation. For example, hypochondriacal patients who may display worry and ward off the concern that their minds are failing can focus the concern instead on the body.)
1. It is closely allied to symbolization (see the discussion of symbolization later in this chapter).
2. It is normal, as when hostile feelings are transferred from an employer to some member of the family or some other object, or when various feelings are displaced onto political figures or certain minority groups.
3. Feelings of hostility toward parents are also often transferred to parent surrogates or other authority figures.
4. It also occurs in the transference-countertransference relationship in psychiatric treatment.
5. It is found in phobic disorders, where there is transference of anxiety from an unconscious conflict to an external focus.
6. It is frequently found in obsessive-compulsive disorders. For example, handwashing may result from feelings of moral uncleanness. These feelings are displaced onto dirt, which must be continually cleansed away.

R. Isolation

*Isolation* is the separation of an unacceptable impulse, act, or idea from its memory origin, thereby removing the emotional charge associated with the original memory.

1. The idea is set apart from its attached original affect, by countercathexis.
2. Isolation differs from repression proper, in which the idea as well as the feeling tone is kept out of awareness.
3. Although the individual consciously retains, or can recall, the painful memory of a traumatic incident, the feeling that originally accompanied it has become detached.
4. This mechanism is commonly seen in obsessive-compulsive disorder. Characteristically, the obsessive-compulsive person remains emotionally aloof from loaded situations. For example,
    a) An obsessed person feels he or she might hurt or kill someone but does not have the accompanying hostile or aggressive feelings.
    b) It is the basis of many compulsive rituals.
5. It is found in the compartmentalization of two ideas that are antithetical as, for example, in the devoutly religious person who shows racial prejudice.

S. Undoing

*Undoing* is a primitive defense mechanism in which some unacceptable past behavior is symbolically acted out in reverse, usually repetitiously. It is also called *symbolic atonement*. (Undoing expresses both the impulse and its opposite, as in being very domineering one minute and then offering obsequiously to defer to another.)

1. It is nullification by counteraction.
2. It is treating an experience as if it had never occurred.
3. It is closely related to reaction formation (magical expiation).
4. Examples of undoing
    a) An executive who has recommended that an employee not be promoted later makes complimentary remarks to the person.
    b) A person with an obsessive-compulsive disorder may undo the hostility shown at the beginning of an interview by being ingratiating at the end of the interview.
    c) Handwashing may represent expiation for antisocial or asocial activities. Repetition compulsion represents an attempt to reenact earlier unacceptable emotional experiences in order to be freed from their original unconscious meaning.

T. Dissociation

*Dissociation* is the unconscious detachment of certain behavior from the normal or usual conscious behavior patterns of an individual, which then function alone (compartmentalization). It is seen

1. In the executive who keeps his or her business from interfering with family life.
2. In sleepwalking, or somnambulism, sleeptalking, and automatic behavior such as automatic handwriting.
3. In the dissociative disorders, such as psychogenic amnesia, psychogenic fugue, and depersonalization disorder.
4. In multiple personalities, for example, in *Dr. Jekyll and Mr. Hyde* or *The Three Faces of Eve*. Generally, the primary character is proper and moral, whereas the secondary personality is hedonistic and impulse-ridden.
5. In schizophrenia, where there is a splitting of affect from mental content.

U. Symbolization

*Symbolization* is the unconscious mechanism by which a neutral idea or object is used to represent another idea or object that has a forbidden aspect.

1. There is a displacement of emotion from the object to the symbol.
2. Symbolization is based on similarity and association. The symbols protect the individual from the anxiety attached to the original idea or object.
3. Symbolization is the language of the unconscious.
4. Examples of symbolization
   a) Dreams are the most common examples of symbolization. In dreams, for example,
      (1) Elongated or projecting objects are often phallic symbols.
      (2) Openings or shrubbery may represent female genitalia.
      (3) A ship, ocean, or mothering figure may represent the mother.
   b) Affectations of speech, dress, or gait may be symbolizations.
   c) Certain psychotic symptoms such as hallucinations, muteness, posturing, and stereotypy may have symbolic meaning.

V. Idealization

*Idealization* is the overestimation of admired qualities of another person or desired object. It is normally seen in

1. Young persons who exaggerate the intelligence and attractiveness of their friends or lovers.

2. Precinct workers who overevaluate the assets and underestimate the limitations of a political candidate.
3. Freud said it was "the origin of the peculiar state of being in love."

W. Fantasy

*Fantasy* is a fabricated series of mental pictures or sequence of events; daydreaming.

1. Fantasy may provide the basis for creative activities.
2. Daydreams can express unconscious conflict, gratify otherwise unattainable wishes, and provide an escape from reality.
3. A disproportionate preoccupation with fantasy may lead to harmful distortion of reality.

## VII. Special defense mechanisms

A. Because of the current interest in borderline and narcissistic personalities (see chapter 16), two additional defense mechanisms are of importance. They are primitive or psychotic defenses that support denial much in the way that displacement, introjection, sublimation, and the other defenses support repression. These defenses are

1. Splitting

*Splitting* is the inability to unite and integrate the hating and loving aspect of both one's self-image and one's image of another person. The loving, fantasied relationships and the hating ones are internally "split." When the individual develops positive fantasies, the negative feelings are dissociated or "split off"; when the person is frustrated, the negative fantasies are elaborated.

2. Projective identification

*Projective identification* is the association of uncomfortable aspects of one's own personality with their projection onto another person, resulting in identification with the other person.

3. For further discussion of these concepts, see Shapiro (1978).

B. *DSM*-III-R also includes the following as defense mechanisms:

1. *Acting out:* A mechanism in which a person acts without reflection or apparent regard for negative consequences. For example, adolescents may "act out" expressions of underlying depression through truancy, running away, aggressiveness, and so forth.
2. *Autistic fantasy:* A mechanism in which a person substitutes excessive daydreaming for pursuits of human relationships, more direct and effective action, or problem solving.
3. *Passive aggression:* A mechanism in which a person indirectly and unassertively expresses aggression toward others.

4. *Somatization:* A mechanism in which a person becomes preoccupied with physical symptoms disproportionate to any actual physical disturbance.

VIII. **Other defense mechanisms**

　A. Altruism: In this mechanism one deals with emotional conflicts or external or internal stress by dedicating oneself to fulfilling the needs of others instead of one's own (in psychiatric literature altruism and morality seem to be closely related).

　B. Devaluation: In this mechanism one deals with emotional conflicts or external or internal stress by attributing exaggerated negative qualities to oneself or others.

　C. Exaggeration: To protect self-esteem and/or emotional balance, certain meanings can be assigned exaggerated values.

　D. Humor: One might deal with external or internal stress by employing humor and emphasizing the ironic or amusing aspects of the stress or conflict.

　E. Minimization: Revaluing a topic as a means of reducing stress, for example, minimizing blame for behavior to avoid shame and guilt.

IX. **Summary**

The foregoing describe the majority of the principal defense mechanisms found in day-to-day adjustments of normal persons as well as in the major psychiatric syndromes.

## References

American Psychiatric Association. *Diagnostic and Statistical Manual of Mental Disorders.* 3d ed., rev. Washington, D.C.: APA, 1987.

Blum, G. S. *Psychodynamics: The Science of Unconscious Mental Forces.* Belmont, Calif.: Brooks/Cole, 1966.

Carson, R., J. Butcher, and J. Coleman. *Abnormal Psychology and Modern Life.* 8th ed. Glenview, Ill.: Scott, Foresman, 1988.

Eaton, M. T., Jr., M. H. Peterson, and J. A. Davis. *Psychiatry.* 4th ed. Garden City, N.Y.: Medical Examination Publishing, 1981.

Freud, A. *The Ego and the Mechanisms of Defense.* New York: International University Press, 1953.

Goldberger, L., and S. Breznitz, eds. *Handbook of Stress.* New York: The Free Press, 1982.

Horowitz, M. "Stress and the Mechanism of Defense." In *Review of General Psychiatry.* 2d ed., edited by H. Goldman. Norwalk, Conn.: Appleton & Lange, 1988.

Horowitz, M. J. *Introduction to Psychodynamics: The New Synthesis.* New York: Basic Books, 1988.

Kaplan, H. I., and B. J. Sadock. *Modern Synopsis of Comprehensive Textbook of Psychiatry/V.* 5th ed. Baltimore: Williams & Wilkins, 1989.

Kolb, L. C., and H. K. H. Brodie. *Modern Clinical Psychiatry.* 10th ed. Philadelphia: Saunders, 1982.

Selye, H. *The Stress of Life.* rev. ed. New York: McGraw-Hill, 1976.

Shapiro, E. R. "The Psychodynamics and Developmental Psychology of a Borderline Patient: A Review of the Literature." *American Journal of Psychiatry* 135 (November 1978): 135.

Solomon, P., and V. D. Patch, eds. *Handbook of Psychiatry.* 2d ed. Los Altos, Calif.: Lange Medical Publications, 1971.

# 7 Symptoms, Diagnosis, and Classification

The diagnosis of disease is often easy, often difficult, and often impossible.

Peter Mere Latham, *Collected Works.*

I. **Introduction**
   A. A medical model, on which the discipline of psychiatry is patterned, is based on a number of assumptions:
      1. Mental disorders are to be eventually understood as specific disorders with characteristic indications of the onset, course, and outcome of the manifestation of the disorder in individuals.
      2. A specific pattern of signs and symptoms will identify each disorder.
      3. Understanding each disorder will reveal a characteristic etiology with identified causative factors.
      4. The pathology of each disorder will be understood so that specific therapies can be applied with predictable outcomes.
   B. A major step toward the fulfillment of the idealized medical model in psychiatric practice is the achievement of a common language of diagnosis based on a system of classification, the categories of which define the ''true'' underlying structure of mental disorders.
   C. While the assumptions on which the medical model is based have not yet been convincingly supported in psychiatric practice, considerable progress has been made in the attempt to develop a descriptive system of classification that can be applied with reasonable confidence in psychiatric diagnosis.

II. **Symptoms**
   A. In clinical diagnosis it is conventional to make a distinction between signs and symptoms.
      1. Signs refer to those indications that are observed by the clinician.

2. Symptoms refer to subjective concerns expressed by the patient.
3. For example, using the preceding distinctions, crying would be a sign, while depressed mood would be a symptom.
4. In practice, the distinction is usually ignored, and both signs and symptoms are referred to as "symptoms."

B. From the biopsychosocial perspective, symptoms are expressions of the person and can be expressed in any of the dominant spheres of human experience: biological, psychological, behavioral, interpersonal, and social.

C. Some symptoms may be nonspecific such as autonomic arousal, sleep disturbance, or mood changes. Most psychiatric symptoms are not pathognomonic, that is, not in and of themselves sufficient to make a specific diagnosis.

D. A syndrome is a cluster of symptoms that occur together as part of a recognizable condition.
1. A syndrome is less specific in meaning and reference than a disorder or a disease.
2. Most psychiatric disorders are, more properly, syndromes.

E. Psychological symptoms are usually an outcome of multiple influences, some originating in the environment (extrapsychic) and some originating in the individual (intrapsychic).

F. Some symptoms may represent a person's attempts to cope with the problems created by other symptoms or to defend against their emotional consequences.

G. Symptoms can have meaning when interpreted in the context of a person's life history, personality development, and current circumstances.
1. Clinicians may see significance in a symptom depending on their orientation (e.g., an organically oriented clinician may be more attuned to interpretations of physiological malfunction while a psychodynamically oriented clinician may be sensitive to indications of conflict or developmental crisis).
2. To illustrate:
   a) Reported somatic (physical) symptoms may indicate autonomic nervous system reactions of acute stress.
   b) Reported somatic symptoms may reflect conscious attempts to receive attention or sympathy.
   c) Reported somatic symptoms may reflect underlying psychological problems but are not under voluntary control (as in some somatoform disorders).
   d) Reported somatic symptoms may be symbolic expressions of psychodynamic conflicts as might occur in a hysterical paralysis as a defense against taking assertive action.

H. Knowledge of symptoms is important in assessing the mental status of a psychiatric patient and in establishing a working diagnosis and treatment plan.

I. Psychological symptoms may be manifested in many ways and may be expressed in a number of psychological processes that are rooted in normal human behavior. An account of the most commonly referred to psychiatric symptoms is presented in the Appendix.

## III. Diagnosis

A. Diagnosis is the procedure by which a patient's presenting clinical picture of complaints, concerns, and disturbances is assessed and compared with that of other patients with similar presentations for the purpose of identifying an underlying disorder or disease.

B. While symptoms and syndromes serve as indicators and expressions of a disorder, they are not usually sufficient to make a diagnosis, since similar symptoms or syndromes might be produced by different disorders and the same disorder might be expressed in somewhat different syndromes.

C. Diagnosis must be based on a variety of sources of information, which include presenting symptoms, life history information, an account of current circumstances, and a variety of specialized assessment techniques.

D. Ideally, diagnosis should point the direction to the etiological factors of a disorder, but pragmatically, diagnosis should be able to at least suggest a choice of treatment strategies.

E. Two general approaches to diagnosis have been used in psychiatry.

1. The descriptive approach is based on an objective description of the signs, symptoms, and history of the clinical presentation of a patient.

2. The inferential approach considers descriptive information to be the expression of inner factors (e.g., psychodynamic mechanisms), which must be interpreted properly by the clinician.

3. The history of psychiatric diagnosis displays periods of relative dominance of either the relatively atheoretical, descriptive approach or the more theoretical, inferential approach.

## IV. Classification

A. Introduction

1. Diagnosis is essentially an act of classification in which a judgment is made that a patient's inferred disorder is a member of a category of disorders with characteristics that differentiate it consistently from other categories of disorder.

2. Nosology is the technical term used to refer to the science of classification of disorders.
3. Functions of classification (Blashfield and Draguns 1976)
   a) Classification provides a universal language or nomenclature for clinicians and researchers.
   b) Classification provides a basis for organizing experimental and clinical research and assists in the search for information about such matters as particular symptoms, effects of treatment, and etiological research.
   c) Classification assists in the description of the important similarities and differences between clinical presentations so that the clinician, with a provisional diagnosis, may be alert to other symptoms or factors that are most likely to be seen in a patient.
   d) Classification can yield predictions of outcome or prognosis and can be used to relate specific treatments to efficacy with specific disorders.
   e) Classification can provide a conceptual basis for theories of pathology and can guide basic research into causation.
4. The history of psychiatry reveals a number of attempts at unifying classifications of disorders, of which the current official example is found in the most recent edition of the *Diagnostic and Statistical Manual of Mental Disorders* (*DSM*-III-R).
5. A "bootstraps" effect occurs with classifications in which the adoption of a common language for talking about diagnoses and common criteria for making diagnoses lead to the accumulation of more reliable information and relevant research, which in turn can lead to more refined and etiologically based classifications. Diagnostic classifications, then, are best viewed as "work in progress."
6. Diagnostic classifications are based on the assumption that there are underlying disorders or disorders that form independent categories. Some clinicians and researchers question this "medical model" assumption as it is applied to some or most of the kinds of clinical patterns that are presented in practice.

B. Historical notes
1. Classification appears to be a strong human intellectual tendency; examples of classifications in early civilizations reveal some categories that are recognizable today (e.g., mania, melancholia, hysteria).
2. Historical classifications reveal a trend toward greater complexity and an underlying issue about whether a single

pathology is the origin of all disorders or there are multiple disorders, each with its own origin and course.

3. The dominant somatogenic view of nineteenth century psychiatry spurred many classification schemes for use in the institutions of the era and eventually led to a call for a single uniform system. The European Congress of Mental Medicine in 1885 agreed on eleven categories of mental disorder:
   a) Mania
   b) Melancholia
   c) Periodical insanity
   d) Progressive systematic insanity
   e) Dementia
   f) Organic and senile dementia
   g) General paralysis
   h) Insane neuroses
   i) Toxic insanity
   j) Moral and impulsive insanity
   k) Idiocy

4. The modern era of classification began with the work of Emil Kraepelin, whose organization provided the basis for current nosologies.
   a) His system was the basis of the organization of his textbooks of psychiatry, which came to be used in the training of most European psychiatrists.
   b) While Kraepelin was committed to the position that there was an underlying organic cause to all mental disorders, his approach was objective and descriptive.
   c) His classification scheme was based on symptom patterns, precipitating circumstances, course of the condition, and outcome. Of these, course was his major organizing principle.
   d) Kraepelin introduced several new concepts in his nosology.
      (1) He combined the old concepts of mania and melancholia into a single category of manic-depressive insanity, which he subdivided into agitated, elated, and retarded forms.
      (2) He introduced the category of dementia praecox as distinct from paranoia and subdivided it further into catatonic, hebephrenic, and paranoid forms.
      (3) He differentiated psychological disorders from dementias and used such concepts as psychogenic neurosis and psychopathic personality.

5. Eugen Bleuler later changed the name of dementia praecox to schizophrenia and departed from the descriptive approach of Kraepelin to base his classification on inferred psychopathological processes.
6. The American Psychiatric Association, in 1917, developed a classification based on Kraepelin's, which was revised in 1934 as *The Standard Classified Nomenclature of Diseases*. It was used primarily in diagnosis and record keeping for chronic inpatient (institutionalized) psychiatric practice.
7. In the 1920s, psychoanalysis became the dominant psychiatric perspective in the United States, and interest in Kraepelinian diagnosis and classification faded.
8. During and after World War II, the army, navy and Veterans Administration each found the 1934 classification unsuitable for many of the disturbances in servicemen, and each service developed its own classification.
9. This confusion led the American Psychiatric Association to form a task force, which eventually produced the first *Diagnostic and Statistical Manual for Mental Disorders* (*DSM*-I) in 1952.

C. *DSM*-I
1. *DSM*-I was an etiologically based classification based in large part on the Adolph Meyer's psychobiologic theory of mental disorders as reactions of the individual's personality to biological, psychological, and social factors (e.g., schizophrenic reactions, psychoneurotic reactions).
2. *DSM*-I also reflected the influence of psychoanalysis in its use of anxiety and defense mechanisms in describing psychoneurotic and personality disorders.
3. The basic distinctions in the classification were:
   a) Disorders caused by or associated with impairment of brain tissue function
      (1) Chronic
      (2) Acute
   b) Mental deficiency
   c) Disorders of psychogenic origin or without clearly defined physical cause or structural change in the brain
      (1) Psychotic disorders (e.g. manic-depressive reaction)
      (2) Psychophysiologic autonomic and visceral disorders (e.g., asthma)
      (3) Psychoneurotic disorders (e.g., anxiety reaction)
      (4) Personality disorders (e.g., sociopathic personality disturbance)
      (5) Transient situational personality disorders

D. *DSM*-II
1. In 1968 a new version was written, primarily to bring the system into closer conformity with the World Health Organization's *International Classification of Diseases.*
2. *DSM*-II dispensed with the term *reaction* and generally tried to minimize any implication of a specific theoretical perspective, although it did retain the anxiety and defense interpretation of the neuroses.
3. It also expanded the number of major classificatory headings by including categories for behavior disorders of childhood and adolescence, special symptoms (e.g., disorders of sleep) and conditions without manifest psychiatric disorder (e.g., marital maladjustment).
4. While *DSM*-I discouraged multiple diagnoses, *DSM*-II encouraged them.
5. *DSM*-II represented a number of compromises and received criticism from a variety of sources.
   a) There was no major organizing principle, so some disorders were defined by etiology, some by age, some by symptoms, and some apparently by arbitrary decision (e.g., sexual deviation).
   b) Specific symptoms required for a particular diagnosis were not clearly defined.
   c) Some categories (e.g., childhood disorders) were only broadly defined.
   d) Reliability studies did not achieve a very high level of agreement.
   e) Some critics viewed the entire classification process as dehumanizing to some degree by emphasizing the attachment of a label (diagnosis) to a person instead of the understanding of an individual's life situation.
E. *DSM*-III
1. The dissatisfactions with DSM-II, together with a major revival of interest in objective descriptive diagnosis and renewed confidence in the somatogenic hypothesis (neo-Kraepelinians), led to a call for a new and more scientifically developed classification.
2. A new, broadly based task force was established by the American Psychiatric Association, and in 1980 *DSM*-III was published.
3. *DSM*-III represented major departures from its predecessors in form, methodology, and underlying assumptions.
   a) *DSM*-III is organized around operational criteria for diagnosis, which indicate both what must be included and

what must be excluded in arriving at a particular diagnostic decision.

b) Criteria are largely based on descriptive characteristics rather than on any inferences about causation or etiology.

c) The system was field tested for reliability before appearing in its final published form.

d) A multiaxial system of diagnosis was introduced, which permits multiple diagnoses that reflect not only the person's primary clinical condition but also personality characteristics and conditions of life.

e) *DSM*-III can represent levels of diagnostic certainty.

f) *DSM*-III deletes the category of neurotic disorders.

   (1) The position was taken that there was no consensus about how to define neurosis.

   (2) In its avoidance of etiological categories, *DSM*-III was not compatible with the psychodynamic view of anxiety and defense as the basis of neurotic disorders.

   (3) While no longer a diagnostic classification, many clinicians still find the psychodynamic view of neurosis a useful one in evaluating and treating some patients.

g) Other changes include a basic revision of what is included as sexual disorders (e.g., removal of homosexuality as a category), reclassification and expansion of the personality disorders, and elimination of the major category of psychophysiologic disorders (a category is provided for psychological factors affecting physical conditions).

4. *DSM*-III was revised again in 1987 (*DSM*-III-R) and it is this version that is followed in the sections on diagnostic groups that follow in this outline.

## V. *DSM*-III-R

A. Most of the revisions of *DSM*-III-R were modifications that tightened operational criteria, refinements of subtypes, and adding material based on intervening research with the system. Sleep disorders were added as a category, and developmental disorders were shifted from Axis I to Axis II. No major category designations were changed.

B. The major categories of *DSM*-III-R are:

1. Disorders usually first evident in infancy, childhood, or adolescence (including developmental disorders that are coded on Axis II)

2. Organic mental disorders

3. Psychoactive substance use disorders

4. Schizophrenia

5. Delusional (paranoid) disorder
6. Psychotic disorders not elsewhere classified
7. Mood disorders
8. Anxiety disorders
9. Somatoform disorders
10. Dissociative disorders
11. Personality disorders (coded on Axis II)
12. Sexual disorders
13. Sleep disorders
14. Factitious disorders
15. Impulse disorders not elsewhere classified
16. Adjustment disorder
17. Psychological factors affecting physical condition
18. In addition there are codes for conditions not attributable to a mental disorder that are a focus of attention or treatment (Code V).

C. There are five diagnostic axes, the first three of which would normally include all appropriate diagnoses that would be made.
1. Axis I includes all mental disorders except the two that are included on Axis II.
2. Axis II includes developmental disorders and personality disorders.
3. Axis III is operationally defined as potentially including all of the diagnoses of physical disorders and conditions in the *International Classification of Diseases* (*ICD*-9–CM) that lie outside the section on mental disorders. Some might have a direct etiological relation to Axis I; others may be significant in the overall management of a case.
4. Axis IV rates the severity of psychosocial stressors from "none" to "catastrophic."
5. Axis V is a global assessment of functioning that evaluates both current functioning and the highest level of functioning during the past year.

D. A typical descriptive section for a diagnostic type in *DSM*-III-R includes:
1. A description of the essential features of the disorder
2. A description of associated features
3. Information about the course of the disorder
4. When available, information about age of onset, predisposing factors, prevalence, sex ratio, and complications
5. Differential diagnosis (other conditions with some similar features that must be ruled out)
6. Detailed diagnostic criteria

## VI. Evaluation of *DSM*-III-R

A. While reliability measures show that *DSM*-III-R achieves considerably more agreement than *DSM*-II, the general level of reliability still falls short of what would be considered necessary for effective clinical use.

   1. Reliabilities are highest for mental retardation, substance use disorders, organic disorders, and schizophrenia.
   2. Reliabilities are lowest for personality disorders and somatoform disorders.

B. Validity is hard to establish, but studies indicate that some of the categories reflect natural groupings.

C. Some of the criteria still reflect clinical intuition and acumen rather than empirical determination of contribution to diagnosis.

D. The multiple axes do not contribute as much to the overall accuracy of diagnosis as was anticipated.

E. The classification of childhood disorders has not satisfied many clinicians who work primarily with children and families.

F. The classification of personality disorders lacks clear boundaries between different disorders and between the disorders and normality. There is no substantial agreement that the groupings reflect natural clusters of personality types.

G. Some critics view the system as too long and cumbersome for efficient clinical use.

H. There is concern that *DSM*-III-R is being viewed as a code to be rigidly adhered to rather than as an evolving system to be modified and corrected by the influence of research and clinical utility.

I. Despite such criticisms, there is general agreement that *DSM* -III-R has achieved an improvement in reliability, has reorganized categories in a way that has improved consistency, and has made classification more responsive to contemporary research.

J. *DSM*-III-R has shown how the development of a classification can be self-corrective.

## VII. Prospects for *DSM*-IV

A. In 1988 a task force was appointed to begin work on *DSM*-IV.

B. The anticipated publication of the tenth edition of the *International Classification of Diseases* (*ICD*-10) in 1993 will include major changes in the mental disorders section, and the planning groups for *ICD*-10 and *DSM*-IV are collaborating to reduce differences in the two systems.

C. Principles and working plan

   1. Major emphasis in the new edition will be on documentation and review of the evidence for any changes that are made.
   2. Special attempts are being made to emphasize utility for clinical practice in a variety of settings. This may lead to

some simplification of categories and resistance to adding new diagnoses unless thoroughly documented and rationalized.

3. While sensitivity must be shown to the political and economic impact of the diagnostic system (e.g., in determination of criminal responsibility or professional liability), the intent is to give highest priority to clinical uses and research foundations.

4. The task force has enlisted a broad base of participation in the planning including communication with other professional and scientific groups interested in the development of *DSM*-IV.

D. Conceptual issues

1. While the preference for a descriptive approach will continue, the contributions of psychodynamic and family systems to classification will be examined.

2. A question remains about whether multiple diagnoses, which are encouraged in *DSM*-III-R, are really independent or may reflect more complex syndromes (e.g., co-occurrence of anxiety and depression).

3. In practice, *DSM*-III-R has followed a categorical approach that emphasizes sharp boundaries and demarcation of discrete patterns. A more prototypic approach in which heterogeneity and borderline uncertainty are recognized is being considered for *DSM*-IV.

E. Work groups have been formed to examine and revise each major diagnostic category, with the major emphasis on accumulation of empirical evidence to support changes rather than relying on expert consensus.

F. Generally, the approach to *DSM*-IV is conservative, and any new diagnoses will be required to meet stringent tests.

# References

American Psychiatric Association. *Diagnostic and Statistical Manual of Mental Disorders*. 3d ed., rev. Washington, D.C.: APA, 1987.

Blashfield, R., and J. Draguns. "Evaluative Criteria for Psychiatry Classification." *Journal of Abnormal Psychology*, 85 (1976).

Davison, G., and J. Neale. *Abnormal Psychology*. 5th ed. New York: Wiley, 1990.

Frances, A., H. Pincus, T. Widiger, W. Davis, and M. First. "*DSM*-IV: Work in Progress." *American Journal of Psychiatry*, 147, no. 11 (1990).

Goldman, H., ed. *Review of General Psychiatry*. 2d. ed. Norwalk, Conn.: Appleton & Lange, 1988.

Hersen, M., A. Kazdin, and A. Bellack, eds. *The Clinical Psychology Handbook*. New York: Pergamon Press, 1983.

Kaplan, H. I., and B. J. Sadock, eds. *Comprehensive Textbook of Psychiatry/V*. Vol. 1, 5th ed. Baltimore: Williams & Wilkins, 1989.

Maxmen, J. *Essential Psychopathology*. New York: Norton, 1986.

Nicholi, A., ed. *The New Harvard Guide to Psychiatry*. Cambridge, Mass.: Belknap/ Harvard, 1988.

# 8 Assessment of the Psychiatric Patient

False facts are highly injurious to the progress of science, for they often endure long; but false views, if supported by some evidence, do little harm, for everyone takes salutory pleasure in proving their falseness.

**Charles Robert Darwin, *The Descent of Man* (1871)**

I. **Purposes of assessment**
   A. Assessment procedures play an important role in establishing a working diagnosis and in planning and evaluating a treatment program for a psychiatric patient.
   B. Systematic assessment contributes to establishing the probable etiology and course of the patient's disorder, designing the form of intervention, predicting and monitoring response to treatment, evaluating results of treatment, and following up the patient when intervention is terminated.

II. **Areas of investigation**
   Assessment procedures elicit information about the following areas of the patient's condition and experience.
   A. Current psychological functioning and symptom expression
   B. Current physical condition
   C. Current life situation and sources of stress
   D. Personal history, including critical developmental incidents
   E. Medical history
   F. Family history
   G. Personality structure and defenses (psychodynamics)
   H. Strengths, competencies, and abilities
   I. Relationships and sources of support

III. **Methods of diagnostic assessment**
   A. The interview
      1. The interview is the most widely used assessment technique in psychiatric practice.
      2. The interview provides not only factual information about the patient but also an opportunity to observe such personal

characteristics as appearance, manner, speech, and mode of interpersonal response.

3. Interviews with informants other than the patient provide independent information that may corroborate the patient's report or indicate important omissions and inconsistencies. This source of information is particularly important when patients may be without insight, delusional, confused, or otherwise inaccessible or uncooperative.

4. In psychiatric interviewing, the following points of inquiry are usually included:
   a) The presenting complaint
   b) History of present illness
   c) Nature of previous adjustment
   d) Family and marital history
   e) Educational, social, and occupational history
   f) Past medical history

5. A number of general and specialized structured interview formats are available, including some specially designed to assess *DSM*-III-R Axis II, IV, and V dimensions.
   a) The Schedule for Affective Disorders and Schizophrenia (SADS) was designed to elicit responses to standardized questions in making *DSM*-III diagnoses.
   b) The Diagnostic Interview Schedule (DIS) is a structured interview that can be administered by nonprofessionals to obtain information relevant to *DSM*-III diagnoses together with other information about personal history and demographic variables. It has been used in epidemiological studies and has been translated for cross-national and cross-cultural studies of prevalence and risk.
   c) The Structured Clinical Interview for *DSM*-III-R (SCID) is the successor to the SADS and provides information and a decision tree format for making diagnoses using *DSM*-III-R criteria.

6. Standardized interview schedules not only assist in making rapid diagnostic judgments but also improve the reliability of diagnoses using the criteria of a diagnostic system.

B. Mental-status examination

1. The mental-status examination is a special form of assessment often conducted in conjunction with the history-taking interview. It provides the following kind of outline for recording the interviewer's descriptions of the patient's behavior.
   a) Attitude, manner, and behavior
      (1) Appearance, dress, facial expression, activity, posture, and demeanor are noted.

        (2) Disturbances include deviations of degree of activity, mannerisms, distortions of motility, and uncooperativeness.

   b) Mental content
        (1) Mental content refers to the thoughts, concerns, and trends that are uppermost in the patient's mind.
        (2) Disturbances of content include delusions, hallucinations, obsessions, and phobias.

   c) Sensorium and intellect
        (1) The degree of the patient's awareness and the level of his or her functioning are assessed.
        (2) Disturbances of orientation, memory, retention, attention, information, and judgment can be elicited with standardized questions and test materials.

   d) Stream of thought (as manifest in stream of speech)
        (1) Information is obtained about the quantitative and qualitative aspects of the patient's verbal communication.
        (2) Disturbances include over- and underproductivity, disconnectedness, unintelligibility, and incoherence.

   e) Emotional tone
        (1) Both the patient's report of subjective feelings (mood or affect) and the examiner's observations of facial expression, posture, and attitude are noted.
        (2) Disturbances include both quantitative deviations (elation, depression, apathy) and incongruence (disagreement among the patient's subject report, behavior, and mental content).

   f) Insight
      This means the degree to which the patient can appreciate the nature of his or her condition and the need for treatment.

  2. Instruments have been developed to standardize the mental-status examination.
   a) The Mental Status Schedule is used by a trained interviewer, guided by a standard interview schedule.
   b) The Inpatient Multidimensional Psychiatric Scale provides a systematic way for rating the behavior of severely disturbed psychiatric patients who may be difficult to interview.

C. Physical and neurological examination
  1. A routine physical and neurological examination is an essential part of general psychiatric assessment.
  2. Since many psychiatric disorders have symptoms that include disturbances of physiological functions (e.g.,

depression, anxiety, conversion disorder), and since many patients have unusual concerns about their health or present themselves as physically ill (e.g., somatoform disorders), it is important to make a careful differential diagnosis.

3. Some psychiatric problems are symptomatic of brain abnormalities, so a careful evaluation of neurological symptoms is particularly important.

4. Recent advances in general medical imaging techniques have contributed to diagnostic assessment in psychiatry as well.

    a) Computerized axial tomography (CAT) uses a moving X-ray detector system to construct successive cross sections of the brain to reveal differences in tissue density, which may indicate tumors, blockage of blood vessels, and shrinking of tissue.

    b) Nuclear magnetic response imaging (NMR) produces images of the brain that are superior to those obtained by CAT scan and permit the detection of small variations or deviations in brain structure.

    c) In positron emission tomography (PET), radioactive isotopes are injected into the bloodstream and permit detection of regional differences in the metabolic activity of the brain.

        (1) PET scans have revealed different patterns in the activity of the brain of patients diagnosed as schizophrenic or depressed.

        (2) PET scans have helped target specific areas of the brain that may be involved in panic disorder and obsessive-compulsive disorder.

5. The electroencephalograph (EEG) is used to obtain records of general brain wave activity or responses to some types of stimuli (evoked potentials).

    a) Traditionally, the EEG has been used to diagnose disturbances of brain rhythms (e.g., seizures) and patterns of sleep.

    b) Computer analysis of patterns of brain waves and evoked potentials in research have revealed some differences in some psychiatric patients that may prove useful in diagnosis.

6. Laboratory tests are particularly important in evaluating chemical use and initiating and monitoring drug therapies.

D. Psychosocial history

1. The psychosocial history provides a biographical account of a person, with particular attention to circumstances, events, and reactions that put the presenting concerns in a historical perspective.

2. Of particular importance are the stresses and supports of the circumstances in which a person is living, the nature and quality of important personal relationships, and the competence and skills displayed in educational and work experiences.
3. When possible, it is beneficial to obtain history information from a spouse or parent as well as from the patient.
4. The general categories of information that are included in a psychosocial history interview are:
   a) General identifying (demographic) information
   b) Parental family information
   c) Developmental history
   d) Educational history
   e) Marital history and current family circumstances
   f) Occupational history and current occupational and financial situation
   g) Military history
   h) Legal and criminal history
   i) History of physical illnesses and treatments
   j) History of psychiatric symptoms, diagnoses, and treatments
5. Structured history interview schedules are available including some, such as the Giannetti On-Line Psychosocial History (GOLPH) and the IPS Social History, that can be administered, scored, and reported by a computer.

## IV. Psychological testing

The development of psychological measurements of human characteristics has provided many tools for psychiatric assessment.

A. Variability from person to person is a commonly acknowledged aspect of many characteristics of human behavior. Psychological testing is based on the assumption that this variability can be measured.

B. Technically, a test is a systematic way to compare the behavior of two or more persons.

C. The development, administration, and interpretation of the tests most widely used in psychiatric assessment require special skill and training. The American Psychological Association has established ethical standards for the distribution and use of psychological tests.

D. Criteria for evaluation of psychological tests. Although psychological tests vary in content, purpose, and range of application, they are generally evaluated by the following criteria:
   1. *Reliability,* the consistency with which a test measures what it proposes to measure.

2. *Validity,* the accuracy with which a test fulfills its purpose of prediction, selection, or classification.
3. *Standardization,* the establishment of responses of reference groups so that individual performance may be compared with the performance of an appropriate group.
4. When test results are used to predict outcomes or to classify individuals, attention must be given to errors of classification and the risks associated with them.
   a) False positives refer to the classification of persons as having a disorder when in fact they don't.
   b) False negatives refer to the classification of persons as not having a disorder when in fact they do.
   c) The significance of classification errors depends on the risk associated with misdiagnoses and treatment or failure to treat.
   d) Since assessment measures are seldom error-free, the relative costs of errors of classification must be weighed against the benefits of correct classification.
E. Other characteristics of tests
   1. Individual versus group
      Some tests can be administered to only one person at a time (individual tests); others are administered to a number of persons at one time (group tests).
   2. Standardization of administration
      Tests vary in the degree to which the tester must follow a prescribed procedure.
   3. Objectivity
      Tests vary in the degree to which interpretation is required in the scoring of responses. An objective test is one whose scoring minimizes differences among different scorers.
   4. Form of response
      Some tests require a specific form of response (e.g., true-false); others permit open-end responses (e.g., sentence completion).
F. There are various kinds of psychological tests. In the ensuing sections, we shall describe the most important of the following types:
   1. Intelligence tests
   2. Personality tests
      a) Objective personality tests
      b) Projective techniques of measuring personality
   3. Behavioral assessment
   4. Neuropsychological tests
   5. Vocational and educational tests

## V. Intelligence tests

A. The theoretical concept of intelligence is a matter of some dispute among psychologists, particularly as to whether intelligence is primarily a general intellectual aptitude or a composite of specific and somewhat independent cognitive functions.

B. The "intelligence" measured by intelligence tests is considered to be a general, relatively stable capacity to learn and deal effectively with one's environment.

C. Intelligence is assumed to be normally distributed in the population.

D. The results of intelligence tests are frequently reported in terms of an IQ (intelligence quotient) score.

   1. The IQ score indicates the position of a person's intelligence test performance relative to the average performance of his or her age group. The average IQ is 100.

   2. A commonly used classification of intelligence translates IQ scores as follows:

      a) Very superior, IQ 130 or more

      b) Superior, 120–129

      c) Bright-normal, 110–119

      d) Average, 90–109

      e) Dull-normal, 80–89

      f) Borderline, 70–79

      g) Mental defective, 69 or less.

   3. The American Association of Mental Deficiency and *DSM-III-R* list four categories of mental retardation:

      a) Mild (IQ 50–69)

      b) Moderate (IQ 35–50)

      c) Severe (IQ 20–35)

      d) Profound (IQ 20 or below)

E. In psychiatric practice, the intelligence test is used to

   1. Aid in establishing the diagnosis of mental retardation

   2. Assess the effects of brain damage

   3. Assess effective intellectual performance in psychiatric disorders

   4. Define a patient's intellectual resources for educational and vocational adjustment

   5. Define efficiency of application of intellectual resources (e.g., when limited by anxiety, depression, etc.)

   6. Show patterns of performance, which are viewed as expressions of personality characteristics by some clinicians

F. Since intelligence is, to a substantial degree, defined culturally, tests of intelligence reflect competencies and achievements that are considered important for success in the culture.

1. The questions and problems of major intelligence tests presume a familiarity with language and problem solving derived from shared childhood experience, particularly in schools.
2. Interpretations of intelligence test results should be made with full consideration of the appropriateness of the test for the particular person who is tested.
3. Special attention should be given to cultural and/or language differences that might influence test performance.

G. Major intelligence tests in current usage
1. The Revised Stanford-Binet (1973)
   a) This is a widely used, individually administered intelligence test for children and for the assessment of mental retardation.
   b) It has served as the standard for comparison with other tests of intellectual ability.
   c) It is composed of various tasks and problems organized by year levels arranged from two years to superior adult.
   d) The problems successfully solved at each year level are totaled, and the sum is expressed as a Mental Age Score and has an IQ score equivalent.
   e) The test has proved useful in the prediction of school achievement.
   f) Examples of types of tasks include vocabulary, memory span for digits, words, and sentences, reasoning, comprehension, and copying geometric figures; verbal ability is strongly emphasized.
   g) The test is of limited usefulness with adults except where mental retardation may be involved, because it was standardized primarily with children and is composed of tasks that are more appropriate for children.
   h) This is the test of choice for reliable assessment of the extreme ranges of intelligence, both low and high.
2. The Fourth Edition of the Stanford-Binet (1986)
   a) This revision introduced some major changes in the organization and content of the scale.
      (1) Fifteen individual tests are organized into content areas of verbal reasoning, abstract/visual reasoning, quantitative reasoning, and short-term memory.
      (2) Test items are arranged in order of increasing difficulty but not according to age levels, as was the case in earlier editions.
   b) The new edition has not been in use long enough to develop the research necessary to evaluate its clinical

utility and advantages over the scale it is designed to replace.

3. The Wechsler Adult Intelligence Scale (WAIS-R) (1981)
   a) This is the most widely used individually administered intelligence test for adults and the standard against which other adult intelligence tests are compared.
   b) It is composed of a series of subtests organized into a verbal scale and a performance scale.
   c) Verbal subtests are information, comprehension similarities, arithmetic, digit span, and vocabulary.
   d) Performance subtests are picture arrangements, picture completion, block design, object assembly, and digit symbol.
   e) The test yields three IQ scores: Verbal Scale IQ, Performance Scale IQ, and Full Scale IQ.
   f) Differences between verbal and performance IQ scores may sometimes be of diagnostic value. Many hypotheses have been proposed about ways in which patterns of subtest scores might be related to specific diagnoses, but no widely accepted pattern analysis has been developed.
   g) Two forms of the test have also been developed for children.
      (1) The Wechsler Intelligence Scale for Children (WISC-R) is a 1974 revision of the original WISC. It is designed for children ages five to fifteen and is the most widely used intelligence test for children.
      (2) The Wechsler Preschool Primary Scale of Intelligence (WPPSI-R) has been developed for children ages three to six and one-half.

4. Special individually administered intelligence tests have been devised for use with illiterate, blind, deaf, and other handicapped persons who would not be accurately tested on the standard tests.

5. Group tests
   a) Large numbers of paper-and-pencil group tests of intelligence are available and are used primarily in schools and personnel departments in business and industry.
   b) Although these tests generally yield IQ scores, it may be more meaningful to reserve the use of the term *IQ* for the results of individually administered intelligence tests.

VI. **Personality tests**
   A. There is a great variety of personality measures that differ in form, content, purpose, and interpretation.

B. Some personality measures are attempts to assess personality traits or characteristics; others are attempts to reveal a pattern of personality dynamics (e.g., motives, defenses, conflicts).

C. Objective personality tests

1. Objective tests usually take the form of questionnaires or rating scales; subjects respond to the items according to how characteristic they are of their experience and behavior.

2. Tests are administered and scored in a standardized way; the results are expressed in numerical scores.

3. Since objective tests are a form of self-report, they are open to faking and dissimulation. However, their ease of administration permits the testing of large numbers of persons by staff other than special clinical personnel.

4. The Minnesota Multiphasic Personality Inventory (MMPI) is the most widely used objective personality test in psychiatric practice in the United States. It consists of 566 true-false items.

   a) Validity scales

   There are four special scales that are scored to indicate response tendencies and test-taking attitudes that might make interpretations of the test doubtful.

   b) Clinical scales

   (1) Responses are scored in terms of correspondence to the responses of diagnosed psychiatric groups. The clinical scales can be scored for hypochondriasis, depression, hysteria, psychopathic deviate, paranoia, psychasthenia, schizophrenia, and mania.

   (2) Two other scales, masculinity-femininity and social introversion, are typically used in connection with the clinical scales.

   c) Other scales

   In addition to the clinical scales, many research scales have been developed for special purposes or to measure other personality characteristics (e.g., dependency, ego strength).

   d) Interpretation

   Interpretation of the test is based on the pattern of scores.

   (1) In recent years, standardized interpretations have been developed for common patterns.

   (2) Computer programs can be used to score the test and produce analyses of the profiles of the scores.

   e) Evaluation

   A sizable literature (several thousand articles and books) has developed around the MMPI, which indicates that the test is sufficiently reliable and valid for many clinical applications.

5. The MMPI-2
   a) A major revision of the MMPI was completed in 1989.
      (1) Some items were altered or excluded because they had been outdated by changes in language use since the origin of the inventory in 1940.
      (2) New items were introduced to provide content that was not represented on the original test.
      (3) The new version was restandardized on a more heterogeneous normal group than the "Minnesota normals" of the original standardization.
      (4) New content scales were developed in addition to the revision of the traditional scales.
      (5) A separate adolescent form of the inventory is being developed.
   b) Preliminary studies indicate differences in profile types for the two versions of the test when given to the same person in about one-third of the cases.
   c) Further research will be needed to provide the rich documentation and clinical application that made the original inventory a valuable clinical instrument.

6. Other objective personality tests in clinical use
   a) Although hundreds of personality tests and scales have been developed to evaluate and extend particular theories of personality or for other research purposes, most of them are not directly useful as diagnostic or descriptive instruments in clinical practice.
   b) Other multiple-scale objective tests that have been found useful in psychiatric practice include the following:
      (1) Cattell's Sixteen Personality Factor Scale (16 PF)
      (2) The Differential Personality Inventory (DPI) developed by Jackson
      (3) The Millon Clinical Multiaxial Inventory (MCMI-R)
      (4) Gough's California Psychological Inventory (CPI)
      (5) The Myers-Briggs Type Indicator, which is based on Jung's theory of personality types
   c) None of these tests has as yet rivaled the wide range of clinical application and research of the MMPI, but they may prove to be valuable additions to clinical assessment techniques.

7. A number of short, objective, self-response scales have been developed to assess patterns of behavior that have clinical significance. Some examples are:
   a) The Fear Survey Schedule (FSS)

b) The State-Trait Anxiety Inventory

c) The Beck Depression Inventory

d) The Maudsley Obsessional-Compulsive Inventory

D. Projective techniques of measuring personality

1. The term *projective* implies that the patients "project" their personalities into the responses they make.

   a) The materials of most projective methods are unstructured or ambiguous; thus, they require that the patient organize them in some imaginative way.

   b) Patients have considerable freedom in their responses.

   c) It is assumed that the way the patients respond reveals emotional and motivational factors that are characteristic of them, though perhaps unconsciously.

   d) The interpretation of the responses is subjective and is usually based on the theoretical assumptions of the interpreter. This leads to less consistent interpretation than is obtained with objective tests.

   e) Both the administration and interpretation of projective tests require special training and experience.

2. The Rorschach is the best known and most widely used of the projective techniques.

   a) Hermann Rorschach (1884–1922), a Swiss psychiatrist, initiated the use of inkblots for diagnostic and descriptive purposes. His students introduced the Rorschach test to the United States. Beginning in the 1930s, the United States became the major source of research on the Rorschach.

   b) Several systems, or approaches to the test, have been developed. Among the best-known systems are those of Samuel Beck, Marguerite Hertz, Bruno Klopfer, Zygmut Piotrowski, and David Rappaport, together with Roy Schafer.

   c) There have been many differences of opinion and controversies among these systematizers. Each system has its own position on administration, scoring (including scoring symbols), and interpretation, but there are some general similarities among them.

   d) Administration and scoring

      (1) The materials consist of ten "inkblots." Although there are differences in instructions from system to system, in general, patients are asked to describe what each one looks like. They may offer as many responses to each card as they wish.

      (2) Following the administration of the test, the examiner questions the subject about the response made,

asking him or her to indicate the location on the inkblot that prompted the response, and to say what about the blot (e.g., shape, color, texture) contributed to the response. Again, there are some differences among the five approaches as to how much detail and elaboration are elicited in this inquiry.

e) Responses are scored according to
   (1) Content (e.g., human, animal, object, X ray)
   (2) The area of the blot included in the content (whole blot or a particular section of it)
   (3) The characteristics of the blot (e.g., color, shading, and shape) that determined the content

f) Interpretation is based on the assumed personal significance of the responses, as well as on characteristic ways in which the patients organize their responses.
   (1) Theories about Rorschach responses relate such factors as location, use of color, texture, and movement, as well as content and sequence to personality characteristics, psychopathology, and special strengths.
   (2) In most systems, interpretation rests heavily on psychoanalytic theory. The Klopfer system is strongly Jungian in its interpretive emphasis.

g) A tremendous literature (several thousand articles and books) pertaining to the Rorschach has developed.
   (1) The complexity of the technique (administration, scoring, and interpretation) and the existence of different systematic approaches to the test have made research difficult.
   (2) Although some of the research has been rigorous, much of it has not met high standards of research design.
   (3) Reviews of the Rorschach literature over the years have consistently raised serious questions about the reliability and validity of this instrument.

h) The Exner Comprehensive System
   (1) J. E. Exner has integrated the various approaches to the Rorschach into a comprehensive system of scoring and interpretation.
   (2) The elements of the Exner system are empirically based and amenable to research validation.
   (3) The development of indices and the correlation of Rorschach variables with clinical variables have provided measures that allow the criteria of objective tests (reliability, validity) to be assessed more appropriately in the Rorschach while retaining its

capacity to elicit a wide range of personal responses.

   i) The Exner approach has been productive in stimulating research and has been instrumental in new and widespread interest in the Rorschach as a clinical assessment procedure.

3. Thematic Apperception Test (TAT)

   a) This test consists of twenty illustrations. The patient is asked to tell a story about the content of each picture.

   b) Stories are interpreted in terms of their themes, the handling of motivational states, the resolution of conflicts, the ways in which interpersonal relations are presented, and the extent to which patients identify themselves with the characters they describe.

   c) Several complete methods of scoring have been developed that require special training.

   d) The TAT now tends to be used more in personality research than in clinical assessment.

4. Other projective techniques

   a) A large number of other techniques, involving word association, sentence completion, drawing, and storytelling, have been devised.

   b) They have in common the assumption that imaginative productions and fantasy yield important clues to personality.

VII. **Behavioral assessment**

A. The increase in the application of behavioral concepts and methodology to clinical practice has been accompanied by the elaboration of techniques of assessing behavior.

B. In behavioral assessment, emphasis is placed on the objective description of behavior and on the environmental events and contexts that were antecedent and consequent to the behavior being investigated.

C. Although some behavioral assessment is similar to traditional methods of investigation, the purpose is to elicit information about characteristic reactions to situations with a minimum of inference, rather than to elicit information about psychodynamic determinants.

D. The emphasis on objective descriptions of current behavior makes behavioral assessment useful to the eclectic practitioner.

E. Techniques of behavioral assessment include:

1. Interviewing

   a) The interview is used to obtain self-reported information about problem behavior and the circumstances that influence it.

b) The interview also provides an opportunity to raise and test hypotheses about the events that may interfere with or support attempts to modify the patient's behavior.
2. Inventories and scales
   a) Self-reported information can be obtained with questionnaires and "behavior-and-situation" checklists.
   b) A large and continually increasing number of special-purpose devices have been developed, and information about reliability and applicability is accumulating.
3. Observation
   a) Both direct and indirect techniques have been used to obtain information about behavior.
   b) Although indirect methods are preferred because they do not, in themselves, influence behavior, they may not be feasible in most clinical situations.
4. Simulation
   a) This technique is also called role playing.
   b) "Real-life" situations are constructed, and patients are asked to assume a role.
   c) By observing how the role is played, the therapist is enabled to observe the patient's characteristic modes of response.
   d) Investigation of similarities in behavior in natural and simulated situations suggests that there is a fair degree of consistency.
5. Assessment of therapeutic change
   a) All the methods described in this section contribute to the modification of problem behavior by directing the patient's attention to the frequency with which it occurs and the contexts in which it is most likely to occur.
   b) Assessment of preferences for reinforcing situations and activities also can be used in the planning of programs for behavioral change.
   c) Self-observation and simulation provide the patient as well as the therapist with opportunities to modify and monitor changes in behavior.
   d) In behavior therapy, the problems are formulated in terms of behavior that is to be altered. Thus, techniques of behavioral assessment can be used to determine the frequency and consistency of behavioral change and, thus, provide an index of success of treatment.
6. The integration of data from various assessment sources may yield a more comprehensive analysis of patient behavior, which emphasizes behavioral interrelationships rather than focuses on specific classes of behavior.

## VIII. Neuropsychological tests

A. The assessment of intellectual deficit and the differentiation of organic brain conditions is often a problem in psychiatric diagnosis.

B. More accurate assessments of deficits due to brain damage can be made if earlier test scores, with which present performance can be compared, are available. This is seldom possible.

C. There are some tests that compare performance that is more sensitive to brain damage (e.g., abstract reasoning) with performance that is less affected (e.g., vocabulary).

D. Other tests have been designed to assess specific aspects of brain function, such as memory, perception, language use, and motor coordination.

E. The Halstead-Reitan and the Luria-Nebraska are two widely used comprehensive neuropsychological test batteries.

F. Neuroscientists and cognitive scientists have been making rapid advances in the localization of brain activity and the assessment of cognitive functioning. Techniques that have been developed for research purposes may also have great value in the clinical assessment of neurological deficits and potential for recovery.

## IX. Vocational and educational tests

A. Since the problems faced by some patients involve vocational maladjustment and dissatisfaction, vocational testing can contribute important information to a total treatment program. In general, vocational tests are of two types: measurements of aptitude and measures of interests.

B. Aptitude tests
   1. Available tests measure a variety of special aptitudes and abilities, such as clerical ability, mechanical ability, spatial reasoning, hand-and-finger dexterity, and rate of manipulation.
   2. Norms permit comparison of individual scores with scores of representative occupational groups.

C. Achievement tests
   1. Achievement tests, which measure the outcome of learning experiences, can yield useful information on the level and extent of a person's attainment of educationally based skills.
   2. Achievement tests can be classified in three general categories:
      a) Survey batteries that contain various individual subject matter or skill tests
      b) Specific subject or area tests
      c) Diagnostic tests that are designed to help determine someone's strengths and weaknesses in particular areas

3. There is an extremely large variety of achievement tests, most of which are designed for classroom use or that require the administrative and interpretive skills of an educational specialist.

4. Although achievement cannot usually be explored in detail in most psychiatric assessment, some appraisal of achievement is useful, since level of achievement is often involved in referral.

5. A useful achievement test for psychiatric assessment is the Wide Range Achievement Test (WRAT).
   a) WRAT scores indicate a person's current level in word recognition, spelling, and arithmetic computation.
   b) The WRAT helps determine weaknesses in areas that are essential as background for academic learning, and results can suggest the need for further evaluation and remediation.

D. Interest tests
   1. Interest tests permit the comparison of the individual's interests with the interests of persons representative of a number of professions and occupations.
   2. The most commonly used vocational interest test for adults is the Strong-Campbell Interest Inventory (SCII).
   3. The correlation of the individual's interests with those of representative members of particular occupations has been shown to be strongly related to job satisfaction.

E. Professional and managerial tests
   1. The assessment of aptitude for professional and managerial occupations is more complex.
   2. It involves the assessment of a variety of factors, including information, intellect, personality, attitudes, and interests.
   3. These tests are not considered as valid as the simpler tests of aptitudes and interests.

X. **Trends in psychiatric assessment**
   A. While emphasis in the use of assessment remains on establishing a diagnosis and providing a personality description of the patient, attention is now also given to defining problems and developing a program of intervention.
   B. *DSM*-III and *DSM*-III-R, by emphasizing behaviorally based criteria for making diagnoses, have contributed to the development and use of assessment procedures that are directed to specific criteria or clinical conditions.
   C. Emphasis is also shifting from the assessment of psychopathology or deficiencies to an inclusion of areas of competency.
   D. Insofar as much behavior seems to be influenced by special characteristics of the environment, more attention is being paid

to the assessment of situations and the way the person responds to and influences them.

E. As patients play a more active role in their own treatment and management, self-assessment procedures assume importance.

F. Assessment is becoming an essential component of therapeutic intervention, from its initial stages through follow-up.

G. In the multiaxial classification proposed in *DSM*-III-R, assessment is not only of symptoms (Axis I), personality (Axis II), and physical disorders (Axis III), but also of experiential and situational sources of stress (Axis IV) and competence or level of adaptive functioning (Axis V).

H. Assessment in hospital-based programs is conducted by each discipline of adjunctive therapies (e.g., occupational therapy, art therapy, etc.) and by nursing. The problems of each patient are identified, sometimes through structured tests and tasks (as in occupational therapy) and sometimes through observing the patient's characteristics, movements, and ways of relating to others (as in movement therapy and nursing). Interventions and possible rehabilitation and growth plans are then developed.

I. Programs and institutions are now assessed, so that the progress of the individual patient is viewed in relation to the effectiveness of programs in medical and social institutions.

## References

Anastasi, A. *Psychological Testing*. 6th ed. New York: Macmillan, 1988.

Barlow, D., ed. *Behavioral Assessment of Adult Disorders*. New York: Guilford Press, 1981.

Davidson, G., and J. Neale. *Abnormal Psychology*. 5th ed. New York: Wiley, 1990.

Goldman, H., ed. *Review of General Psychiatry*. 2d ed. Norwalk, Conn.: Appleton & Lange, 1988.

Goldstein, G., and M. Hersen, eds. *Handbook of Psychological Assessment*. 2d ed. New York: Pergamon Press, 1990.

Graham, J. *MMPI-2*. New York: Oxford University Press, 1990.

Hersen, M., A. Kazdin, and A. Bellack, eds. *The Clinical Psychology Handbook*. New York: Pergamon Press, 1983.

Kaplan, H. I., and B. J. Sadock, eds. *Comprehensive Textbook of Psychiatry/V*. Vol. 1, 5th ed. Baltimore: Williams & Wilkins, 1989.

Neitzel, M., D. Bernstein, and R. Milich. *Introduction to Clinical Psychology*. Englewood Cliffs, N.J.: Prentice-Hall, 1991.

Wetzler, S. *Measuring Mental Illness*. Washington, D.C.: American Psychiatric Press, 1989.

# 9 Treatment In Psychiatry: Psychotherapy

The light that a man receiveth by counsel from another is drier and purer than that which cometh from his own understanding and judgement, which is ever infused and drenched in his affections and customs.

**Francis Bacon, "Of Friendship,"** *Essays* **(1625)**

## I. Introduction
  A. In the presentation on etiology in chapter 5 of the outline, attention was given to possible causative factors. The possible sources were loosely classified as:
    1. Psychological and developmental
    2. Social and environmental
    3. Biological
  B. Similarly, treatment can be classified according to the presumed causative factors that are being treated.
    1. Individual psychotherapy presumes the importance of factors in the personality dynamics and experiential history of the patient.
    2. Group, family, activity, and expressive therapies presume the importance of factors in the social relationships and social communications of the patient.
    3. Pharmacological and somatic therapies presume the importance of genetic, physiological, and neural factors.
  C. This chapter will be concerned with individual psychotherapy and with group, family, and adjunctive therapies. Pharmacological and somatic therapies will be considered in the following chapter.

## II. Definition
  A. In the broad sense, many things that are done to or for a patient may have a psychotherapeutic effect.
  B. As defined in the more traditional sense in *A Psychiatric Glossary,* psychotherapy is "a process in which a person who wishes to relieve *symptoms* or resolve problems in living or is seeking

personal growth enters into an implicit or explicit contract to interact in a prescribed way with the psychotherapist."[1]

C. Traditionally, distinctions have been drawn between the practice of psychotherapy and the practice of counseling in terms of differences in professional training of practitioners, type of patient or client treated, and setting in which treatment takes place. Currently, these distinctions are somewhat blurred or have been defined in terms of licensing and certification practices of individual states.

### III. Types of psychotherapy

A. There are many variants of individual psychotherapy and the array of approaches can certainly be confusing to students and consumers.

B. Although psychotherapies can be classified in various ways according to historical traditions, goals of treatment, theoretical orientations, and stated principles of method, the organization in this chapter will be a descriptive one that is representative of the most widely used approaches.

   1. Psychoanalysis
   2. Expressive and insight-oriented psychodynamic therapies
   3. Supportive therapies
   4. Interpersonal therapies
   5. Behavior therapies
   6. Cognitive therapies
   7. Humanistic therapies (phenomenological and existential)

C. Common elements in psychotherapy
Marmor (in Sipe and Rowe 1984) lists seven elements that are common to all forms of psychotherapy.

   1. Relationship—both the therapist and patient contribute something to the therapeutic experience.
     a) The patient has a perceived need to change. This must be accompanied by an element of motivation and expectancy of getting help.
     b) The therapist brings to the relationship knowledge (this includes adequate training, discipline, and the capability of "understanding"), objectivity (the "fair neutrality" that allows the patient to be himself or herself), empathy (warm understanding), and integrity.
   2. Emotional release (usually brought about by verbalizing).
   3. Cognitive learning (each psychotherapist, regardless of his or her orientation, conveys therapeutic objectives and in some way offers an explanation about how change is going to occur).

---

1. American Psychiatric Association, *A Psychiatric Glossary*, 6th ed. (Washington, D.C.: APA, 1988)

4. Conditioning (all forms of therapy, regardless of orientation, have some element of conditioning, even if it is covert and implicit, e.g., the therapist conveys a certain set of values and what is healthy and unhealthy).
5. Identification (modeling or "social learning").
6. Suggestion (persuasive and suggestive elements are either implicit or explicit in all forms of therapy).
7. Reality testing (also referred to as "rehearsal," or "practicing" of the new ways of coping that are learned in therapy).

IV. **Psychodynamic view of therapeutic relationships**

Of the common elements in psychotherapy, the nature and quality of the therapist-patient relationship is often cited as of particular significance. While the special features of the therapeutic relationship may be identified by a variety of terms, the following psychodynamic concepts give an idea of its special nature.

A. Rapport
1. *A Psychiatric Glossary* defines *rapport* as "the feeling of harmonious accord and mutual responsiveness that contributes to the patient's confidence in the therapist and willingness to work cooperatively. It is to be distinguished from *transference,* which is unconscious."[2]
2. Rapport is important in any treatment relationship, regardless of whether the patient is being treated for an emotional or a physical illness.
3. It is probably the single most effective therapeutic tool a physician has.
4. Some therapists speak of the "therapeutic alliance," which involves the primarily conscious and rational aspects of the treatment relationship. It is an agreement to work toward a mutual therapeutic goal.
5. Whatever treatment modality is used, *confidentiality* is an essential element of the relationship.

B. Transference and Countertransference
1. *Transference* is the patient's unconscious attachment to the therapist (or others involved in the patient's treatment) of feelings and attitudes that were originally related to important figures (e.g., parents, siblings) in early life.
2. Transference can become so intense that it leads to the development of a "transference neurosis," a state in which early feelings and attitudes make up the bulk of the patient's feelings toward the physician.
3. *Countertransference* is the therapist's unconscious or conscious emotional reaction to the patient.

2. Ibid.

a) Feelings arising from the therapist's unresolved underlying conflicts may at times become intense and interfere with an understanding of the patient.

b) It is especially important that a therapist recognize any underlying negative countertransference.

c) Sometimes countertransference can be used diagnostically and therapeutically. For example, irritability or hostility in a therapist may be induced by fear in the patient; if the therapist is aware of the countertransference, he or she may more directly and correctly help the patient identify the underlying conflicts, recognize the fear, and resolve the issues behind it.

4. Both positive and negative feelings are involved in transference and countertransference.

C. Resistance

1. Resistance arises from the conscious or unconscious psychological forces in the patient that oppose bringing repressed (unconscious) material into consciousness.

2. Resistance is encountered in all forms of therapy, but is especially noted in individual psychotherapy.

3. It represents a mobilization of underlying defenses to resist treatment.

4. In any given situation, the physician must decide whether to leave the patient's resistance intact or to try to reduce it.

D. Many variables may affect outcomes in psychotherapy, but the personality of the individual psychotherapist as it influences the relationship must be considered an important determinant.

V. **Psychoanalysis**

A. As noted in chapter 2, *psychoanalysis* means a theory of personality development, a method of research, and a system of treatment. It was originally developed by Sigmund Freud.

B. As a treatment technique, it is defined in *A Psychiatric Glossary* as follows: "Through analysis of *free associations* and *interpretation* of dreams, emotions and behavior are traced to the influence of *repressed instinctual drives* and *defenses against them in the unconscious.*"[3]

C. Because it involves a large expenditure of time, feeling, and money, psychoanalysis has only a limited place in the treatment of most mental disorders. However, the insights gained from it have been extremely helpful in the other forms of psychotherapy.

D. Characteristics of psychoanalytic therapy

1. As used by psychoanalysts, uncovering involves the exploration of the unconscious, chiefly through free association, which *A Psychiatric Glossary* defines as "the spontaneous

3. Ibid.

uncensored verbalizations by the patient of whatever comes to mind."[4]

2. Dream material is often evaluated for clues to unconscious feelings, and interpretations are made to the patient.

3. Resistance (see section C) must be recognized and dealt with.

4. Of major importance in this type of therapy is the therapist's ability to be a meaningful listener.

5. Interpretation is an integral part of this type of therapy. Interpretations may be made either of currently operating psychodynamic factors or of psychogenic forces. (The latter is focused on the relationship between current reactive states and past emotion.) Interpretation also helps to reduce resistance.

6. The interpretation and analysis of transference provide a substantial framework on which psychoanalytic therapy is developed.

7. Correlation (reconstruction) is also employed to help relate past, repressed conflicts to current situations.

8. "Working through" follows the development of insight and constitutes a major portion of the treatment time. It includes repeated exploration of the insight gained through interpretation.

VI. **Psychodynamic psychotherapy**

A. Psychoanalytic theory has influenced the procedures of many psychotherapists who themselves are not practitioners of psychoanalysis.

B. The general purpose of psychodynamic therapy is to produce insight by uncovering emotional conflicts, chiefly unconscious, so that they can be dealt with in a way that does not hamper current relationships and activities.

C. Psychodynamic psychotherapy is based on assumptions that are derived from psychoanalytic theory.

1. Patients' symptoms are expressions in current relationships of "neurotic" conflicts.

2. Current conflicts are manifestations of patterns of conflict established in childhood.

3. Recognition of the conflict and its childhood relevance is difficult because of unconscious factors.

4. Therapeutic change occurs as a result of insight into the connections between current maladaptive behaviors and their relation to "neurotic" conflict.

5. Interpretation of transference and resistance is an important contributor to progress in treatment.

4. Ibid.

D. Brief dynamic psychotherapy
   1. A current trend in psychodynamic psychotherapy is to work on focused problems in a delineated time frame.
   2. This approach was first developed in detail by Chicago psychoanalysts Franz Alexander and Thomas French.
   3. Features of brief dynamic psychotherapy
      a) Psychoanalytic principles are applied to the solution of a patient's specific problems rather than to the full array of the patient's personality characteristics.
      b) The initial diagnosis determines the appropriateness of time-limited psychotherapy for the patient.
      c) The focus of treatment is usually the manifestation of a long-standing personality problem that has emerged in the circumstances of a current interpersonal difficulty.
      d) Since time is limited, as part of the therapeutic approach it is considered very important to establish an effective therapeutic alliance (rapport) as quickly and efficiently as possible.
      e) The significant phase of treatment is "working through" that is specifically directed toward the resolution of the focal problem.
      f) Though termination is anticipated from the beginning of treatment, special attention is given to the dynamic significance (attachment and separation) of the ending of the therapeutic relationship.
   4. Hans Strupp (1984) has developed a guide to time-limited dynamic psychotherapy (TLDP), which provides a systematic basis for training and the evaluation of therapeutic processes.
E. The following three case examples illustrate some of the features of psychodynamic therapy.
   1. A forty-five-year-old widower complained of impotence. After three interviews, it became obvious that his symptom resulted from two important factors: (a) his guilt over having rejected his wife because she was physically unattractive; (b) the guilt was reactivated when he was sexually aroused.

      His impotence was a protection against a second marriage to a woman he was dating but did not wish to marry. In this case, the conflicts were relatively superficial and readily accessible to the therapist. His symptom cleared up when he recognized the dynamic factors and broke off his relationship with the woman.
   2. A twenty-five-year-old man had consulted many physicians for palpitation, tachycardia, precordial pain, and apprehension. Each time, physical and laboratory examinations

revealed no evidence of cardiac disease. Although he worried about his heart, his symptoms were typical of anxiety disorder.

During the first interview, it became apparent that his symptoms were related to his feelings about his father, but it was not until he had been seen for twelve sessions that he was able to see the relationship between his own symptoms and his father's heart attack a year earlier. When he did see that the onset of his own symptoms followed his father's heart attack and that his anxiety was being perpetuated by his guilt over his unconscious wish for his father's death, his symptoms disappeared.

3. A thirty-year-old housewife had repeated episodes of paresthesia, dizziness, and pains in her arms. These had begun shortly after marriage and seriously handicapped her. After about fifty hours of psychotherapy, she was able to recognize that these symptoms always developed when she felt rejected by her husband. This rejection awakened the underlying feelings that she had had when her father rejected her. When she recognized this, her symptoms cleared up.

The conflict here was unconscious and hence not as immediately available. Uncovering therapy brought the conflict to light.

## VII. Supportive psychotherapy

A. Supportive psychotherapy deals predominantly with conscious material and is centered chiefly on bolstering the individual's strengths and assets (enhancing self-esteem and ego strength). It reinforces healthy defenses (enhances the patient's defensive functioning) and is based primarily on the therapist-patient relationship (thus, it fosters and maintains a positive transference), including the therapeutic alliance. Unlike uncovering psychotherapy, the focus tends to be on current problems; probing into the unconscious past is avoided. It usually requires an active "giving of self" by the therapist (e.g., it may require extra time, availability, and the giving of advice). As a matter of fact, many patients receiving supportive therapy have had such extreme difficulty with interpersonal relationships that the therapist must be more of a "real object" and less of an anonymous neutral figure, as is necessary in more intensive or interpretative therapies.

B. The treatment objectives are usually limited. It is usually indicated for patients with acute emotional upheavals (e.g., anxiety disorders, depressive disorders) or for patients with acute psychotic decompensation, or it is often appropriate for chronically severely ill patients (especially those who are trying to live in the community and especially for those with prominent, primitive defense mechanisms of projection and denial).

C. Techniques include reassurance, unburdening, environmental modification, persuasion, and clarification. Interpretations are usually avoided.

1. Reassurance

   *Reassurance* is the imparting or restoration of confidence and freeing the patient from fear and anxiety. It does not mean false reassurance. Reassurance cannot be imparted if the therapist is not herself or himself assured.

   a) Physical, laboratory, and X-ray examinations may relieve a person's anxiety about significant organic illness, and hence be reassuring.

   b) Examples of psychological reassurance include assuring panicky or obsessive-ruminative persons who fear serious mental breakdown that they will not lose their minds; assuring parents that the hostile and aggressive feelings they occasionally have about their children are not abnormal and will not lead to physical abuse; explaining to acutely depressed persons that their illness will be resolved.

2. Unburdening

   a) *Unburdening* is the therapeutic release of feelings through conscious, free expression. This is "getting it off the chest." It is also called *ventilation* and *catharsis.*

   b) It serves two purposes: sharing, which helps "dilute" the feelings; and self-punishment, by revealing oneself.

   c) For example, a sixty-year-old woman was finally able to tell the doctor how she had been emotionally clutching onto her thirty-five-year-old married daughter. After unburdening herself of this fact, which she had never before been able to verbalize, she was able to take the first major steps to release the hold on her daughter.

3. Environmental modification

   a) *Environmental modification,* also called *environmental intervention* or *environmental manipulation,* means altering the environment so as to relieve the patient's symptoms and distress.

   b) Caution must be exercised lest this type of treatment be misused.

   c) Examples are providing a temporary homemaker or housekeeper for an anxious or depressed mother whose symptoms are aggravated by her responsibility for her young children; placing a patient in the relatively neutral environment of a hospital; placing a runaway child in a foster home until the parents can work out the marital conflicts that contributed to the running away; advising a vacation for a widower whose grief has been unduly prolonged.

4. Persuasion
   a) *Persuasion* is direct suggestion, inducement, or entreatment in an effort to influence a patient's behavior.
   b) Examples include asking a person who seems to be becoming psychologically dependent on alcohol for relaxation to try jogging, bicycling, or some other kind of physical exercise; asking a spouse to modify his or her behavior and attitudes if the patient for some reason is unable to do this (this example also includes the element of environmental modification).

5. Clarification
   a) *Clarification* is a process by which the physician helps patients to understand their feelings and behavior and to gain a clearer picture of reality.
   b) Examples include pointing out to an agitated and depressed patient that a period of hospitalization will not worsen the condition; showing a paranoid patient how he or she is projecting; pointing out to a married person the rejecting behavior of a spouse who is really seeking a dissolution of the marriage.

## VIII. Interpersonal therapies

A. Interpersonal approaches to psychotherapy have features similar to both psychodynamic and cognitive therapies.

B. The interpersonal perspective is derived from the work of Harry Stack Sullivan, who viewed personality development as the outcome of the "recurrent interpersonal situations which characterize a human life."

C. A system for organizing and diagnosing forms of interpersonal behavior was developed by Timothy Leary. This conceptual system has provided the basis for diagnostic inventories and scales (e.g., Lorr's Interpersonal Behavior Inventory, Wiggins's Interpersonal Adjective Scale).

1. The diagnostic scheme is based on two primary dimensions of power (dominance-submission) and affiliation (love-hate), which define quadrants of a circle.

2. Interpersonal styles of interacting with others are ordered on the circle, with complementary styles occupying adjacent positions and antagonistic styles occupying opposite positions on the circle.

D. Disorders of behavior occur when rigid or extreme patterns of interpersonal behavior are used, which lead to repeated unhappiness, distress, or significant failure in a person's relationships and work.

    E. Therapeutic intervention is directed toward eliciting and developing interpersonal action that is on the opposite side to the maladaptive style on the interpersonal style circle.

        1. Since, according to the theory, a person will try to evoke responses from a therapist (and others) that are complementary to the person's style, the therapist must work to disengage from the patient's expectations, shift to responding in a noncomplementary manner, and eventually respond in an anticomplementary manner, thereby exerting pressure for change.

        2. This approach requires care in establishing a working alliance (rapport) early and timing properly the progressive behavioral shifts on the part of the therapist.

        3. Interpersonal therapy, in principle, can develop specific strategies to apply to distinctive maladaptive styles.

    F. The interpersonal approach has been directed particularly to the interpretation and treatment of *DSM*-III-R personality disorders.

    G. Klerman has developed a set of techniques and a training manual for the treatment of depression, which has achieved success in a major study of effectiveness.

## IX. Behavior therapy

    A. *Behavior therapy* has a specific meaning when used by some writers, but it will be used here as a general term that refers to all therapy that is derived from principles of learning (see chapter 3).

    B. Historical notes

        1. Ivan Pavlov, late in his career, attempted to give an account of human psychiatric disorders in terms of excitation and inhibition, the concepts that had so successfully accounted for data from his animal laboratory. His clinical interpretations were less successful, but he did stimulate other experimental scientists of learning to apply their analyses to clinical disorders.

        2. In the 1920s John Watson and Mary Jones demonstrated how a focal fear or phobia could be learned and extinguished by classical conditioning, but these demonstrations had no significant impact on the practice or theory of clinical psychiatry.

        3. Psychologists working with children with poor "habits" (e.g., nail biting, bed-wetting, temper tantrums) during the 1920s and 1930s developed practical techniques that are now viewed as forms of behavior therapy.

4. Learning theorists such as O. H. Mowrer, Neal Miller, and John Dollard in the 1950s attempted to interpret psychoanalytic theory and therapy in terms of the systematic learning theory of Clark Hull (1943); their writings renewed the interest of some experimental psychologists in psychiatric problems.
5. B. F. Skinner and his student Ogden Lindsley applied operant analysis of learning to the behavior of schizophrenics, and this incursion into the realm of psychiatric disorder was rapidly followed by the application of the same methods to treatment or, in operant conditioning terminology, behavior modification.
6. The publication by Joseph Wolpe in 1958 of his book *Psychotherapy by Reciprocal Inhibition* attracted widespread attention to developments in therapy in several countries and signaled the beginning of the modern era of behavior therapy.
7. Hans Eysenck encouraged a systematic approach to the theory and practice of behavior therapy by emphasizing the main points of difference from traditional psychotherapy.

C. General principles
1. Behavior therapy can be defined as the modification of responses through the application of experimentally established principles of learning.
2. Maladaptive behavior is viewed as either deficient or excessive. Thus, therapy involves increasing the incidence of appropriate behavior and decreasing behavior that is inappropriate in frequency, duration, or place of occurrence.
3. Maladaptive responses may be covert as well as overt. Thus, such traditional cognitive symptoms as hallucinations, delusions, and fantasies are not, in principle, recalcitrant to behavior therapy.
4. Psychiatric disorders are viewed primarily, though not exclusively, as the result of faulty learning.
5. Treatment is directed toward the removal of the inappropriate target behavior (symptoms) and toward learning new, more effective patterns of behavior.
6. Emphasis in treatment is placed particularly on the social environment as a source of stimuli that support symptoms but that can also support changes in behavior.
7. The experimental study of learning and the clinical practice of behavior therapy are viewed as mutually supporting activities that together can contribute to a unified understanding of learned behavior.

D. Types of behavior therapy

There are many variants of behavior therapy, but the examples that follow typify the most widely used techniques.

1. Systematic desensitization

a) This technique was developed by Joseph Wolpe as a means of associating anxiety-eliciting stimuli with relaxation.

b) Since anxiety and relaxation are incompatible reactions, the increase in the strength of relaxation responses will inhibit the anxious responses to the same stimuli.

c) Wolpe's approach consists of three stages.

(1) Relaxation training similar to the procedures introduced by Edmund Jacobson in 1938, in which the subject is taught to identify and control localized tension and relaxation of muscle groups.

(2) Construction of hierarchies of anxiety-producing stimuli by the subject; these threatening stimuli or events in the subject's life are ranked by the reactions they produce, from the weakest to strongest.

(3) Desensitization proper. The subject, in a deep state of relaxation, is presented with a stimulus from the weak end of the hierarchy and then with successively stronger ones as he or she is able to maintain relaxation.

d) Variations of this "gradual approach" method have been used to rehearse adequate behavior in an anxiety-inhibiting context (e.g., assertiveness training).

2. Aversion therapy

a) This is the oldest of the procedures outlined in this section, but it was used for many years with little systematic attention to the principles of learning that were applied.

b) This therapy is based on straightforward classical (Pavlovian) conditioning procedures. Stimuli are associated with some strong, unacceptable responses such as nausea, pain, or extreme disgust.

c) The noxious stimuli that are used to produce the response of aversion may be chemical (e.g., apomorphine), electrical, or visual (including imaginal).

d) Aversion therapy has most often been used in the treatment of habitual excesses (e.g., overuse of alcohol) and compulsive unacceptable or criminal social behavior (e.g., shoplifting, exhibitionism).

e) Considerable controversy has been generated both about the effectiveness of aversion therapy and about the social appropriateness of aversive control of socially deviant behavior.

f) Both operant conditioning analyses of the effect of aversive stimuli and the exploration of the effect of aversive imagery are attempts to find less unpleasant and more socially acceptable alternatives to aversion therapy.

3. Behavior modification
   a) *Behavior modification* is conducted by the application of operant conditioning principles to the interpretation and management of behavior problems.
   b) The basic principle of behavior modification is the control of the reinforcing consequences of behavior. *Reinforcing consequences* range from physical reinforcers (e.g., food) to social reinforcers (e.g., approval, tokens of exchange).
   c) Behavior modification has been used in a variety of institutional settings and on a great variety of problems. Striking examples include language training of autistic children, self-care training of intellectually retarded children and adults, socialization of regressed psychotic patients, and management of self-injurious behavior.
   d) Some chronic wards of psychiatric hospitals, some training schools and institutions for mentally retarded children and adults, and day-care and residential programs for mentally ill and mentally retarded adults have been managed according to operant conditioning principles in a "token economy." That is, appropriate changes in behavior are rewarded with tokens that can be exchanged for food, activities, and privileges.
   e) Operant principles, combining rehearsal and modeling with reinforcement, have been used not only to modify maladaptive behaviors in chronic mentally ill individuals but also to train social skills toward a level of improved social adequacy and appropriateness.
   f) Self-regulation techniques, by which patients learn to distinguish the environmental stimuli that evoke their maladaptive behavior and to manage their own reinforcing consequences, have grown in popularity among behavior therapists and have become a significant part of the popular literature of self-treatment (e.g., weight regulation, reduction of smoking, etc.).
   g) Biofeedback techniques are a form of self-regulation based on operant methods. Subjects monitor their own physiological processes (muscle tension, brain waves)

and, using the information they receive (feedback), learn to control them within limits.

    h) Behavior modification is an active, rapidly expanding, and enthusiastically professed learning approach to therapy.

4. Exposure treatments

    a) This approach requires actual exposure to feared or avoided situations.

    b) The degree of exposure may vary from low levels with general accommodation to direct confrontation with a most feared situation (flooding).

    c) Accompaniment by a supportive, reassuring person may be used in early stages of exposure.

    d) Agoraphobia, social phobias, and simple phobias have been shown to be responsive to exposure techniques.

5. Covert techniques

    a) Cautela asserts that self-defeating behaviors are maintained by complex covert processes (e.g., images) that can be modified by covert conditioning.

        (1) Patients are taught first to use "thought-stopping" imagery at the onset of maladaptive thought sequences.

        (2) Desensitization is used to establish relaxation imagery when unwanted thoughts emerge.

        (3) Patients learn to reinforce themselves with pleasurable images when they are successful in controlling their thoughts.

    b) Following Bandura's (1986) examples of vicarious learning through observing a model perform a target behavior, patients are instructed to imagine an ideal model enacting the behavior and to imagine obstacles that might arise and how they might be overcome.

6. Trends and appraisal

    a) Although behavior therapy was initially developed for and applied in the treatment of phobias and compulsions, it does not appear to be limited to reactions (symptoms) that obviously fit a learning interpretation.

    b) Since the emphasis in treatment is on modification of symptoms, the question of substitution has been raised by some critics (i.e., the removal of one symptom may lead to another if the underlying cause is not also treated). However, according to proponents of the therapy, substitution does not usually occur.

    c) Some enthusiastic supporters of behavior therapy, such as Hans Eysenck, claim that their evaluations show behavior therapy to be clearly superior to other forms of psychotherapy, particularly psychoanalysis.

d) More moderate and well-controlled evaluations indicate that behavior therapy is useful, that it is at least as effective as traditional psychotherapy, and that it may have particular benefits.

e) Since experimental investigations of learning and clinical applications of behavior therapy make use of similar concepts and sources of evidence, a consistent association between laboratory and clinic is maintained in this approach to treatment.

f) Since behavioral approaches are directed toward changing behavior, the benefits of treatment can be assessed objectively by observing the increases or decreases in the rate of targeted behaviors.

## X. Cognitive therapy

A. Early approaches to behavior therapy minimized or excluded from consideration such cognitive or mental variables as images, thoughts, expectations, or beliefs.

B. Many practitioners of behavior therapy, however, now assume that self-statements provide a basis for inferences about cognition and accept the idea that the beliefs and expectations that mediate much maladaptive behavior can be modified by behavior therapy.

C. Albert Ellis

1. Ellis names his approach "rational-emotive therapy" (RET).

2. This approach assumes that patients are maladaptive in their behavior because they act on irrational beliefs about themselves, about others, and the relationship between activating events on experiences and their consequences.

3. The goal of therapy is to eliminate or reduce the "irrational consequences" of irrational belief systems, which in turn reduces anxiety and hostility.

4. Through confrontation and active interpretation, patients are helped to restructure behavior by adopting more rational beliefs and altering the things they tell themselves.

D. Aaron Beck

1. Beck, in his cognitive therapy, also assigns major importance to correcting the faulty thinking about oneself and about the rewarding opportunities in one's present or future environment.

2. The approach focuses on helping the patient overcome faulty perceptions, distortions in self-concept, and false judgments about relationships in the world.

3. The therapist may begin at a behavioral level of working toward reduction of abnormal symptoms, but the underlying distorted attitudes must also be identified and challenged.

4. Active testing of assumptions through a variety of problem-oriented tasks leads to engaging in new activities based on cognitive modification.

E. Donald Meichenbaum

1. Meichenbaum developed his cognitive approach to behavior modification by treating cognitions as internal verbalizations (self-talk) and images that in distressed persons may interfere with performance.

2. In treatment patients learn to identify and then replace the self-statements and self-instructions that are maladaptive.

3. Treatment is also directed toward providing means of desensitizing tension-producing conditions and producing more successful coping behavior through reinforcing self-comments and reassuring imagery.

4. As in the other cognitive therapies, a cognitive restructuring is the desired outcome of treatment.

F. Trends and appraisal

1. As with behavioral therapies, cognitive therapies are most frequently applied where problems and desired outcomes can be specified.

2. Cognitive approaches lend themselves to research outcomes, and evaluation of cognitive therapies has been associated with positive outcomes.

3. Beck's procedures have been intensely investigated and have been shown to be effective with depression when compared with other treatment approaches.

4. Behavioral and cognitive approaches, by specifying methods of application, are seen as accessible and more possible to be applied in a uniform way; training manuals have been developed for some of the approaches.

5. To some practitioners, the integration of cognitive and behavior treatment modes is still controversial because they believe that concern with inferred mental states reduces the effectiveness of direct manipulation of the environment.

XI. **Humanistic therapies**

A number of therapeutic approaches characterized by their phenomenological or existential assumptions about human experiences or by their opposition to traditional psychoanalysis or behavior therapy have come to be loosely referred to as "humanistic" therapy. While *humanistic* is a word with many connotations, it is used here merely as a conventional label for these approaches. (See the section on humanistic perspectives on personality in chapter 2.)

A. Principles

1. A person's world is a product of individual perceptions. Therefore, what one says about one's personal world should be accepted as subjective truth.

2. Each person is unique. Therefore, individual dignity must not be affronted by the attempt to label, categorize, or reduce a person to some set of generalizations about human character or behavior.

3. Individuals are processes, rather than products of influences. Thus, each person has, in principle, the capacity to realize his or her potentialities and to live the life suited to those potentialities.

4. Individuals are free, capable of choice, and responsible for the choices, fulfilling or unfulfilling, that they make.

5. The goals of treatment are those that the patients choose freely and that are congruent with their understanding of themselves and their interests.

6. The role of the therapist is to provide a supportive, understanding, and accepting context for the exploration of opportunities for personal growth and development.

B. Variants

There are many variants of humanistic therapy, both individual and group. The following have achieved wide recognition.

1. Client-centered therapy

   a) The chief proponent of client-centered therapy is Carl Rogers.

   b) Rogers believes that there is a strong innate tendency to develop and realize one's potentialities. Nevertheless, a person may adopt a set of values or attitudes that limits experience or blocks development.

   c) The therapist offers total acceptance (unconditional positive regard), which is the necessary condition of change.

   d) The therapist uses techniques of recognition and clarification of the client's feelings, and encourages honesty in communication.

   e) In a therapeutic context of this kind, the client can reassess his or her self-perceptions and make constructive choices.

2. Existential analysis

   a) Exponents include Medard Boss, Viktor Frankl, and Rollo May.

b) They believe that people define themselves in terms of interpersonal relationships and that the relationships must be honest and open (authentic) to give existence its value and meaning.

c) Patients' symptoms reflect evasions of responsibility for their own choices, for their dysphoria, or for their unstable or incoherent set of values (meaninglessness).

d) The therapist encourages the patient to accept responsibility for symptoms as self-chosen and to decide on ways of dealing with life that are active, authentic, and meaningful.

e) Since individuals (and therapists) are unique, no particular techniques and procedures can be formulated as general principles.

3. Gestalt therapy

a) Fritz Perls is the leading proponent of Gestalt therapy.

b) Disordered behavior is viewed as the result of unresolved past conflicts, but its resolution occurs in the action and decisions of the here and now.

c) Emphasis is placed on the identification and acceptance of one's needs and one's personal responsibility for meeting them by selecting effective strategies.

d) Gestalt therapy is more technique-oriented than other humanistic therapies, using reenactment of dreams, role-played conversations with one's own feelings or with other persons or objects, cathartic "acting out," and interpersonal confrontation in groups.

e) The Gestalt therapist is also more direct and manipulative in treatment sessions, but the patient is responsible for defining the changes to be made and for exploring change.

f) The goal of Gestalt therapy (the German word *Gestalt* means "whole") is the unification of feeling and action into a new configuration of decisive and fulfilling experience.

C. Trends and appraisal

1. There has been little evaluation of humanistic therapy by practitioners. Evaluation is viewed as a violation of the humanistic emphasis on the uniqueness and integrity of the individual. Carl Rogers's research program is an exception.

2. Concern with individual responsibility and choice is not the exclusive domain of humanistic approaches, though these approaches have led to a reevaluation of the role of self-determination in other types of therapy.

3. It is doubtful that any therapeutic situation is as free from the therapist's influences as the humanistic therapists claim theirs are.
4. The humanistic perspective is viewed by some critics as reflecting an unscientific and even antiscientific approach to the understanding and treatment of human problems.
5. Nevertheless, humanistic therapy has achieved popular acceptance and has had a major role in the development of alternatives to traditional psychiatric and psychological treatment.

## XII. The assessment of therapeutic outcomes and processes

A. In the past, much treatment has been evaluated only in clinical reports and case histories or in studies lacking appropriate comparison groups.
B. The proper evaluation of psychotherapy is very difficult because there are so many patient, therapist, and method variables to sort out and control; also, no clearly reliable measures of improvement exist, so various subjective patient and observer judgments must be used.
C. It is hard to draw conclusions about the benefits of one therapy compared to another because most achieve similar rates of reported success with general patient groups.
D. Psychotherapy research currently is directed toward either the study of outcomes (the traditional study of efficacy) or the study of process (what activities and events in psychotherapy contribute to change).
E. With greater precision of diagnosis and the development of specific problem-oriented techniques, outcome research has shifted from the general evaluation of success of a therapeutic method to evaluation of the relative success of procedures applied to particular diagnostic conditions of symptoms.
F. Some investigators have attempted analogue research in which clinical variables associated with subject characteristics, problems, therapist characteristics, and treatment techniques are investigated in controlled experimental settings that simulate as many relevant clinical conditions as possible.
G. The technique of metanalysis has been used to combine results of many studies. While the use of metanalysis is not without severe critics of its methodology and applications, there have been some consistent findings:
1. The average person who receives psychotherapy is better off at the end of treatment than the large majority of the people who do not receive treatment.
2. Effects of psychotherapy are still maintained over periods of six- to eighteen-month follow-ups.

3. A small percentage of patients become worse after psychotherapy.
4. School or theory of psychotherapy does not seem to be a major factor in overall estimates of effectiveness, but if there is an advantage it usually goes to cognitive and behavioral treatments.
5. When cognitive and behavioral therapies are directed toward fairly specific outcomes, they show a consistent (although small) advantage over other therapies.

H. The National Institute of Mental Health (NIMH) conducted a Treatment of Depression Collaborative Research Program (TDCRP) beginning in 1977, the results of which are being reported by Elkin and associates.
1. The study compared Beck's cognitive therapy with Klerman's interpersonal psychotherapy and pharmacological treatment.
2. Therapists were selected and trained in the therapeutic techniques they were to employ.
3. Patients were selected to meet the *DSM*-III-R criteria for Definite Major Depressive Disorder.
4. A variety of assessment techniques were used to evaluate changes in depressive symptomatology, overall symptomatology and life functioning, and functioning related to particular treatment approaches.
5. Results are still being analyzed and reported, but some of those published so far show:
   a) All three approaches achieved significant and equivalent degrees of success.
   b) A placebo plus clinical management control group also showed significant improvement.
   c) Pharmacological treatment was faster in reducing depressive symptoms at first, but the initial advantage was matched in a few weeks by the psychotherapies.
   d) Severely depressed patients did not do as well in the placebo condition as those in the treatment modes.

I. A current NIMH study, The Depression Awareness, Recognition, and Treatment Program, is adding clinical trials with short-term dynamic psychotherapy to trials with cognitive, interpersonal, and pharmacological therapies to explore further the effectiveness and appropriateness of individual therapies and combinations of therapies for specific patient characteristics.

## XIII. The future of psychotherapy
A. For many decades psychotherapy was based on Freudian psychoanalytic theory. It was basically a medical treatment performed by psychiatric physicians, was frequently the "core

treatment'' for the emotionally disordered, and was the central focus of residency training programs in psychiatry.

B. With the advent of biologic psychiatry, the growth in research focused on biological determinants, and the development of psychotropic drugs in the 1950s, there has been a simultaneous shift away from the practice of psychotherapy by psychiatrists.

C. There has also been a shift away from therapies directed toward achieving insight into historical causal factors in behavior toward problem-solving approaches to contemporary dilemmas with systematically selected therapeutic interventions.

D. The proliferation of therapies (one study reports over four hundred varieties) has led some therapists to seek common features that might produce a more integrative and less ideological personality-theory-based approach to psychotherapeutic practice.

E. The development of detailed training guides such as those provided in Beck's cognitive therapy and Klerman's interpersonal therapy contribute to systematic training and evaluation.

F. As nonmedical practitioners (including psychologists, social workers, family and marriage counselors, and nurse practitioners) began doing psychotherapy, they at first adhered to the psychodynamic model but ultimately developed treatment techniques based on their own training and experience.

G. Counseling is emerging as a profession that provides assistance in dealing with nonpsychiatric problems of living and relationships. The professional status of this form of human service in relation to more traditional psychiatric and psychological therapies is as yet undetermined.

H. For many decades psychotherapy was paid for primarily by the patient (out-of-pocket). Psychiatric treatment, especially outpatient psychotherapy, was not covered by health insurance plans. Even now the health-care providers often place limits on the amount of coverage they will provide and often have a dollar limit on what they will cover. Since health insurance is usually provided by employers, governmental bodies, or welfare agencies, the practice of psychotherapy has become increasingly driven by the marketplace with the (1) increased external influence of clinical practices by the control of third-party reimbursement, (2) the shifting of costs to the consumer (patient) through higher deductible, higher coinsurance, and top dollar limits, (3) the availability of an ever-increasing array of different therapeutic options, and (4) an explosive increase in the number of nonmedically trained mental health professionals practicing psychotherapy. (Gibson, 1984, 1986)

I. Psychotherapy is now affected—for better or for worse—by the economics of the overall health care system.

## XIV. Group psychotherapy

A. Disorders of behavior, experience, and relationship develop and are expressed in a social context.

B. All psychotherapeutic approaches recognize this obvious point, but some therapeutic strategies emphasize the social environment as the source of opportunities to initiate and reinforce change.

C. *Group psychotherapy* is defined in *A Psychiatric Glossary* as the "application of psychotherapeutic techniques to a group, including utilization of interactions of members of the group."[5]

D. Although it is sometimes used as the sole psychotherapeutic modality, it is most commonly used in conjunction with individual psychotherapy and other types of psychiatric treatment.

E. The groups are usually composed of one therapist and six or eight patients, who may be homogeneous in some way or heterogeneous. The sessions last about ninety minutes.

F. This type of psychotherapy has its origins in observations made by Sigmund Freud, who noted the dynamics of the interplay between individuals in a group setting. In the 1920s psychoanalytic therapists began applying their techniques in group.

G. The group provides an opportunity for developing personal insights as well as testing out new methods of coping and relating in a controlled type of environment.

H. The group process
Three stages characterize the life of the group, bringing specific issues into focus and dominating group interaction.

   1. In the first phase, the patient is concerned about whether she or he will be accepted as a part of the group.

   2. In the second phase, the patient is concerned with issues of autonomy, that is, becoming an independent person within the group.

   3. In the third stage, the patient deals with the issues of sharing and equality.

I. There was a time when group psychotherapy was considered an expedient, a way to involve a greater number of patients, but this is no longer believed to be true.

   1. For many patients, it is superior to individual psychotherapy.

   2. The techniques used closely parallel those used in individual psychotherapy, and they vary with the aims of the therapist and the type of patient.

   3. Some group therapists are relatively nonparticipating and mostly summarize what is going on in the group; others are very active and confrontive, suggesting subject material,

5. Ibid.

making interpretations, setting up role-playing situations, and so forth.

4. Patients who have fragmented into psychosis need more supportive, reality-oriented therapy, whereas those with greater ego strength may use more insight-oriented therapy.

J. Factors that induce therapeutic change in groups

1. Groups can develop a sense of cohesiveness and provide an experience of social solidarity and belonging.

2. Group membership can have important motivational consequences by supporting and encouraging (rewarding) some kinds of behavior and by implicitly or explicitly developing rules and standards of conduct within the group.

3. In a cohesive and supportive group, a member may be able to experience, express, and release strong feelings and beliefs.

4. A group provides a basis for self-definition both by defining a social reality for members and by affirming insights and improvements.

K. There are many types of groups that vary in goals of participation, role of therapist, and assumptions about the nature of problems. Almost every variant of individual psychotherapy has a counterpart in group therapy (e.g., psychoanalytic, interpersonal, Gestalt, existential, cognitive-behavioral).

1. Since 1960, a number of variations of group therapy have emerged. They emphasize the usefulness of social processes in increasing self-understanding, improving relationships, and developing human potentialities; such procedures can be useful adjuncts to psychiatric treatment (human potential groups).

2. However, the variety of group procedures that is available may be confusing to many people; no "consumer's guide" is available, and care must be exercised in evaluating the appropriateness of a group for oneself.

L. Self-help groups

1. *Self-help,* or support groups without professionally trained leaders, in which the group experience does not uncover basic conflicts but does offer new shared experiences to the patient.

2. Alcoholics Anonymous (AA) and the substance abusers group are effective self-help groups, as are groups for persons and families of persons living with chronic or fatal illness.

3. Consciousness-raising groups provide support to people who experience difficulties related to social biases and neglect.

## XV. Family therapy

A. Description
1. Family therapy is a form of group therapy, wherein the nuclear family is the unit, that has developed during the past three or four decades.
2. Family therapists view the family as a behavioral system with unique properties. Emotional disturbances of individual members are therefore regarded as outgrowths of conflicts between family members.
3. One or more therapists deal with an entire family unit (or sometimes with a part of the family) during the therapeutic sessions. The goal of treatment is to resolve or reduce the pathogenic conflicts and anxiety within the unit.
4. Forms of family therapy vary in the same characteristics as do other group therapies and individual psychotherapies.

B. Scope
1. In the past, in certain experimental situations, entire family units were hospitalized so that the genesis of schizophrenia and other emotional disorders could be studied.
2. Family therapy may be used as the sole treatment, or it may be used in conjunction with other types of therapy.
3. It has been recommended for marital conflict and child-parent conflicts.

C. Difficulties
1. The therapist often finds it difficult to keep the family group intact for sessions (siblings resist, parents have to work, and so forth).
2. Another difficulty is keeping the focus on the family process and related to the family as a functioning unit rather than shifting to individual members.

D. Current trends in family therapy represent a movement away from psychodynamic interpretations of family organization and pathology to an emphasis on active interventions in family behaviors.
1. Structural family therapy (Minuchin 1974)
   a) The main emphasis of this approach is on current functioning.
   b) The family is viewed as a structural organization with hierarchical arrangements and relationships among the family members.
   c) In functional families there is a clear differentiation between the boundaries and functions of parents and children in the decision-making and problem-solving activities of the family.

d) The dysfunctional family has distorted or chaotic distributions of power in its structure, and its boundaries are either too rigid or too weak.
e) The goal of treatment is to modify relationships and boundaries, which will allow the family to return to a functional status.

  2. Strategic family therapy
a) The central emphasis in this approach is on inducing rapid change by quickly defining problems and devising strategies for intervention.
b) Families are often given direct charges to take particular actions.
c) The directions may be straightforward or may be paradoxical if the family is rigid or resistant and the contradiction of a paradoxical direction might lead to positive change.
d) The approach may sometimes put the therapist in a dramatic and potentially manipulative role.

## XVI. Marital therapy

A. Current marital therapies have developed from family therapeutic approaches where it was recognized that the dynamics of parent-child interactions often reflected problems in the marital relationship.
B. Since not all living arrangements involve marriage or are heterosexual, a more appropriate term for therapy that focuses on the close relationship of two persons is "couples therapy."
C. Conjoint therapy refers to the practice of both members of a couple seeing the same therapist in the same sessions.
D. In couples therapy the emphasis of treatment is on the disturbance of the relationship rather than on the disturbed individual. ("The relationship is the client.")
E. While couples therapy can reflect a variety of perspectives, depending on the orientation of the therapist, most approaches have in common an emphasis on problem solving and communication.
  1. Couples learn to identify their own problems and cooperate in strategies to solve them.
  2. Communication refers not only to what couples say to each other but also to what they say to themselves about the relationship.
F. The most effective role of the therapist is not that of neutral arbiter but rather that of a participant who can move from side to side in a way that develops a productive alliance with each partner.

G. The difficulties for the therapist often reside in the context of grievances and blame that characterize relationship problems.

XVII. **Adjunctive therapies** (therapies used in psychiatric inpatient, day treatment, and partial hospital programs)

A. A wide spectrum of therapies is available for use in psychiatric and inpatient settings. These therapies can be classified into three groups: activity therapies, expressive (or creative arts) therapies, and verbal therapies.

1. Activity therapies include occupational therapy and therapeutic recreation.

a) Historical notes

(1) Concerned observers of the institutionalized mentally ill in the nineteenth century recognized the value of structured activity in reducing maladaptive behavior, and industrial and/or agricultural activities were developed in most state hospitals.

(2) During World War I, the reconstruction aides demonstrated their effectiveness through activity programs and were the immediate forerunners of occupational therapy.

(3) After World War II, therapeutic recreation developed out of occupational therapy and physical education.

b) Activity therapies are concerned with the adaptation of the individual in the community. They provide evaluation and treatment of the patient's independent living skills—for example, physical and psychological skills, work and play leisure skills, and the sensorimotor, cognitive, and psychosocial components that influence these skills.

c) The assumption is made that through structured activities, persons can learn a range of interpersonal attitudes and behaviors as well as new skills that will help them in coping with life tasks, in controlling their own resources, and in maintaining increased self-esteem.

d) Activity therapists provide here-and-now experiences in which individuals can acquire and practice skills, learn how their behavior affects not only the task, recreational event, or activity, but also the members of the participating group and, consequently, how it affects their roles in the community. Occupational therapists and therapeutic recreation professionals are trained in activity analysis and group process. They adapt activities to meet the needs of the patients involved and provide feedback to the treatment team.

(1) The occupational therapist evaluates the patient's performance and plans treatment to remediate deficits in independent living skills and/or performance components. Techniques used may be individual or group craft activities, task groups, homemaking or child/parenting sessions, or prevocational skill development. In addition, for the more severely impaired, self-care activities, such as use of public transportation, budgeting and check writing, and time organization, may be utilized to increase functional independence.

(2) The therapeutic recreation professional uses recreation to promote personal growth and development. Some examples are the use of such activities as volleyball or creative writing to promote opportunities for the expression and release of feelings; the use of individual or group recreation to facilitate the development of leadership, self-confidence, cooperation, and social skills; the use of programs to facilitate and practice behavior changes (feeling charades for the appropriate expression of affect); leisure education to aid in the development of new interests and to provide balance in the patient's daily life; and training in the use of recreation for relaxation and anxiety reduction.

e) Occupational therapy has the longest history and is the most widely accepted and utilized of all the therapies in inpatient settings. Both occupational therapy and therapeutic recreation have specific educational curricula and internship programs leading to certification. Both fields have well-developed, articulated standards and codes of ethics.

2. Expressive (creative arts) therapies include music therapy, art therapy, and movement (or dance) therapy.

a) Historical notes

(1) Expressive therapies have emerged over the past three decades. The roots of each therapy are in the arts (e.g., music, art, or dance) from which it has developed and in the field of special education.

(2) Teachers of emotionally disturbed children discovered that the arts often provided a way of communicating and provided information that could not be obtained in structured activities or in attempts at verbal exchanges.

b) Expressive therapists are concerned with maximizing the possibilities of communicating and the media through which persons can express and communicate their feelings, conflicts, personal characteristics, and creative potential. Expressive therapists provide evaluation of these expressions and give feedback to patients, the patients' primary therapists, and the treatment teams.

c) The assumption is made that through participation in creative processes and using a variety of media, materials, instruments, tools, and body motions, persons can express themselves in ways that provide information, communication possibilities, and a sense of personal productivity that leads to the reduction of disturbing symptoms, increased trust in interpersonal relationships, and raised self-esteem.

d) Each of the expressive therapies uses materials and methods associated with the art from which it has developed.

   (1) In art therapy, a patient provided with clay may construct figures and place them in positions in relationship to one another that reveal information about family dynamics and the patient's relationship to them. This may lead to communication with the therapist and provide information that can also be utilized by other members of the treatment team.

   (2) In music therapy, an anxious patient may learn to relax and experience increased comfort through listening to music or by participating in the making of music.

   (3) In dance and movement therapy, body language that a person uses in movement in interactions with others (movements that may express resistance, withdrawal, manipulation, etc.) becomes apparent to other members of the group and to the therapist and is noted and processed by the therapist, patient, and group members.

e) Since the expressive therapies are relatively new, the educational, internship, and credentialing process is not as completely developed as it is for the activity therapies. There are, however, now an American Art Therapy Association, a National Association of Music Therapy, and an American Dance Therapy Association. These groups are working to professionalize their disciplines, have established some criteria for training and credentialing, and are developing professional standards and ethics.

3. Verbal therapies include individual psychotherapy, group therapy, and family therapy.

   a) Most patients in psychiatric hospitals or treatment programs have a primary therapist, usually a psychiatrist, but sometimes a psychologist, social worker, or nurse, who works in collaboration with a psychiatrist.

   b) The primary therapist provides individual psychotherapy for his or her patients, is usually the head of the treatment team, and is responsible for taking leadership in the development of the treatment plan.

   c) Other members of the treatment staff may also provide individual psychotherapy. It is, for example, usual for patients to have one-to-one sessions with members of the nursing and therapy staff. Often these sessions are of a supportive nature but sometimes are directed toward a particular problem identified in the treatment plan.

   d) Group and family therapy have already been discussed and are essentially the same in inpatient and outpatient settings. For the more disturbed patients in inpatient settings, group therapy should be supportive and reality oriented.

   e) Group and family therapists come from a variety of educational and professional backgrounds, including psychiatry, psychology, social work, and psychiatric nursing. In order to function as group and family therapists, such persons should have special training in group and family therapy. Credentialing programs are not yet uniformly applied.

B. The treatment plan

  1. Each of the previous adjunctive therapists makes an evaluation of the patient, which is the basis for the setting of goals or the suggesting of interventions.

  2. These are then presented to the treatment team, which is usually under the leadership of a psychiatrist.

  3. Often, the patient attends the treatment plan review and participates in the development of the treatment plan.

  4. At any rate, the treatment *team* formulates an overall treatment plan for the patient.

# References

Bandura, A. *Social Foundations of Thought and Action: A Social Cognitive Theory*. Englewood Cliffs, N.J.: Prentice-Hall, 1986.

Beck, A., A. Rush, B. Shaw, and G. Emery. *Cognitive Therapy of Depression*. New York: Guilford Press, 1979.

Bellack, A., M. Hersen, and A. Kazdin, eds. *International Handbook of Behavior Modification and Therapy*. New York: Plenum, 1982.

Beutler, L., and J. Clarkin. *Systematic Treatment Selection.* New York: Brunner/Mazel, 1990.

Davison, G., and J. Neale. *Abnormal Psychology.* 5th ed. New York: Wiley, 1990.

Dobson, K., ed. *Handbook of Cognitive-Behavioral Therapies.* New York: Guilford Press, 1988.

Freeman, A., K. Simon, L. Beutler, and H. Arkowtz, eds. *Comprehensive Handbook of Cognitive Therapy.* New York: Plenum, 1989.

Gibson, R. W. "The Future of the Practice of Psychotherapy," *The Psychiatric Hospital,* 16-4, 155–9, (October 1984).

Gisbon, R. W. "The Future of Psychotherapy," *The Psychiatric Times,* 3(7):1 (July 1986).

Goldfried, M., L. Greenberg, and C. Marmar. "Individual Psychotherapy." In *Annual Review of Psychology,* vol. 41. Palo Alto: Annual Reviews, 1990.

Goldman, H., ed. *Review of General Psychiatry.* 2d ed. Norwalk, Conn.: Appleton & Lange, 1988.

Gurman, A., and D. Kniskern, eds. *Handbook of Family Therapy.* New York: Brunner/Mazel, 1981.

Hersen, M., A. Kazdin, and A. Bellack, eds. *The Clinical Psychology Handbook.* New York: Pergamon Press, 1983.

Kaplan, H. I., and B. J. Sadock, eds. *Comprehensive Textbook of Psychiatry/V.* Vol. 2, 5th ed.

Baltimore: Williams & Wilkins, 1989.

Kiesler, D. "Interpersonal Methods of Diagnosis and Treatment." In *Psychiatry,* edited by A. Cooper, A. Frances, and M. Sacks. Vol. 1, *The Personality Disorders and Neuroses.* New York: Basic Books/Lippincott, 1986.

Minuchin, S. *Families and Family Therapy.* Cambridge, Mass.: Harvard University Press, 1974.

Neitzel, M., D. Bernstein, and R. Milich. *Introduction to Clinical Psychology.* 3d ed. Englewood Cliffs, N.J.: Prentice- Hall, 1991.

Nicholi, A., ed. *The Harvard Guide to Modern Psychiatry.* 2d ed. Cambridge: Belknap Press, 1989.

Sipe, A. W. R., and C. J. Rowe. *Psychiatry, Ministry, and Pastoral Counseling.* 2d ed. Collegeville, Minn.: St. John's University Press, 1984.

Strupp, H., and J. L. Binder. *Psychotherapy in a New Key.* New York: Basic Books, 1984.

Yalom, I. *Existential Psychotherapy.* New York: Basic Books, 1980.

Yalom, I. *The Theory and Practice of Group Therapy.* 2d ed. New York: Basic Books, 1983.

Zeig, J., ed. *The Evolution of Psychotherapy.* New York: Brunner/Mazel, 1987.

# 10 Treatment in Psychiatry: Pharmacological and Somatic Treatment

Canst thou not minister to a mind diseas'd;
Pluck from the memory a rooted sorrow;
Raze out the written troubles of the brain;

And, with some sweet oblivious antidote,
Cleanse the staff'd bosom of that perilous matter
Which weighs upon the heart?

**Shakespeare, *Macbeth* (c. 1606)**

## I. Introduction
A. Assumptions
1. It is assumed, in the treatment of psychiatric disorders by pharmacotherapy, that the effectiveness of the drug is achieved by action on the central nervous system; in turn, it is implied that at least some psychiatric disorders, especially psychoses, involve defective functioning of the central nervous system.
2. Although the effectiveness of pharmacotherapy and somatic therapies in relieving symptoms of psychiatric disorders may be taken as support of the somatogenic hypothesis, the relation between effects of drug treatment and underlying pathology is not clear for most conditions.
3. Pharmacotherapy can relieve symptoms of anxiety or depression that arise from psychological or social conditions.
B. Historical notes
1. Historically, attempts have been made to use chemical or medicinal means to modify abnormal behavior and emotional pain. Alcohol and opiates have been used for many centuries.

2. Prior to the early 1950s, drug treatment in psychiatry consisted primarily of attempts to sedate excited and overactive patients or to stimulate withdrawn or underactive patients.
3. The history of drug treatment in psychiatry has been dated from 1949, when the antimanic effects of lithium were discovered, or from 1952, when reserpine was isolated and chlorpromazine (Thorazine) was discovered.
4. The history of drug treatment reveals many examples of initially promising effects that did not persist. In some cases the drugs themselves produced additional problems of dependency and misuse (e.g., opium, cocaine, barbiturates).
5. In the early 1950s new groups of drugs were introduced in the treatment of psychiatric disorders, and the outcome has been characterized as the "third psychiatric revolution." (The freeing of patients from prisonlike conditions and the use of "moral" treatment by Phillipe Pinel signaled the first "revolution," and the second revolution was the development of psychoanalytic theory and therapy by Sigmund Freud.)
6. Developments in pharmacological therapy and research into underlying neural mechanisms have transformed institutional treatment and pointed the way to a much more sophisticated but still incomplete understanding of brain functions in mental illness.

## II. Major classes of psychoactive drugs in psychiatric practice
A. Reasonably safe and effective medical treatment is available for most of the major mental disorders.
B. A limitation to developing uniquely specific therapeutic agents is the lack of knowledge of the biological basis of most major mental disorders.
C. Psychoactive drugs used in psychiatric practice
  1. Antipsychotics (neuroleptics)
  2. Mood modifiers (antidepressants, lithium)
    a) Antidepressants
    b) Antimanics
  3. Antianxiety agents
D. Other psychoactive drugs not used primarily in psychiatric practice
  1. Analgesics
  2. Stimulants
  3. Sedative-hypnotics
  4. Psychedelics

## III. Pharmacological principles
A. Route of administration and absorption

1. Most psychiatric drugs are produced in forms to be taken orally.
2. Intravenous (IV) and intramuscular (IM) injectable forms of some drugs are available for special uses.
3. Rate of absorption of a drug by the body is in part a function of the route of administration and in part a function of the form in which the drug is administered (e.g., liquid, solid, coated, etc.).
4. Some drugs are prepared to be absorbed slowly or released over a period of time.

B. Distribution and elimination
1. Absorption of a drug into the bloodstream distributes it over the entire body. This means that at any given time, just a fraction of the total drug administered is at the therapeutic site of action.
2. The blood-brain barrier determines the ease or difficulty with which drugs enter the brain. Most psychiatric drugs pass the blood-brain barrier fairly easily.
3. Drugs (and their metabolites) are ultimately excreted from the body, primarily by the kidneys.

C. Each drug has a characteristic time course of action. This refers to the magnitude of action as a function of the length of time the drug is in the body. Some long-acting drugs may accumulate in the body if they are taken more frequently than the time they take to be metabolized and excreted.

D. Drug effects are also dependent on dose size in relation to body size (dose dependency).

E. Side effects and toxicity
1. Some effects of drugs may be undesirable or harmful depending on the nature of the drug, the dosage, and the individual characteristics of the recipient (e.g., allergic reactions or other signs of individual sensitivity).
2. Toxicity may be a general side effect of some drugs at high dosage or may be a special effect for some sensitive recipients.
3. Some drugs may interact with each other in beneficial, harmful, or unpredictable ways. Many drugs do not interact in any way that would be considered clinically significant.

F. Placebo effects refer to reactions to pharmacologically inert substances. These psychologically mediated responses are related to social factors and expectations and probably operate to a degree in all pharmacological treatment.

G. Drug tolerance refers to a decreasing responsiveness to a drug with continued use. If a person develops tolerance, a larger dose is required to achieve the original effect of a smaller dose.

H. Physical dependence on a drug is indicated if a person develops dysfunctional physiological symptoms when the drug is reduced or withdrawn (withdrawal effects).

I. Psychological dependence is not a precisely defined term, but usually refers to a degree of loss of control in drug self-administration which does not entail physical dependence.

J. Addiction refers to a compulsive pattern of drug use even at the expense of physical harm and psychosocial deterioration. (See chapter 19 for the way in which the terms *dependence* and *addiction* are used in *DSM*-III-R.)

IV. **Antipsychotic agents**

A. There are a large number of these agents, whose effects are characterized more by their similarity than by their differences.

1. They produce emotional calmness and mental relaxation ("tranquilizing effects").

2. They effectively control symptoms of both acutely and chronically disturbed psychotic patients.

3. They show some effectiveness in treating *positive* symptoms of schizophrenia, such as thought disorders, hallucinations, delusions, alterations in affect, and bizarre behavior.

4. They are capable of producing reversible "extrapyramidal effects."

a) Dystonias (torsions, twistings, and spasms of muscle groups)

b) Akathisia (motor restlessness)

c) Pseudoparkinsonism (akinesia, rigidity, tremors, etc.)

5. They create little, if any, habituation or dependency.

6. They have revolutionized the treatment of psychiatric patients by allowing psychotic patients to be managed as outpatients with reduced periods of hospitalization.

B. Types of antipsychotic agents

1. Phenothiazines

a) Aliphatic

(1) Chlorpromazine (Thorazine)

(2) Triflupromazine (Vesprin)

b) Piperidines

(1) Mesoridazine (Serentil)

(2) Thioridazine (Mellaril)

c) Piperazines

(1) Acetophenazine (Tindal)

(2) Fluphenazine (Prolixin)

(3) Perphenazine (Trilafon)

(4) Trifluoperazine (Stelazine)

2. Thioxanthenes

a) Chlorprothixene (Taractan)

b) Thiothixene (Navane)

3. Butyrophenones

a) Haloperidol (Haldol)

4. Diphenyl-butylpiperidines

a) Pimozide (Orap)

5. Dibenzoxazepines

a) Loxapine (Loxitane)

b) Clozapine (Clozaril)

6. Dihydroindolones

a) Molindone (Moban)

7. The rauwolfia alkaloids, forms of reserpine (Serpasil), were once part of the "third revolution" but are rarely used in the treatment of psychotic disorders now because of their relative ineffectiveness and tendency to induce depression.

C. Indications

1. The antipsychotics are most effective for patients with acute symptoms and good prognosis.

2. The symptoms that respond best include tension, hyperactivity, hostility, combativeness, negativism, acute delusions, hallucinations, anorexia, and sleep disturbances.

3. The "positive" symptoms of schizophrenia are more responsive to treatment than the "negative" symptoms.

D. Side effects and toxicity

1. In general these agents are safe, although they do produce a number of annoying, though mostly mild, side effects.

2. Anticholinergic side effects include dry mouth and blurred vision.

3. Neurological side effects include the extrapyramidal syndrome of rigidity, tremors, dystonia, and akathesia.

4. In some instances in prolonged therapy, they produce the sometimes nonreversible effects of *tardive dyskinesia.*

a) Symptoms include choreiform involuntary movements and dyskinesia of the face and mouth, which produce such things as smacking lips, protuberances of the tongue, and grotesque facial grimaces.

b) Prevalence may be as high as 20 percent in chronically treated patients.

c) Some symptoms considered as indications of tardive dyskinesia may be manifestations of movement disturbances associated with the disorder being treated (e.g., schizophrenia, senile disorders).

d) Often, continued use of antipsychotics must be considered despite tardive dyskinesia if the patient is to be free of disabling psychotic symptoms.

5. Neuroleptic malignant syndrome (NMS), the rare, sometimes fatal, complication of treatment with high-potency neuroleptics, consisting of hyperthermia, sweating, neuromuscular rigidity, abnormal blood pressure, and usually some disturbance of consciousness. (It is possible that some cases that have been described as lethal catatonia in the past would now be attributed to NMS. Further research is indicated.)

6. Treatment of extrapyramidal side effects
   a) Most of the general extrapyramidal effects respond to anti-Parkinson drugs such as:
      (1) Benzotropine (Cogentin)
      (2) Diphenhydramine (Benadryl)
      (3) Trihexyphenidyl (Artane)
      (4) Biperiden (Akineton)
   b) There is no adequate treatment of tardive dyskinesia though lithium, and diazepam (Valium) may provide some relief of symptoms in some cases. Anti-Parkinson drugs may actually worsen symptoms in some cases, as may reducing antipsychotic medication.

E. Mechanisms of action
   1. The major effects of antipsychotic agents are attributed to the blockade of dopamine receptors.
      a) Most antipsychotic agents vary in the range of dopamine receptors affected (D1 and D2) and the strength of binding to receptors.
      b) The relative effectiveness of agents, appears to be a function of the degree of blockade of D2 receptors.
      c) Dopamine blockade also accounts for the extrapyramidal effects of antipsychotic agents since they block dopamine transmission in the basal ganglia system.
      d) Tardive dyskinesia is attributed to supersensitivity of dopamine receptors in the affected person.
      e) Some "atypical" antipsychotics such as clozapine (Clozaril) appear to be more selective for D1 receptors and also appear to be more selective for limbic system binding sites than for basal ganglia binding sites.
   2. Antipsychotics have anticholinergic (muscarinic) actions, which account for some of the side effects of treatment, but central nervous system anticholinergic action has not been clearly implicated in the reduction of psychotic symptoms.
   3. Some antipsychotics may also interfere with storage and transmission of the other biogenic amines, serotonin and norepinephrine.
   4. The "dopamine theory" of schizophrenia has enjoyed some popularity as a hypothesis, but the treatment success of

some drugs that are relatively weak in dopamine system effects and the involvement of many antipsychotic agents in serotonin and norepinephrine transmission suggest that the precise role of dopamine transmission in schizophrenia is still to be determined.

## V. Mood modifiers

A. Antidepressants
1. Antidepressant agents include the following groups:
   a) Stimulants
   b) Cyclic antidepressants
   c) Monoamine oxidase inhibitors (MAOI)
2. In the past, stimulants were the primary treatment for depression but have a limited place in the current treatment of depressive disorders.
   a) In the last century, cocaine was considered a promising antidepressant (Sigmund Freud was an early champion of its therapeutic use), but it failed to beneficially affect clinical depression, and its associated side effects and potential for misuse were soon recognized.
   b) Amphetamines (e.g., Dexedrine and Methydrine) have also been used in the past but are not now considered to be effective antidepressants.
   c) Methylphenidate (Ritalin) is sometimes prescribed in the treatment of mild depressions but is most frequently used in the treatment of attention-deficit hyperactivity disorder in children and adults.
3. Cyclic antidepressants
   a) Tricyclics are the most commonly employed of the cyclic antidepressants. This group includes:
      (1) Amitriptyline (Elavil)
      (2) Clomipramine (Anafranil)
      (3) Desipramine (Norpramin)
      (4) Doxepin (Sinequan)
      (5) Imipramine (Tofranil)
      (6) Nortriptyline (Aventyl)
      (7) Protriptyline (Vivactil)
      (8) Trimipramine (Surmontil)
   b) Tetracyclics
      (1) Maprotiline (Ludiomil)
   c) Two recently developed cyclics of significance are:
      (1) Bupropion (Wellbutrin), a monocyclic
      (2) Fluoxetine (Prozac), a bicyclic
   d) Sertraline (Zoloft)
   e) Paroxetine—an investigational selective serotonin reuptake inhibitor

4. Monoamine oxidase inhibitors
   a) Isocarboxazid (Marplan)
   b) Phenelzine (Nardil)
   c) Tranylcypromine (Parnate)
5. Other agents used in the treatment of depression
   a) Amoxapine (Asendin) is a dibenzoxazepine; tardive dyskinesia is a rare side effect of this antidepressant.
   b) Trazodone (Desyrel) is a triazolopyride.

B. Indications for the use of antidepressants
1. Tricyclics are used in the treatment of major depressions and in the treatment and maintenance of patients with the recurrent depressions of unipolar affective disorder. They are less effective with milder or reactive depressions.
2. Monoamine oxidase inhibitors are less effective than tricyclics in the treatment of endogenous depression but have some special applications.
   a) They are effective with certain "atypical" depressions.
   b) They should be considered with depressions that are not responsive to tricyclics.
   c) They appear to have a special use in patients who have both anxiety and depression as prominent features.
3. Amoxapine and trazodone have more rapid action in the improvement of depressive symptoms than tricyclics.

C. Side effects and toxicity of antidepressants
1. Both tricyclics and MAO inhibitors may have anticholinergic effects such as dry mouth, blurred vision, sweating, constipation, etc.
2. Central nervous system effects include drowsiness, weakness and lethargy, insomnia and other sleep disturbances, fine tremors, and occasionally restlessness or agitation.
3. Orthostatic hypotension may occur initially in the use of MAO inhibitors, particularly in elderly patients.
4. MAO inhibitors pose a risk for hypertensive crisis, and users must avoid foods that contain elevated levels of tyramine (e.g., cured and aged cheeses) and certain other sympathomimetic amines.
5. Trazodone has fewer anticholinergic effects.
6. Amoxapine may produce tardive dyskinesia (previously noted).

D. Mechanisms of action
1. MAO inhibitors act by inhibiting the action of monoamine oxidase, an enzyme that breaks down and regulates the supply of biogenic amines in axon terminals, effectively increasing the availability of serotonin, norepinephrine, and dopamine.

2. Tricyclics and other antidepressants also increase the availability of biogenic amines, primarily through blocking the reuptake of released neurotransmitter from the synaptic cleft.
   a) Agents vary in the neurotransmitters affected and the strength of the effect.
   b) Most tricyclics and tetracyclics affect both serotonin and norepinephrine transmission but have limited effects on dopamine.
   c) Amoxapine affects dopamine as well as serotonin and norepinephrine.
   d) Bupropion and fluoxetine appear to affect only serotonin.

E. Antimanic agents (mood stabilizers)
   1. The two major classes of antimanic agents are:
      a) Lithium carbonate (Lithane, Lithonate, Eskalith, Lithobid)
      b) Carbamazepine (Tegretol)
   2. Lithium is the major agent used in the treatment of mania.
   3. Carbamazepine is an anticonvulsant, structurally related to tricyclics, which may be used alone or in combination with lithium.

F. Indications for use of antimanic agents
   1. Lithium is used in the management of acute mania and hypomania.
      a) It is effective in 80 percent of acute manias in one to two weeks.
      b) It can be used prophylactically to minimize recurrent attacks of mania in bipolar disorders.
   2. Some schizoaffective patients respond to lithium but not as well as manic patients.
   3. There are reports of schizophrenics who respond to lithium ("lithium responders"), but there is diagnostic uncertainty about some schizophrenics, schizoaffectives, and manic-depressives.
   4. Sometimes lithium is prescribed for depressives where it is presumed to potentiate the action of antidepressants.
   5. Carbamazepine is used in the treatment of acute mania, particularly in lithium nonresponders and in rapidly cycling bipolar disorders.
      a) It is reported to achieve up to 76 percent response in acute mania.
      b) In combination with lithium, it is effective in the prophylaxis of bipolar disorder.

G. Side effects and toxicity of antimanic agents

1. Some side effects may vary with the plasma level of lithium and include irritation of the gastrointestinal tract, muscular weakness, restlessness, and dizziness.
2. Some more persistent effects (which are reversible) are tremor, weight gain, and effects on fluid balance (edema, thirstiness, frequent urination).
3. Since lithium is toxic at levels close to therapeutic doses, serum levels must be monitored regularly and users must be alert to symptoms of toxicity.
4. Carbamazepine may produce dizziness, drowsiness, headache, and tremors in the initial stage of treatment. It may also produce side effects similar to those seen with the use of antidepressants.

H. Mechanism of action
1. The exact mechanism of action of lithium is unknown, but it is presumed to regulate catecholamine receptors (dopamine and norepinephrine) and may particularly block release or facilitate reuptake of norepinephrine.
2. Lithium may also alter calcium-mediated intracellular functions.
3. Carbamazepine may act through binding with the gamma-aminobutyric acid (GABA) receptor complex and amplifying inhibitory neurotransmitter effects.

**VI. Antianxiety agents (anxiolytics)**
A. Historical notes
1. For centuries, alcohol has been used in many cultures as a nonspecific ''treatment'' of anxious discomfort.
2. In the early twentieth century, bromides were used as sedatives and were present in over-the-counter ''nerve remedies'' until their toxic effects were acknowledged.
3. Subsequently barbiturates replaced bromides as sedatives but also were later acknowledged to have accompanying risks of dependence and addiction.
4. In the 1950s meprobamate largely replaced the barbiturates as a widely prescribed sedative.
5. Currently benzodiazepines are the popular anxiolytic agents.

B. Common characteristics of anxiolytics
1. They produce calmness and relaxation but of a quality different from that of antipsychotic agents.
2. They are not useful in reducing psychotic reactions but are helpful in relieving anxiety and tension.
3. With the exception of antihistamines, they have little direct effect on autonomic functions.

4. All have depressant effects on the central nervous system; many act as sedative-hypnotics and are used to induce or assist sleep.
5. Many have muscle relaxant and anticonvulsant properties.

C. Indications
1. The chief use of antianxiety agents is in the treatment of disabling forms of anxiety.
2. They are used in other conditions in which anxiety, tension, or agitation play a part.
3. They are commonly employed as preoperative sedatives and in the management of pain syndromes, especially those accompanied by muscular tension.

D. Commonly used antianxiety agents
1. Barbiturates
   a) In spite of their strong sedative effects, barbiturates are seldom used as anxiolytics because of their potential for physical dependence, withdrawal symptoms, capacity for tolerance, and dangerous effects of toxic doses.
   b) Use of barbiturates to assist sleep has largely been replaced by benzodiazepines.
2. Meprobamate (Equanil, Miltown) is of historical importance as one of the "minor tranquilizers" but is not commonly used at present.
3. Antihistamines have sedative side effects
   a) Diphenhydramine (Benadryl)
   b) Hydroxyzine hydrochloride (Atarax)
   c) Hydroxyzine pamoate (Vistaril)
4. Benzodiazepines
   a) Short-acting types
      (1) Alprazolam (Xanax)
      (2) Halazepam (Paxipam)
      (3) Lorazepam (Ativan)
      (4) Oxazepam (Serax)
   b) Long-acting types
      (1) Chlordiazepoxide (Librium)
      (2) Chlorazepate (Tranxene)
      (3) Diazepam (Valium)
      (4) Prazepam (Centrax)
   c) For many years, Valium was the most commonly prescribed of all drugs.
   d) Some of the newer anxiolytics, such as alprazolam, are considered to be particularly effective in the treatment of severe anxiety associated with panic.

5. A new anxiolytic, buspirone (BuSpar), is an azaspirode-canedione, which is not a benzodiazepine and not sedative in its action.
E. Side effects and toxicity
1. Annoying side effects are relatively rare and are primarily expressions of a general sedative effect (e.g., drowsiness, fatigue).
2. Prolonged use can lead to dependence, tolerance, and withdrawal symptoms.
3. Anxiolytics potentiate the effects of alcohol.
4. Anxiolytics are frequently used in conjunction with alcohol by people who are dependent on alcohol.
5. Buspirone does not interact with alcohol and seems to have a low potential for habituation or dependence.
F. Mechanisms of action
1. Benzodiazepines bind to receptor sites that are part of the GABA receptor complex and amplify the inhibitory action of GABA.
2. Buspirone appears to achieve its effect by interacting with serotonin receptors.

## VII. New and supplemental agents
A. Adrenergic agents stimulate or block norepinephrine receptors.
1. Clonidine inhibits norepinephrine transmission and has been used in the treatment of anxiety, mania, and schizophrenia.
2. Propranolol is a noradrenergic beta-blocker that is used in treating the autonomic effects of anxiety; it has also been used in the treatment of aggressive behavior, mania, and schizophrenia.
B. Other anticonvulsants (in addition to carbamazepine) have been used in the treatment of anxiety, mania, and schizophrenia because of their serotonin-potentiating and GABA-like inhibitory characteristics.
C. Calcium channel blockers such as verapamil have been used to supplement lithium in the treatment of mania and antipsychotics in the treatment of schizophrenia. Calcium has important and far-reaching effects on the synthesis and release of neurotransmitters and on the regulation of excitatory receptors.
D. A number of agents are coming into use because of their specific effects on acetylcholine, serotonin, dopamine, and endorphin transmitter systems.

## VIII. Five drugs that have been recently developed or recently released for use require special attention
A. Fluoxetine (Prozac)

1. Prozac has recently become one of the most widely prescribed antidepressants in use.
2. In clinical studies, fluoxetine has been shown to be as effective as tricyclics and appears to have fewer side effects.
3. As a selective serotonin reuptake inhibitor, fluoxetine appears to have a mechanism of action that is different from most of the other antidepressants.
4. Because of its persistent antiobsessional effect, it is being prescribed for obsessive-compulsive disorder and other disorders in which obsessional craving plays a part.

B. Bupropion (Wellbutrin)
1. Like fluoxetine, bupropion is an "atypical" antidepressant.
2. It also appears to have fewer side effects than traditional antidepressants and has no sedative side effects.
3. It neither blocks amine reuptake nor inhibits MAO activity but does affect the availability of norepinephrine and dopamine.
4. It acts like a stimulant though it does not seem to have a potential for self-administration.
5. It was implicated in producing seizures when used with patients with eating disorders, and as a result was voluntarily withdrawn from the market by its manufacturer for additional studies (it was reintroduced with cautions about administering to patients with seizure disorders, current eating disorders, or other factors that predispose toward seizure).

C. Clomipramine (Anafranil)
1. This tricyclic antidepressant has been shown to be effective in relieving the symptoms of severe obsessive-compulsive disorder (though not because of its antidepressant action).
2. The mechanism of this specific symptom reduction is not known, but it is presumed that it is related to the blocking of serotonin reuptake by the agent.

D. Sertraline (Zoloft)
1. Released in the United States in 1992.
2. Is a potent serotonin uptake inhibitor.
3. Is structurally different from all other antidepressants.
4. Is indicated in the treatment of major depressions, but may be beneficial in some patients with obsessive-compulsive disorders.
5. Its use in other disorders in which serotonin plays a role, is being investigated (Ayd, 1992).

E. Clozapine (Clozaril)
1. Clozapine is an "atypical" antipsychotic.
2. It appears to be selective for D1 receptors and does not have marked extrapyramidal effects.

3. It has a symptomatic effect similar to other antipsychotics but in addition may also relieve the "negative" symptoms of schizophrenia and provide a basis for better social motivation than has been the case with traditional antipsychotics.
4. A frequency of up to 7 percent incidence of agranulocytosis (which drastically reduces white blood cells) makes it necessary that blood condition is monitored closely.

F. None of these agents have been in use long enough to accumulate an extensive clinical or experimental research record, but their atypical structure and/or clinical effects indicate that they may signal another major transition in the pharmacological treatment of psychiatric conditions.

IX. **Evaluation of pharmacological treatment**

A. An assessment of the effectiveness of drugs in the treatment of psychiatric disorders requires special research designs.

B. The response of patients to drug therapy is influenced by a number of variables, only some of which are related to the pharmacological properties of the drug.

1. Taking a drug is a complex social behavior, and social suggestion may operate to produce "placebo effects."
2. Researchers, physicians, and hospital or clinic staff also have expectations and hopes about the benefits of drugs, which may affect their observation.
3. To control for patient and observer expectations that might bias results, the *double-blind* research design is used, which controls for placebo effects in the patient and expectation effects of the researchers by hiding the identity of who is taking the active drug.

C. The results of careful double-blind research, together with research into the mechanisms of drug action, have established the effectiveness of antipsychotic, mood-modifying, and antianxiety agents in relieving the symptoms of many patients.

D. A continuing problem in the evaluation of drugs, however, is the lack of diagnostic precision in identifying treatment groups for research purposes.

E. A "bootstraps" effect may be occurring, where diagnostic classification is improved by paying attention to which patients respond to which drugs.

F. Recently developed agents are targeted to specific receptor subtypes, and in the future drugs may be classified according to identified sites of action and specific symptom effects rather than in terms of the more general and somewhat inconsistent behavioral effects that currently provide the basis of classification.

G. Correlation of drug effects with information from imaging procedures and other studies of brain functions should contribute to more specific application of pharmacotherapy.

X. **Electroconvulsive therapy**

A. Since the introduction of the antipsychotic and antidepressant drugs in the late 1950s and early 1960s, the use of electroconvulsive therapy (ECT) as a treatment for schizophrenic disorders has declined, but it remains a treatment for severe affective illness.

B. It is known that convulsive activity is necessary for effectiveness. Recent neurobiological research suggests that ECT

1. Increases the serotonin levels
2. Increases the turnover rate of norepinephrine
3. Improves the sodium transport system in the red blood cells
4. Decreases serum calcium concentration

C. It is an empirical treatment, in use for over fifty years, that relieves symptoms. Many theories have been proposed yet no satisfactory explanation of why convulsive seizures elicit behavioral improvement has been accepted. Recent neurobiological research suggests that ECT may alter amine metabolism in the central nervous system. (Some researchers have found increased serotonin levels; others have noted a decrease in norepinephrine.) Such a theory seems plausible in light of studies that indicate that catecholamines play a role in affective illnesses. It remains unclear, however, whether any of these agents are related to therapeutic effects in humans. Amnesia is the principal risk, and this usually dissolves rapidly.

D. Techniques

1. Sufficient electrical current is passed through electrodes applied to both temporal areas of the head to produce a grand mal seizure. A series of such treatments is given, the average being six to twelve.
2. In recent years, electrodes have been applied over the nondominant temporal hemisphere. This unipolar technique was thought to produce less postseizure confusion and memory loss. Although at first it was claimed to be as effective as bilateral ECT, this claim has now been questioned. A 1978 study by the American Psychiatric Association Task Force found that 70 to 80 percent of all psychiatrists questioned were still using the bilateral technique at that time.
3. Certain medications are given in conjunction with the treatment to minimize apprehension and physical risk. These are usually administered and monitored by a trained anesthesiologist. The following drugs are given intravenously.
   a) Atropine, to reduce salivation and inhibit vagal action

b) Succinylcholine chloride (Anectine), to modify the muscular contractions of the convulsive seizures

c) Barbiturate anesthesia, usually methohexital (Brevital) or pentothal sodium to put the patient to sleep just prior to treatment; thus, the patient is placed under light general anesthesia for a brief period of time

4. During the procedure, the patient receives oxygen under pressure.

5. According to a recent update (Coffey and Weiner 1990), clinical indications for ECT include:

a) Major depression (this probably accounts for about 90 percent of the patients treated with ECT in the United States). Overall response rates are 80 percent or greater. This is usually better than the response to antidepressant medications.

b) Need for faster onset of action. For example, severe suicidal potential, catatonia, or marked malnutrition and dehydration.

c) Acute mania (it should be considered for those patients who have extreme mania and who require a rapid remission).

d) Schizophrenia—those patients with catatonic or prominent affective symptoms, especially in those who have not responded to drugs.

e) Other disorders. There is no evidence that ECT is effective in the treatment of other mental disorders.

6. Contraindications

a) The physical risk is extremely small, particularly when given with the medications listed previously under Techniques (D.).

b) There are many physical conditions that were thought to increase the risk of the treatment, but as experience with ECT has increased, the number of physical conditions that contraindicate has dwindled to a bare minimum (e.g., the presence of a brain tumor with its accompanying increased intracranial pressure; an acute myocardial infarction; abdominal aneurysm). Many would say there are *no* absolute contraindications, only conditions for which there is increased risk.

c) Cases must be judged individually, however, weighing the possibility of psychiatric recovery against the possible physical risk.

d) Mortality: The mortality rate is very low, ranging from .002 percent to .004 percent per treatment. The mortality rate is at the bottom of the reported range for anesthesia induction alone (.003 percent to .04 percent).

XI. **Psychosurgery**

    A. Although it is usually regarded as beginning in 1936 by Egas Moniz, a psychiatrist collaborating with a neurosurgeon, the initial report of a surgical procedure on the brain with the goal of alleviating psychiatric symptoms appears to have been made by Gottlieb Burckhardt nearly fifty years earlier.

    B. Indications

        1. Patients for whom psychosurgery has been recommended generally have had crippling mental disorders (for example, unusually crippling obsessive-compulsive disorders) that have not responded to adequate trials of other treatment modalities and that have a poor prognosis.

           a) Currently the criteria for consideration for psychosurgery would be a continuous illness for at least three years that has not been responsive to pharmacological, behavioral, somatic, or psychotherapeutic interventions.

           b) The results of modern surgery on such carefully selected cases vary with the series; in general, more than 50 percent of the patients show major improvement, but a few are made worse by the procedure.

           c) Of critical importance in such treatments is the postoperative psychiatric care.

           d) It should be kept in mind that psychosurgery is radical therapy and is used only as a last resort when other methods have failed.

           e) It is performed infrequently in the United States at the present time.

    C. Although this is a radical treatment, it would be premature to abandon it until further evaluation has been made, particularly in light of current developments in brain imaging and microsurgical techniques.

# References

American Psychiatric Association. *A Psychiatric Glossary*. 6th ed. Washington, D.C.: APA, 1988.

————. *Electroconvulsive Therapy*. Task Report No. 14. Washington, D.C.: APA, 1978.

American Psychiatric Association, Task Force on ECT. *The Practice of ECT: Recommendations for Treatment, Training, and Privilege*. Washington, D.C.: American Psychiatric Press, 1990.

Ayd, F. ed. *International Drug-Therapy Newsletter* (March 1992, vol. 27, #3).

Benson, W. M., and B. C. Schiele. *Tranquilizing and Antidepressive Drugs*. Springfield, Ill.: Thomas, 1962.

Bezchlibnyk-Butler, K., and J. Jeffries, eds. *Clinical Handbook of Psychotropic Drugs*. 2d ed., rev. Toronto: Hogrefe & Huber, 1990.

Coffey, C. E., and R. D. Weiner. "Electroconvulsive Therapy."

*Hospital and Community Psychiatry*
41 (May 1990): 515.

Fink, M. *Convulsive Therapy: Theory and Practice*. New York: Raven Press, 1985.

Gilman, A., T. Rall, A. Nies, and P. Taylor, eds. *The Pharmacological Basis of Therapeutics*. 8th ed. New York: Pergamon Press, 1990.

Goldman, H. ed. *Review of General Psychiatry*. 2d ed. Norwalk, Conn.: Appleton & Lange, 1988.

Julien, R. *A Primer of Drug Action*. 5th ed. New York: Freeman, 1988.

Kalinowsky, L. B., and P. H. Hoch. *Somatic Treatment in Psychiatry*. New York: Grune & Stratton, 1961.

Kaplan, H. I., and B. J. Sadock, eds. *Comprehensive Textbook of*

*Psychiatry/V*. 5th ed. Baltimore: Williams & Wilkins, 1989.

Kolb, L. C., and H. K. H. Brodie. *Modern Clinical Psychiatry*. 10th ed. Philadelphia: Saunders, 1982.

Martin, R., and S. Preskorn, eds. "Psychopharmacology I: Present and Future." *Psychiatric Annals* 20, no. 11 (November 1990).

Poling, A., K. Gadow, and J. Cleary. *Drug Therapy for Behavior Disorders*. New York: Pergamon Press, 1991.

Synder, S. *Drugs and the Brain*. New York: Scientific American Books, 1986.

# 11 Anxiety Disorders

My apprehensions come in crowds;
I dread the rustling of the grass;

The very shadows of the clouds
Have power to shake me as they pass;

I question things and do not find
One that will answer to my mind;

And all the world appears unkind.

**William Wordsworth, *The Affliction of Margaret* (1804)**

I. **Definition**
A. The characteristic features of this group of disorders are symptoms of anxiety and avoidance behavior.
1. In panic disorder and generalized anxiety disorder, anxiety is usually the predominant symptom, and avoidance behavior is almost always present in panic disorder with agoraphobia.
2. In phobic disorders, anxiety is experienced if the person confronts or anticipates confronting the dreaded object or situation.
3. In obsessive-compulsive disorders, anxiety is experienced if the person attempts to resist the obsessions or compulsions.
4. Avoidance behavior is almost always present in phobic disorders and frequently present in obsessive-compulsive disorders.
5. The classification of post-traumatic stress disorders is controversial because the predominant symptom is the reexperiencing of the trauma, not anxiety or avoidance behavior. However, anxiety symptoms in avoidance behavior are extremely common, and symptoms of increased arousal are invariably present (*DSM*-III-R, p. 235).

B. Anxiety and fear are universally experienced emotions. Both are felt responses to danger and have similar physiological reactions. In the psychoanalytic sense, the distinction between anxiety and fear, the fortuitous result of an error in translating the word *angst* from Freud's original work into English, has been overdrawn. Apparently Freud himself did not distinguish appreciably between the two terms.

    1. Anxiety as a symptom can be defined as a diffuse, unpleasant uneasiness, apprehension, or fearfulness stemming from anticipated danger, the source of which is unidentifiable.

    2. Fear is a response to a recognized external threat.

    3. Patients often don't talk about these two responses interchangeably.

## II. Prevalence

A. Recent studies suggest that anxiety disorders are those most frequently found in the general population, simple phobia being the most common anxiety disorder in the general population, but panic disorder the most common in people seeking treatment (*DSM*-III-R, p. 235).

B. It is also a common symptom in general medical practice, and the physiological reflections of it are what often cause people to seek medical help.

C. The lifetime incidence of these disorders is not known, but is probably in the range of 15 to 25 percent (Goldman 1988).

## III. Components of Anxiety

The manifestations of anxiety occur at three levels.

A. Neuroendocrine

*Neuroendocrine* refers to the chief hormone adrenaline, or epinephrine, secreted by the medulla of the adrenal glands. It is related to norepinephrine, which, in turn, is related to mood disturbance and depression. It accounts for the physiological responses listed next.

B. Somatic

The *somatic,* motor-visceral, manifestations of anxiety are the result of the physiological responses of the various bodily systems to the increased secretion of epinephrine. These include: the dermatological response, cardiovascular response, gastrointestinal response, respiratory response, genitourinary response, vasomotor response, musculoskeletal response, and the pupillary response.

C. Psychic

The *psychic* manifestation of anxiety is the sensation of apprehension and the cortical perception of discomfort. It thus includes the appreciation of the physical responses as well as the awareness of the apprehension.

1. Although the individual consciously perceives and realizes the apprehensiveness, the cause of the anxiety usually escapes awareness.
2. Anxiety can be divided into degrees:
    a) *Free-floating anxiety* is severe, persistent, generalized, and unattached anxiety. It is typically found in anxiety disorders and is often a precursor of panic.
    b) *Agitation* is a state of restlessness and uneasiness often characterized by mental perturbation and by such muscular manifestations as motor restlessness (anxiety overflows into the muscular system).
    c) *Tension* is tautness, motor and emotional restlessness.
    d) *Panic* is an acute anxiety attack of overwhelming severity that leads to disorganization of ego functions. It produces physiological changes and terror. (The word is derived from Pan, the Greek god who suddenly appeared to unsuspecting travelers in the woods, causing them to "panic.")
    e) *Normal anxiety (stress).* The source of the anxiety is actual and realistic.

**IV. Etiology**
A. Psychodynamics
1. Anxiety occupies a focal position in the dynamics of all human adjustment (regarded as a symptom of the emergence of unconscious conflict).
    a) It is a normal response to threat.
    b) It is the driving force for most of our adjustments. For example, anxiety resulting from concern about financial security may drive one individual to accumulate excessive wealth; stimulate another to plan a realistic investment, insurance, and retirement program; and cause still a third individual to become completely dependent.
    c) The pattern for developing anxiety is inborn and always available. Evidence of this has been noted by child psychiatrists, who have described the underlying *universal* anxieties that are normally associated with the infant's dependency on the mother. There is a wide range of individual differences in infant susceptibility to anxiety-provoking situations.
        (1) *Separation anxiety* is the apprehension noted in infants when they are removed from their mothers or mother surrogates. It is most marked from the sixth to the tenth month.
        (2) *Stranger anxiety* is the apprehension noted in infants when they are approached by strangers.

(3) *Nocturnal anxiety* is the infant's fear of the dark.
  2. The mechanisms for coping with anxiety and the defenses against it form the basis of the psychodynamic theory of psychopathology. (These are discussed in chapter 6.)
B. Biochemical factors
  1. Patients with anxiety disorder have different psychological functioning compared to normals. (for example tachycardia, greater oxygen use during exercise, and higher blood lactate levels).
  2. Patients with panic disorders are more sensitive to substances (e.g., caffeine, lactate), all of which increase the activity of the locus ceruleus, the part of the midbrain that supplies most of the norepinephrine neurons in the central nervous system. Medications that inhibit locus ceruleus functioning reduce anxiety in humans (for example, benzodiazepines and MAOI antidepressants).
  3. The role of other substances (including dopamine, serotonin, acetylcholine, and enkephalins) is also being investigated.
C. Learned behavior
  1. From a learning perspective, anxiety can be viewed as a conditionable component of the autonomic or neurosystem. Fear response can be associated with other stimuli and events or generalize to them.
  2. Such conditioning may be direct and recognized (e.g., anxiety about riding in a car after being in an accident) or may be fortuitous and unrecognized, as may be the case in anxiety stemming from a childhood experience.
  3. Avoidance behavior that is a component of anxiety disorders is interpreted as due to the operation of motive reinforcement, the reinforcing effect of escaping from or avoiding a fear-producing object or situation.
  4. Avoidance behaviors may also be positively reinforced by the attention and concern of others.
  5. Patterns of anxiety and avoidance behavior may also be imitated, modeled, or socially reinforced in families where other members display them.
  6. The inability to control or predict the onset of anxiety can contribute to the condition of "learned helplessness."
  7. The way in which a person anticipates and interprets sources of anxiety and their personal implications can introduce cognitive components (e.g., habits of thought), which complicate and sometimes become focal in anxiety disorders.

D. Genetics

Anxiety disorders are more common among the relatives of the affected proband than among controls; alcoholism and secondary depression may also be over-represented.

V. Types

The anxiety disorders include the following.

A. Panic disorder with agoraphobia and panic disorder without agoraphobia
B. Agoraphobia without history of panic disorder
C. Social phobia
D. Simple phobia
E. Obsessive-compulsive disorder (or obsessive-compulsive neurosis)
F. Post-traumatic stress disorder
G. Generalized anxiety disorder (GAD)

VI. **Panic disorder with agoraphobia**
**Panic disorder without agoraphobia**

A. Definition

1. The essential features of these disorders are recurrent panic attacks, that is, discrete periods of intense fear or discomfort, with at least four characteristic associated symptoms (shortness of breath or smothering sensations; dizziness, unsteady feelings, or faintness; palpitations or accelerated heart rate; trembling or shaking; sweating; choking; nausea or abdominal distress; depersonalization or derealization; numbness or tingling sensations; flushes or chills; chest pain or discomfort; fear of dying; fear of going crazy or of doing something uncontrolled). The diagnosis is made only when it cannot be established that an organic factor initiated and maintained the disturbance (e.g., amphetamine or caffeine intoxication, hyperthyroidism) (*DSM*-III-R).

2. Panic attacks typically begin with the sudden onset of intense apprehension, fear, or terror. Often there is a feeling of impending doom.

3. In most cases seen in clinical settings, the person has developed some symptoms of agoraphobia.

B. Definition of agoraphobia

*Agoraphobia* is the fear of being in places or situations from which escape might be difficult (or embarrassing) or in which help might not be available in the event of a panic attack (as a result of this fear, there are either travel restrictions or a need for a companion—"phobic partner" or "obligatory companion"—when away from home, or there is endurance of agoraphobic situations despite intense anxiety) (*DSM*-III-R).

1. Common agoraphobic situations include being outside the home alone, being in a crowd or standing in a line, being on a bridge, and traveling in a bus, train, or car (*DSM*-III-R).
2. The person often develops varying degrees of nervousness and apprehension between attacks, usually focused on the fear of having another attack. Depressive disorder is often present.

C. Age at onset
   Usually in the late twenties
D. Course
   Typically, recurrent panic attacks several times a week or even daily
   1. It may be limited to a single episode, be recurrent, or become chronic.
   2. Usually occurs as attacks; between attacks the individual may be comfortable, although more commonly he or she is somewhat tense.
   3. If the conflict is not resolved, the individual may utilize one or more of the defense mechanisms and thus develop the picture of one of the other clinical reaction types.
   4. Ordinarily, the prognosis is for recurrent episodes.
   5. Some cases become chronic.
   6. A panic attack may be the precursor of other mental disorders, such as schizophrenia, major depressive disorder, or somatization disorder.
E. Impairment
   Panic disorder without agoraphobia may be associated with only limited impairment in social and occupational functioning. Panic disorder with agoraphobia, by definition, is associated with varying degrees of constriction in life-style.
F. Complications
   Since some people with panic disorder attempt self-treatment, they may develop psychoactive substance use disorders, particularly alcohol and anxiolytics.
G. Predisposing factors
   Separation anxiety disorder in childhood and sudden loss of social supports or disruption of important interpersonal relationships apparently predispose to the development of this disorder.
H. Prevalence
   This disorder is common.
 I. Differential diagnosis
   Disorders that can produce panic symptoms must be ruled out (e.g., hypoglycemia, pheochromocytoma, and hyperthyroidism). Also, panic attacks may be associated with withdrawal from such substances as barbiturates, caffeine, or amphetamines.

J. Etiology and pathogenesis
  1. A combination of psychological, social, and biological factors in a complex causal relationship
     a) Psychological factors include a disturbed childhood or current conflicts.
     b) Biological
        A predisposition to panic and/or depressive disorders may produce hypersensitivities or biochemical and electrophysiologic pathways. Both the noradrenergic and serotonergic pathway may be involved.
     c) A person susceptible to panic attacks may develop "psychological" explanations that may lead to phobic response when confronted with similar circumstances (thus, anxiety results when some conflict is aroused or rearoused either by a weakening of the repressive forces or by strengthening—or reinforcement—of the underlying drive or wish). Thus, repressed conflicts press for reemergence. The symptoms are nonspecific and do not offer any clues to the underlying etiology. However, the precipitating circumstances and the setting in which attacks occur, especially the first attack, usually give some clues to the underlying cause.
K. Treatment
  1. Short-term supportive psychotherapy
     This is usually indicated and includes:
     a) Reassurance and support (not only verbal but attitudinal as well).
     b) Clarification and education, including pointing out various dynamic and stress factors and supporting various positions and recommendations about changes. It could also include attempts to provide the patient with an understanding of panic episodes or other related states of mind. Effort should be made to explore the stimuli that trigger the panic attacks.
     c) Environmental modification, including changing the environment in some way, modifying whatever stresses may be present, and family therapy.
  2. Cognitive therapy has been used with success.
  3. Insight psychotherapy
     Although most psychotherapy is aimed at giving some insight, certain cases of this disorder may require long-term interpretative, psychoanalytically oriented psychotherapy.
  4. Medications
     Reliance is chiefly on benzodiazepines (chlordiazepoxide, diazepam, oxazepam, lorezepam, and so forth). Newer

antianxiety medications, such as alprazolam (Xanax) seem to be especially effective (caution must be exercised in the use of Xanax because of the problem of managing withdrawal as addiction develops). Antidepressant medications such as tricyclics are sometimes effective, especially if depressive symptoms occur. Some studies indicate that monoamine oxidase inhibitors are useful in patients with severe protracted panic disorder. Neuroleptic agents such as chlorpromazine or thioridazine are sometimes prescribed.

5. Behavior therapy
   a) Since much anxiety is a conditioned response, deconditioning through exposure has been tried with some success.
   b) Specific training in prevention of hyperventilation during onset of panic attacks has been useful in helping patients get some sense of control over their panic attacks.

L. Case example

Mrs. J., a thirty-year-old housewife, sought psychiatric treatment because of the following symptoms: irritability, anxiousness, lower abdominal pain, numbness and tingling of her extremities, and fearfulness about her health. Although she had been a "nervous" person most of her life, her presenting symptoms had begun three months earlier and occurred in "attacks."

During a series of interviews, it was learned that the onset of her symptoms occurred the day her sister unexpectedly removed a niece the patient had been caring for in her home while the mother was hospitalized for delivery of a baby. Two factors in her past history were of dynamic significance: she had been the oldest girl in a large family and cared for the other siblings, especially when her mother was in the hospital having babies; and sterility—she had been unable to conceive during ten years of marriage.

Thus, recurrent anxiety attacks were precipitated in a woman desirous of having a family, who in the past had to "give up" children when the mother returned, and who again had been forced to "give up" a child.

From a dynamic viewpoint, the symptoms were manifestations of the patient's conflict between her desire for children and her inability to conceive. The fact that she had to "give up" a child three months earlier reactivated the conflict and precipitated the symptoms.

In this case, the presenting symptoms were panic attacks. The psychodynamic factors seem readily apparent in this case and were the focus of subsequent treatment.

## VII. Agoraphobia without history of panic disorder

A. Definition

The essential feature is agoraphobia without a history of panic attacks.

B. Definition of agoraphobia (see previous section)

C. Common agoraphobic situations include being outside the home alone, being in a crowd or standing in a line, being on a bridge, and traveling in a bus, train, or car.
D. Usually the person is afraid of having a limited symptom attack (developing a single or small number of symptoms, such as dizziness or falling, depersonalization or derealization, loss of bladder or bowel control, vomiting or having cardiac distress) or in other cases the person may fear that the symptoms "could" develop and incapacitate him or her or be extremely embarrassing (*DSM*-III-R).
E. Associated features
   A personality disorder, particularly avoidant personality disorder, may accompany.
F. Age at onset
   Usually in the twenties or thirties
G. Course
   Typically chronic (or persistent)
H. Prevalence
   Rare in clinical practice but said to be the most common anxiety disorder seen in clinics specializing in treating anxiety disorders
I. Etiology and pathogenesis
   1. The cause is not known. There may be multiple interacting factors.
   2. Some studies suggest that agoraphobic disorder may be related to genetic factors.
   3. Some may be predisposed to developing intense anxiety when threat is anticipated.
   4. Anxiety is often found to have a psychological basis (fear of giving way in public to unacceptable wishes). This conflict between impulses and proper social behavior leads to anxiety and thus motivates various psychological defenses such as avoidance, displacement, symbolization, repression, and suppression.
   5. The specific train of thought that leads to anxiety once it becomes conscious yields to repression (and thus is out of one's awareness).
   6. Development of avoidance behavior reduces the anxiety, a reward that thus reinforces that behavior.
J. Treatment
   1. Exposure therapy is the most effective treatment (with and without panic attack).
   2. See K. in previous section.
K. Case example

   Mrs. A. W., the forty-eight-year-old wife of a small-town physician, sought psychiatric treatment because she had a fear of being in church.

Actually, as she unfolded her story, she really feared leaving the home and, before she developed the fear of going to church, had become uneasy while shopping and driving the children to school. It became evident, during exploratory interviews, that the onset of this agoraphobic behavior was related to her husband's heart attack two years earlier. Since he was several years her senior, she was fearful that he might have a second heart attack that would prove fatal.

As she became aware of the relationship of her symptom to her concern about her husband's health, she was able to respond to a combined approach of psychotropic medication and a program of gradual desensitization. She began by forcing herself to attend a church of her own denomination in a nearby town and then, by degrees, finally forced herself to attend her own church and sit in the front row.

## VIII. Social phobia
### A. Definition
The essential feature of this disorder is a persistent fear of one or more situations (the social phobic situations) in which the person is exposed to possible scrutiny by others and fears that he or she may do something or act in a way that will be humiliating or embarrassing. The social phobic fear may be circumscribed, such as fears of being unable to continue talking while speaking in public, choking on food when eating in front of others, being unable to urinate in a public lavatory, or having a hand tremble when writing in the presence of others. In other cases the social phobic fears may involve most social situations, such as general fears of saying foolish things or not being able to answer questions in social situations. If exposed to the specific phobic stimulus, the person develops an immediate anxiety response. Marked anticipatory anxiety occurs if the person is confronted with the necessity of entering into the social phobic situations, and such situations are thus usually avoided (*DSM-III-R*).

### B. Prevalence
Social phobia involving fear of public speaking and social phobia involving a generalized fear of most social situations are common.

### C. Associated features
Panic disorder and simple phobia commonly coexist with social phobia.

### D. Course
Is usually chronic

### E. Complication
Persons with social phobia are prone to abuse alcohol, barbiturates, and anxiolytics. When social or occupational functioning is severely impaired, a depressive disorder may be a complication.

F. Symptoms
1. Aside from the phobia itself, the symptoms are ways of avoiding the feared object, activity, or situation. These obviously restrict the individual's freedom of action. The individual has focalized the anxiety and, as long as he or she can avoid the focalized object, activity, or situation, remains relatively comfortable and free of anxiety.
2. The type of fear is in part culturally determined and, as in some conversion disorders, there is a secondary gain factor. For example, fear of airplanes may develop in a person whose job requires air travel.
3. If confronted with the feared object, activity, or situation, the individual develops anxiety that varies in degree from mild uneasiness to panic.
4. The individual recognizes the unreasonableness of the phobia but is unable to control the behavior or explain the fear.
5. There are numerous types of phobias, since they can develop about almost anything.
6. Counterphobic attitude: At times persons with a phobia seek out the very situation of which they are afraid. There is a striving to master excess anxiety through repeated coping with the danger. (Such repetitive behavior makes possible the transformation of passivity to activity.) Some of the involvement in dangerous sports, such as parachute jumping and racing, may be examples of counterphobic behavior.

G. Etiology
1. The cause of social phobia is unknown.
2. There is often a family history of phobia.

H. Treatment
1. Behavior therapy: Exposure therapy is often helpful.
2. Cognitive approaches using cognitive restructuring have been used with some success.
3. In the past, psychoanalytically oriented or other kinds of psychodynamic therapy were prescribed. Research does not support the effectiveness of such approaches for phobia disorders.
4. Drug treatment
   a) Beta-blocking agents are often helpful in minimizing the peripheral symptoms such as sweating, tremor, and tachycardia.
   b) Benzodiazepine antianxiety agents are sometimes helpful (and sometimes in combination with beta-blockers).
   c) Monoamine oxidase inhibitor (MAOI) antidepressants are thought to be helpful as well.

    d) Sometimes a combination of exposure therapy and beta-blocker drugs works well.

    5. Social skills training can be used to supplement the previous therapies.

I. Case example

A twenty-four-year-old single man consulted a psychiatrist because of his fear of speaking before groups of people, particularly in classrooms. He reported that the first episode occurred in the sixth grade, when he was called on to recite in front of his class and that his fearfulness became more evident in high school and worsened during his college days, when he was in smaller classes where more personal participation was demanded. Whenever he had to speak to a group of people, he became shy, nervous, and short of breath.

On examination, he appeared cooperative, pleasant, but unable to look at himself in a psychological way. He did not exhibit any unusual behavior or thinking pattern throughout the interviews and, although somewhat anxious and uneasy to begin with, related later.

Psychological testing revealed that he had superior intelligence and good ego strengths, but he seemed to view the world about him as a somewhat threatening and conflictual place in which to live. This seemed particularly true of his relationships with men, whom he regarded as competitors. Since his symptoms were not severe and he had good ego strengths, he was urged to return to school, enroll in a course that required classroom participation, and forcibly confront himself with the situation that might make him fearful.

## IX. Simple phobia
  A. Definition

The essential feature of this disorder is a persistent fear of a circumscribed stimulus (object or situation) other than fear of having a panic attack (as in panic disorder) or of humiliation or embarrassment in certain social situations (as in social phobia) (*DSM*-III-R).

    1. Types

The most common simple phobias in the general population involve animals, particularly dogs, snakes, insects, and mice. Others are claustrophobias (fear of closed spaces), acrophobias (fear of heights), fear of witnessing blood or tissue injury, and fear of air travel.

    2. Exposure to the simple phobic stimulus provokes an immediate anxiety response. Marked anticipatory anxiety occurs if the person is confronted with the necessity of entering into a simple phobic situation; such situations are thus usually avoided.

    3. The diagnosis of simple phobia is made only if the avoidant behavior interferes with the person's normal routine or with usual activities or relationships with others, or if there's marked distress about having the fear.

B. Associated features

Unrelated social phobia and panic disorder with or without agoraphobia are often present.

C. Age at onset

Varies, but animal phobias usually begin in childhood; blood-injury phobias usually begin in adolescence or early adulthood; circumscribed phobias of heights, driving, closed spaces, and air travel appear to begin most frequently in the fourth decade of life.

D. Course

Most simple phobias that start in childhood disappear without treatment; those that persist into adulthood rarely remit without treatment.

E. Prevalence

Simple phobias are common in the general population, but since they rarely result in marked impairment, people with this disorder rarely seek treatment.

F. Etiology and pathogenesis

1. The sources of phobias are quite heterogeneous.

2. The usual psychodynamic formulation is selected because of special unconscious symbolic significance to the individual. The meaning is repressed and displaced (see chapter 6). Rarely, unknown biological or psychosocial mechanisms cause phobic patients to acquire an ingrained and unconscious stimulus-response association, which generates fear and subsequent exposure to the phobic stimulus.

3. From a behavioral perspective, phobias can be viewed as outcomes of classical conditioning, however, for such learning may not be present in the history of some phobias.

4. Why certain objects are feared and not others is an unanswered question. Some theorists suggest there is an adaptive predisposition to fear certain objects or situations (biological preparedness).

5. Agoraphobia runs in families; most social and simple phobias do not.

G. Treatment

Exposure therapy works quite well with single phobias.

H. Historical notes

1. Shakespeare described phobic behavior in *The Merchant of Venice:*

> Some men there are love not a gaping pig:
> Some, that are mad if they behold a cat.

2. In 1872, C. Westphal published his classic monograph *Agoraphobia (die Agoraphobia).*

3. In 1909, Freud described the case of ''Little Hans,'' a five-year-old who developed a phobia.

## X. Obsessive-compulsive disorder (or obsessive-compulsive neurosis)

A. Definition

The essential feature is recurrent obsessions or compulsions that are sufficiently severe to cause marked distress, are time-consuming, or significantly interfere with the person's normal routine, occupational functioning, or usual social activities or relationships.

*Obsessions* are persistent ideas, thoughts, impulses, or images that are experienced, at least initially, as intrusive and senseless.

*Compulsions* are repetitive, purposeful, and intentional behaviors that are performed in response to an obsession, according to certain rules, or in a stereotyped fashion (*DSM*-III-R).

B. Prevalence

1. Fleeting obsessions or compulsions are more or less universal.
2. Obsessive-compulsive traits are not uncommon in children and adolescents.
3. Recent community studies indicate the mild forms may be relatively common.
4. Once considered rare, this disorder may now be affecting as much as 2 to 3 percent of Americans.
5. The incidence may be somewhat higher because people with this disorder often conceal their symptoms and avoid consulting a physician about them.
6. It is said that a large number of obsessive-compulsive people remain unmarried.
7. Some studies indicate that the disorder is more common among people in the upper socioeconomic class and those of high IQ.
8. Gender is apparently not a factor.

C. Symptoms

1. The symptoms may take many forms. Doubt and vacillation are prominent (*folie du doute*).
2. Obsessions

These recurring ideas or impulses can be about anything, but the most common themes are about violence, contamination, and doubt. Other themes are sexuality, obscenities, and religion or religious subjects (scrupulosity).
3. Compulsions

These are recurrent, compelling acts that develop in the attempt to relieve obsessions or fears. They are of two types: a) reactions to or attempts to control the underlying obsession, and b) direct expressions of the underlying obsessive urges. The second type is rare and similar to counterphobic measures in phobic patients.

    (1) The most common compulsions involve handwashing, counting, checking, and touching.

    (2) Another common compulsion is self-mutilation, for example, self-inflicted excoriation as a compulsive punishment for guilt about masturbation.

4. As can be seen from the foregoing, the obsessions are mainly asocial in nature and the compulsions are mainly "caricatures of morality." In fully developed cases, there is a 50:50 ratio between the obsessions and compulsions. Such a state of dynamic equilibrium explains the underlying indecision, uncertainty, and ambivalence of these patients.

5. Sometimes the symptoms are less specific, being manifested as a compulsive and ritualistic quality that pervades all of the individual's behavior. Thus, some individuals perform certain rituals on arising in the morning, dress according to a certain pattern, or perform daily tasks and duties in a fixed and exact sequence.

6. Sometimes the compelling idea may be neutral or indifferent, and the term *obsessive-ruminative state* is then used. The central rumination is often of a religious or philosophical nature. The matter is repeatedly meditated upon, consideration is given to the pros, cons, and imponderables, but no resolution of the matter is achieved.

7. The patient is often embarrassed about the compulsions and rituals and may go to great lengths to disguise them from others. If they become more severe or chronic, the person's ability to hide the acts becomes progressively less successful.

8. Depression and anxiety symptoms are common.

9. Frequently there is a phobic avoidance of situations that involve the content of the obsessions. For example, a person with obsessions about dirt may avoid public rest rooms; a person with obsessions about contamination may avoid shaking hands with strangers (*DSM*-III-R).

D. Course and prognosis

1. The onset of obsessive-compulsive disorder may occur at any period of life, but commonly begins in adolescence or early adulthood. From a psychodynamic point of view, this is probably because this is the period when there is increased sexual awareness, conflict about dependency and independence, and so forth.

2. Obsessive-compulsive traits found in childhood often clear up or respond promptly to treatment.

3. Some episodes are transitory and relatively circumscribed. Such patients frequently have a good prognosis if they undergo psychotherapy.
4. Unfortunately, some of these reactions tend to become chronic and follow an unremitting course. As such, they are often resistant to treatment.
5. In general, the prognosis is more favorable when
   a) The symptoms are of short duration.
   b) Environmental stressors are prominent.
   c) There is a good environment to return to following treatment.
   d) Interpersonal relationships are good.
6. Complications include major depression and the abuse of alcohol and anxiolytics.
7. This disorder is equally common in both males and females.

E. Etiology and pathogenesis
1. Psychodynamic (psychoanalytic) perspective
   a) Obsessive-compulsive disorder is dynamically much more complicated than any of the other anxiety disorders.
   b) Obsessions and compulsions arise in three phases: (1) an internally perceived dangerous impulse, (2) the threat of what would occur if the impulses were acted upon, and (3) the defense to avert the threat. The threat is the danger of actually harming others, fear of punishment, and the pain of guilt.
   c) Repression, for some reason, is unsuccessful or only incompletely successful, and the individual makes use of other defenses to reinforce the repression. These subsequent defenses are isolation, reaction formation, undoing, and displacement (see chapter 6).
   d) *Ambivalence,* coexistence of two opposing feelings toward the same individual or object, is very prominent in obsessive-compulsive patients. The feelings are usually love and hate. Ambivalence is also evident in undoing.
   e) Psychopathology generally and obsessions specifically are found in the families of obsessives.
   f) The premorbid personality typically has obsessional characteristics. That is, he or she is rigid, restricted, orderly, meticulous, cautious, deliberate, conscientious, and dependable. The person who possesses such compulsive qualities is also referred to as an *anankastic personality,* or *anal character* (an individual who needs to feel in control of himself or herself and of the environment). The presence of these traits does not constitute abnormality. Most of the people who have obsessive-

compulsive traits do not become obsessive-compulsive patients.

According to psychoanalytic theorists, such anal qualities develop in the infant during the period of toilet training (the anal phase of infantile sexuality). The development of obsessive-compulsive disorder represents fixation at, or regression to, this anal phase of development—a period when the superego is harsh, demanding, and punitive.

g) The function of the compulsive act is to allay (relieve) and bind (tie down or focalize) anxiety.

h) The acts are symbolic, and the symbolic nature is often only discovered during psychotherapy.

i) Pathogenesis of the obsessive-compulsive disorder may be clarified by biochemical and neurophysiological studies now under way. (The capacity to regulate anxiety depends in part on the ability to maintain repression as a defense, and impairment of that function interferes with the ability to suppress unacceptable ideas and feelings. Although the mechanism of this impairment is unknown, it could conceivably have a neurobiologic component.)

2. Behavioral perspectives

Behaviorists regard obsessions and compulsions as *learned* behavior. For example, compulsive behavior relieves the obsessional preoccupations with obsessions.

3. Biological perspective

a) The biological models have centered on the role of serotonin and to a lesser extent norepinephrine and other neurotransmitter systems.

b) Neurological models of this disorder have been suggested and are based on the onset of obsessive-compulsive disorder following nervous system damage.

c) PET (positron emission tomography) studies of patients with severe obsessive-compulsive disorders show differences in activity in regions of the basal ganglia and frontal lobe (Rappaport 1989).

F. Treatment

1. Only a small number of obsessive-compulsive people enter treatment. Of the treatments available—psychotherapy, behavioral therapy, and pharmacotherapy—none is ideal. (However, recent reports indicate that clomipramine (Anafranil) is particularly effective in the treatment of severe obsessive-compulsive disorder.)

2. Psychotherapy
   a) Intensive psychoanalytically oriented psychotherapy was at one time thought to be the treatment of choice. However, it would appear that only a small number of people with this disorder respond to such treatment. (Even the most optimistic of psychoanalytic writers are unenthusiastic about insight-oriented therapy.)
   b) Supportive psychotherapy is often helpful. However, it should be kept in mind that responses to psychotherapy will often last only a matter of hours, and then the individual's doubts recur.
3. Behavior therapy
   a) Behavior therapy has been tried recently. Rather than attending to the underlying complexities of the disorder, attempts are made to focus on the person's behavior.
   b) The treatment is similar to behavioral treatment of phobias. The most widely used and accepted behavioral approach to compulsive rituals entails exposure with response prevention (Davison and Neale 1990).
4. Pharmacotherapy
   a) Anxiolytics, neuroleptics, and antidepressants have been used in attempts to treat obsessive-compulsive disorder for many years.
   b) Recently, however, new drugs have been introduced which seem to have specific antiobsessional effects. These are:
      (1) Clomipramine (Anafranil), which was recently released in the United States for the treatment of obsessive-compulsive disorder (it had previously been approved for depressive disorders).
      (2) Fluoxetine (Prozac) seems to offer a persistent antiobsessional effect. Patients on this medication seem to relapse less frequently following twelve months of therapy than patients treated with clomipramine; and fluvoxamine, which is a potent and selective serotonin reuptake inhibitor, has been an effective treatment in some published studies (so far this drug has not been released in the United States).
5. Somatic therapy
   a) Electroconvulsive therapy has been used in the past, often with disappointing results.
   b) Psychosurgery, specifically stereotactic lympic leukotomy, has been performed on some patients who have had chronic crippling disorders.

G. Case example

Mrs. B., a thirty-three-year-old housewife, consulted a psychiatrist, complaining of fear of germs and dirt, obsessions about religious ideas, and obsessions about the number 3. These symptoms had begun about three months earlier, following the birth of her second child. She had had a similar episode five years earlier, after her first child was born. This had lasted about six months and finally cleared up during counseling with her pastor.

She was a bright person who was always orderly, methodical, conscientious, and dependable. As a child, she was overly concerned with the "normal" compulsions that children have, such as counting the pickets in fences and avoiding the cracks in sidewalks. At ten she became obsessed with the idea that she would die on a certain Tuesday in October.

In her present episode she had developed a number of compulsions in response to her fears and obsessions. For example, she washed her hands repeatedly and relaundered clothes because of her fear of germs and dirt, and she avoided reading automobile license plates and house numbers because she wished to avoid the number 3. After several weeks in the hospital, she improved enough so that she was able to carry on her housework, although she was still troubled somewhat by her symptoms.

In this case, note the previously compulsive personality and the typical obsessions and compulsions. In view of her compulsive personality and incomplete response to hospital treatment, her prognosis was necessarily poor.

## XI. Post-traumatic stress disorder
A. Definition
1. This disorder was introduced in *DSM*-III in 1980 and assembled together a seemingly disparate collection of entities including battle fatigue, war neurosis, concentration camp syndrome, post-Vietnam syndrome, and post-disaster syndrome, thus emphasizing the ubiquity of the emotional responses manifested by the individuals faced with a psychological trauma of overpowering magnitude (Bowman 1986).
2. In *DSM*-III-R, diagnostic criteria for post-traumatic stress disorder are the following:
   a) The person has experienced an event that is outside the range of usual human experience and which would be markedly distressing to almost anyone—for example, serious threat to one's life or physical integrity; serious threat or harm to one's children, spouse, or other close relatives and friends; sudden destruction of one's home or community; or seeing another person who has recently been, or is being, seriously injured or killed as the result of an accident or physical violence.

b) The traumatic event is persistently reexperienced in at least one of the following ways:
   (1) Recurrent and intrusive distressing recollections of the event (in young children, repetitive play in which themes or aspects of the trauma are expressed)
   (2) Recurrent distressing dreams of the event
   (3) Sudden acting or feeling as if the traumatic event were recurring (includes a sense of reliving the experience, illusions, hallucinations, and dissociative [flashback] episodes, even those that occur upon awakening or when intoxicated)
   (4) Intense psychological distress at exposure to events that symbolize or resemble an aspect of the traumatic event, including anniversaries of the trauma
c) Persistent avoidance of stimuli associated with the trauma or numbing of general responsiveness (not present before the trauma), as indicated by at least three of the following:
   (1) Efforts to avoid thoughts or feelings associated with the trauma
   (2) Efforts to avoid activities or situations that arouse recollections of the trauma
   (3) Inability to recall an important aspect of the trauma (psychogenic amnesia)
   (4) Markedly diminished interest in significant activities (in young children, loss of recently acquired developmental skills such as toilet training or language skills)
   (5) Feeling of detachment or estrangement from others
   (6) Restricted range of affect—for example, unable to have loving feelings
   (7) Sense of a foreshortened future—for example, does not expect to have a career, marriage, or children, or a long life
d) Persistent symptoms of increased arousal (not present before the trauma), as indicated by at least two of the following:
   (1) Difficulty falling or staying asleep
   (2) Irritability or outbursts of anger
   (3) Difficulty concentrating
   (4) Hypervigilance
   (5) Exaggerated startle response
   (6) Physiologic reactivity upon exposure to events that symbolize or resemble an aspect of the traumatic

event (e.g., a woman who was raped in an elevator breaks out in a sweat when entering any elevator)
   e) Duration of the disturbance (symptoms in b, c, and d) of at least one month.
B. Types
   1. Cases in which the symptoms have their onset within six months after the trauma and do not last more than six months are considered acute, and the prognosis with treatment is good. Those in which the symptoms are delayed more than six months or last longer than six months are considered chronic or delayed, and the treatment is usually more difficult.
   2. Kolb and Brodie (1982) point out that 75 percent of acute war neuroses were anxiety reactions and that the survivors of concentration camps of World War II are the largest group of sufferers of chronic stress reaction. The Vietnam experience is a well-known type of delayed stress disorder.
   3. Patients with combat-induced post-traumatic stress disorder (PTSD) commonly experience depersonalization, flashbacks, rage attacks, and fugue states. One case of a Vietnam veteran has been reported in which a multiple personality emerged.
C. Etiology
   Although a psychologically distressing event is the precipitating stressor in this disorder, individual predisposition may play a role in the development of the disorder.
D. Treatment
   1. Early treatment seems to be essential to help resolve the condition.
   2. The usual treatment is short-term psychotherapy (five to sixteen weeks) during which the therapist a) gets a history from the patient, b) gives the patient a realistic appraisal of the event and the patient's reaction to it, c) identifies themes that the patient is still resisting, d) interprets the patient's pathological defenses, e) encourages active confrontation of feared topics and harsh memories, f) begins discussing termination, g) clarifies remaining conflicts and issues, h) summarizes the gains in therapy, i) alerts the patient to future concerns, and j) bids good-bye.[1]

**XII. Generalized anxiety disorder (GAD)**
   A. Definition
   The essential features of this disorder are unrealistic or excessive anxiety and worry (apprehensive expectation) about two or

1. M. Horowitz, "Disasters and Psychological Response to Stress," *Psychiatric Annals* 15 (1985): 161–67.

more life circumstances—for example, worry about possible misfortune to one's child (who is in no danger) and worry about finances (for no good reason), for six months or longer, during which the person has been bothered by these concerns more days than not. In children and adolescents this may take the form of anxiety and worry about academic, athletic, and social performance. When the person is anxious, there are many signs of motor tension, autonomic hyperactivity, and vigilance and scanning. (Symptoms that are present only during panic attacks are not considered in making the diagnosis.) (*DSM*-III-R)

B. Symptoms

The person with generalized anxiety disorder is chronically and persistently anxious and generally shows signs of motor tension, autonomic hyperactivity, and vigilance and scanning.

   1. Motor tension

     Trembling, twitching, or feeling shaky; muscle tension, aches, or soreness; restlessness; and easy fatigability.

   2. Autonomic hyperactivity

     Shortness of breath or smothering sensations; palpitations or accelerated heart rate (tachycardia); sweating or cold, clammy hands; dry mouth; dizziness or light-headedness; nausea, diarrhea, or other abdominal distress; flushes (hot flashes) or chills; frequent urination; and trouble swallowing or "lump in throat."

   3. Vigilance and scanning

     Feeling keyed up or on edge; exaggerated startle response; difficulty concentrating or "mind going blank" because of anxiety; trouble falling or staying asleep; and irritability.

   4. Organic factors that might initiate or maintain the disturbance must be ruled out (e.g., caffeine intoxication, hyperthyroidism).

C. Etiology and pathogenesis

   1. Neurobiologic factors

     Some persons are biologically predisposed to states of anxiousness.

     a) The physiological reflections of anxiety are produced by discharge of the adrenergic division of the autonomic nervous system.

     b) Noradrenergic pathways originating in the locus caeruleus in the upper pons and projecting to the cortex and limbic system are thought to help regulate anxiety.

     c) Central nervous system receptors for the neurotransmitter gamma-aminobutyric acid (GABA) are found to contain a modulating protein that has a binding site for the anxiety-reducing benzodiazepines.

2. Psychological activation of states of anxiousness
   Some individuals actually seek anxiety states. People may deliberately pursue excitement such as roller coaster rides, horror movies, skydiving, and so forth, in order to be stimulated, gain a sense of mastery over a fear, escape from some mental state (boredom, apathy, anger), or achieve the sensation that follows fear ("high," relief, pleasure, and others' admiration and acceptance).

   On the other hand, such anxiety states occur because a person unconsciously anticipates the out-of-control situation; intolerable and dangerous states of mind may occur if conscious thoughts about threatening ideas are pursued to their conclusion.

   Such anxious states of mind may have been experienced or witnessed in the past, with results that may have been psychically traumatic so that the person fears the repetition.

D. Psychoanalytic perspectives consider the source of generalized anxiety as a reaction to underlying unconscious conflict (see chapter 2).

E. Associated features
   Unrelated panic disorder or depressive disorder is often present.

F. Impairment
   Impairment in social or occupational functioning is rarely more than mild.

G. Treatment
   Little is known about specific therapy for generalized anxiety disorder; however, the following principles underlining the therapy for anxiety symptoms (from Maxmen 1986) seem appropriate.
   1. Pharmacotherapy
      Generally, for mild symptoms of anxiety, medication should be avoided. However, when symptoms warrant it, benzodiazepines are the preferred drugs (diazepam, alprazolam, etc.).
   2. Psychotherapies
      Insight-oriented psychotherapy explores the unconscious and symbolic meanings of the patient's anxiety and clarifies its defensive and "signal" functions. It seeks to identify the stressors producing the anxiety and find a better means of handling stress.
   3. Cognitive therapy focuses on particular stress events or circumstances that trigger conscious, dysphoric "automatic thoughts" and then rational ways of responding.

4. Behavior therapy

Relaxation, biofeedback, and meditation are frequently helpful, either by themselves or as supplements to other therapies.

# References

American Psychiatric Association. *Diagnostic and Statistical Manual of Mental Disorders.* 3d ed., rev. Washington, D.C.: APA, 1987.

Barlow, D. H. *Anxiety and Its Disorders.* New York: Guilford Press, 1988.

Bowman, B. "Combat Stress, Post-Traumatic Stress Disorder, and Associated Psychiatric Disturbance." *Psychosomatics* 27, no. 8 (August 1986): 567ff.

Davison, G. C., and J. M. Neale. *Abnormal Psychology.* New York: Wiley, 1990.

Dysken, M. W., and J. M. Davison, eds. "Obsessive-Compulsive Disorder." *Psychiatric Annals* 19, no. 2 (February 1989).

Goldman, H. H. *Review of General Psychiatry.* Los Altos, Calif.: Lange Medical Publications, 1988.

Kaplan, H. I., and B. J. Sadock, eds. *Comprehensive Textbook of Psychiatry/V.* 5th ed. Baltimore: Williams & Wilkins, 1989.

Kolb, L. C., and H. K. H. Brodie. *Modern Clinical Psychiatry.* 10th ed. Philadelphia: Saunders, 1982.

McDoudle, C. J., and S. M. Southwick. "Emergence of an Alternate Personality in Combat-related Post-traumatic Stress Disorder." *Hospital and Community Psychiatry* 41, no. 5 (May 1990): 554–55.

Maxmen, J. S. *Essential Psychopathology.* New York: Norton, 1986.

Nicholi, A. M., Jr., ed. *The New Harvard Guide to Modern Psychiatry.* Cambridge: Belknap Press, 1988.

Rapoport, J. *The Boy Who Couldn't Stop Washing.* New York: Dutton, 1989.

# 12 Somatoform Disorders

For the body at best
There is a bundle of aches,
Longing for rest, it cries when it wakes.

**Edna St. Vincent Millay**

I. **Definition**

The essential features of this group of disorders are physical symptoms suggesting physical disorder (hence, somatoform), for which there are no demonstrable organic findings or known physiologic mechanisms, and for which there is positive evidence, or a strong presumption, that the symptoms are linked to psychological factors or conflicts. Unlike in factitious disorder or malingering, the symptom production in somatoform disorders is not intentional; that is, the person does not experience the sense of controlling the production of the symptoms. Although the symptoms of somatoform disorders are "physical," the specific pathophysiologic processes involved are not demonstrable or understandable by existing laboratory procedures and are conceptualized most clearly by means of psychological constructs. For that reason, these are classified as mental (not physical) disorders (*DSM*-III-R).

II. **Types**

The subtypes of somatoform disorders are listed next. Each will be discussed in turn.

A. Body dysmorphic disorder (dysmorphophobia)

B. Conversion disorder (or hysterical neurosis, conversion type)

C. Hypochondriasis (or hypochondriacal neurosis)

D. Somatization disorder (Briquet's syndrome)

E. Somatoform pain disorder

F. Undifferentiated somatoform disorder

G. Somatoform disorder not otherwise specified

III. **Prevalence**

A. Many patients seen in general medical practice do not have significant organic disease to account for their complaints. Many of these probably have somatoform disorders, but they do not seek psychiatric treatment because they do not perceive themselves as having psychiatric difficulties. Especially primary care doctors, but many specialists—for example, neurologists and cardiologists—should be familiar with these disorders so they can be managed properly.

B. Estimates are that 10 percent of all medical services are provided for patients who have no evidence of organic disease (exclusive of services provided for identified psychiatric patients) (Ford 1986).

## IV. Body dysmorphic disorder (dysmorphophobia)

A. Definition

The essential feature of this disorder is preoccupation with some imagined defect in appearance in a normal-appearing person. The most common complaints involve facial flaws, such as wrinkles, spots on the skin, excessive facial hair, shape of nose, mouth, jaw, or eyebrows, and swelling of the face. More rarely the complaint involves the appearance of the feet, hands, breasts, back, or some other part of the body. In some cases a slight physical anomaly is present, but the person's concern is grossly excessive (*DSM*-III-R).

B. The previous diagnosis of dysmorphophobia seemed to be a misnomer, since the disturbance does not involve phobic avoidance. The term *dysmorphophobia* has also been used to include cases in which the belief in a defect in appearance is of delusional intensity. (''Dysmorphophobia'' was coined in 1886 by Morselli to describe ''a subjective feeling of ugliness or physical defect.'' Actually it is a nonspecific symptom that can appear in several psychiatric disorders including major depression and schizophrenia. Nondelusional dysmorphophobia, a nondelusional belief, is a defect sometimes considered and ''overvalued'').

C. Associated features include history of repeated visits to plastic surgeons and dermatologists for correction of the imagined defect, obsessive personality traits, and depression.

D. The age at onset is most commonly from adolescence through the third decade of life. (Keep in mind normal adolescent concerns with minor defects such as acne.)

E. Treatment

1. Medication: Antipsychotic agents are sometimes helpful in those cases which seem to be delusional (e.g., pimozide). Diphenylbutylpiperidine or antidepressants have been helpful in other cases.

2. Psychotherapy: Dealing with psychosocial factors must be considered.

3. It is difficult to recommend the treatment of choice because the condition is infrequent and only rarely seen by

psychiatrists. A further confounding factor is the inclusion of delusional and nondelusional categories in the diagnosis of body disorders.

V. **Conversion disorder (or hysterical neurosis, conversion type)**
   A. Definition
   1. The essential feature of this disorder is an alteration or loss of physical functioning that suggests physical disorder, but that instead is apparently an expression of a psychological conflict or need. The symptoms of the disturbances are not intentionally produced (as in factitious disorder or malingering) and, after appropriate investigation, cannot be explained by any physical disorder or known patho-physiologic mechanism (*DSM*-III-R).
   2. Psychodynamically, it is a disorder in which unconscious conflict is manifested as disguised and symbolic somatic symptoms. That is, the anxiety arising out of some conflictual situation is converted into somatic symptoms in parts of the body innervated by the sensorimotor system (symbolic somatization). Thus, the conflict is reflected as physical symptoms instead of being expressed directly.
   B. The differentiation from factitious disorder and from malingering is sometimes difficult. Conversion disorder must be distinguished from other illness-affirming states.
   1. *Malingering*: Signs and symptoms of illness are consciously produced and consciously motivated.
   2. Factitious disorder: The intentional production of symptoms to assume the *patient role*. The presentation may be fabricated or self-inflicted, but the motivation is unconscious.
   3. The differentiation of conversion disorder from factitious disorder or malingering is sometimes difficult because
      a) Some behavior may be in part consciously determined and in part unconsciously determined.
      b) Many hysterical and factitious patients are so histrionic about their symptoms, and their secondary gain is so obvious, that one sees them as consciously feigning or simulating disease.
   4. However, whichever the disorder, psychiatrists must approach it therapeutically.
   C. Prevalence
   1. Classical conversion disorder is rarely encountered now.
   2. Conversion symptoms, however, are fairly common.
   3. Conversion elements are commonly seen in compensation cases.

4. Conversion disorder is usually considered to be more common among women, although it is seen in men in the military setting.
5. Classical conversion disorder is rarely seen in ordinary psychiatric practice, but is more commonly seen by neurologists, orthopedic surgeons, and by military physicians, especially in time of war.
D. Predisposing factors
Antecedent physical disorder (which may provide a prototype for the symptoms), exposure to other people with real physical symptoms or conversion symptoms, and extreme psychosocial stress (warfare or the recent death of a significant figure) are predisposing factors (*DSM*-III-R).
E. Persons with histrionic and dependent personality disorders have increased vulnerability for this disorder.
F. Symptoms
1. Somatic symptoms
a) The somatic symptoms can vary widely. Frequently, they simulate organic disease and represent the patient's idea of the disease. The closeness with which the patient's symptoms approximate the symptoms of an organic disease depends in large measure on the patient's medical and psychological sophistication.
b) The somatic symptoms chiefly involve organs that are in contact with the external world.
c) The distribution of the symptoms is unphysiological and nonanatomical.
d) Somatic symptoms can be considered under two headings.
(1) Motor symptoms, such as convulsive states, paralysis, paresis (muscular weakness), or aphonia (inability to produce normal speech)
(2) Sensory disturbances, such as analgesia (diminished sense of pain), anesthesia (absence of feeling), or paresthesia ("tingling feeling")
e) The somatic symptoms associated with conversion disorder tend to be singular rather than multiple (as in somatoform disorder).
f) The onset or exacerbation of the symptoms almost always follows a psychologically meaningful environmental stimulus.
2. Psychological symptoms
a) The mental-status evaluation of the person with conversion disorder reveals no significant abnormalities.

b) The classical psychological symptom in the conversion disorder is the patient's indifference to the illness (*la belle indifférence*). Though the symptoms are obviously disabling, the patient seems unconcerned and shows no anxiety. However, it should be kept in mind that people with serious medical illnesses may also be indifferent.

c) Pseudodementia may be a conversion symptom in elderly people. This is characterized by exaggerated indifference to one's surroundings, without actual mental impairment, and reversible decline of mental functioning, which occurs in depression.

d) Some histories show a preexisting histrionic personality disorder or dependent personality disorder (see chapter 16).

e) This disorder is unique in the *DSM*-III-R classification because specific mechanisms are thought to account for it (see *primary gain* and *secondary gain* under "Psychopathology," which follows).

f) The onset or exacerbation of the symptoms almost always follows a psychologically meaningful environmental stimulus.

G. Historical conceptions of psychopathology

1. Hippocrates believed that conversion disorder resulted from a wandering uterus.

2. In the seventeenth century, hysteria was thought to be due to demoniacal possession.

3. Jean Charcot believed it was a genetic reaction that resulted in degeneration of the nervous system. He demonstrated that the hysterical symptoms could be produced and removed by hypnotic suggestion. (He also believed that normal people could not be hypnotized.)

4. Pierre Janet introduced the concept of dissociated mental processes in the subconscious. He demonstrated that automatisms were of unconscious origin.

5. Both Joseph Babinski and Hippolyte-Marie Bernheim believed that the symptoms resulted from suggestion. (Bernheim's extensive work with hypnosis led him to believe that normal people could be hypnotized.)

6. Breuer and Freud introduced the concept of repressed conflict as the source of conversion. Freud believed that the repressed conflict was the Oedipus complex.

7. Most authorities now feel that any highly charged instinct or impulse may be involved.

H. Psychopathology
  1. Essentially, the psychopathology is repression of a conflict and conversion of the anxiety into a somatic symptom that is symbolic of the underlying conflict.
  2. It was once thought that only sexual conflict produced conversion symptoms. Theorists now believe that all types of instinctual impulses may find expression in this manner.
  3. The premorbid personality is often histrionic. Such individuals are theatrical, shallow, superficial, or insincere. They are often narcissistic and manipulative. They go through the motions of feeling without really experiencing emotion and tend to overreact to minor stimuli.
  4. The precipitating factor may seem trivial but have a special meaning to the person (thus, as in anxiety disorder, it is important to know the setting in which the first hysterical symptoms occurred).
  5. The choice of symptom may be determined in several ways.
     a) Events may tend to focus the conflict in a specific area (e.g., a tonsillectomy or other type of operation on the throat or neck may be a precursor to aphonia that is an expression of some underlying conflict).
     b) The experience of the organ in relation to the conflict may be the determinant (e.g., paralysis of a hand with which the patient has struck someone in anger).
     c) The suitability of the organ to express the conflict symbolically may also dictate the choice (e.g., paralysis of the legs as a defense against meeting a threat by either attack or flight).
  6. In conversion disorder, both primary gain and secondary gain are observed.
     a) The *primary gain* is the relief of anxiety.
     b) The *secondary gain* is the advantage that accrues to the patient by virtue of the illness. Secondary gain is often a factor in illness, both emotional and physical; however, it is most prominent in conversion disorders.
I. Onset, course, and prognosis
  1. A conversion disorder may prolong or exaggerate symptoms that originally resulted from physical illness.
  2. Conversion symptoms may develop following an accident.
  3. In acute cases—in which the onset is abrupt and the duration of symptoms has been short—the prognosis is usually favorable when the patient is treated.
  4. When the symptoms have been allowed to endure for a sustained period, the prognosis is less hopeful.

        a) In such cases, the secondary gain operates to decrease the individual's motivation to get well by giving up the symptoms.

        b) However, active treatment of someone who is well motivated is often successful.

    5. *DSM*-III-R states that the course of conversion disorder (as distinct from conversion symptoms that are parts of other disorders such as somatization disorders) is unknown, but probably is usually of short duration with abrupt onset and resolution. Recurrence of an episode of conversion disorder usually predicts a recurrent course.

    6. Some studies have indicated that in the long term, some individuals with "conversion symptoms" reveal an underlying neurologic disorder.

    7. The relative maturity of the premorbid personality and the intensity of the underlying conflict are factors that must be evaluated in estimating the prognosis.

J. Case example

The twenty-year-old soldier previously mentioned in chapter 6 developed paralysis of his right hand when firing for the first time on the rifle range. This was a defense against repressed hostility to his father, who had been physically abusive of the soldier's mother many times and who often abandoned the family for long periods. Upon the father's return home, shortly before the young man entered the service, he again threatened his wife. At that point, the young man stepped up to his father and said, "If you ever strike my mother again, I'll kill you." However, he had a very well-developed conscience and obviously would have trouble following through on such a threat.

When he first reached the rifle range and saw the target over his gun sights, he recalled the incident and "saw" the face of his father. Because his conscience could not let him "kill" his father, his right hand became paralyzed, thus preventing him from expressing the strong hostile feelings he had for the father.

K. Treatment

    1. During World War II, intravenous barbiturates (such as sodium amytal) were administered to facilitate the recall of traumatic events and emotions associated with the onset of the conversion reaction. This was sometimes called narcosynthesis.

    2. Some patients respond to psychoanalytically oriented individual psychotherapy.

    3. Individual or group supportive therapy aimed at dealing with changes in the psychosocial environment is sometimes helpful.

VI. **Hypochondriasis (or hypochondriacal neurosis)**

A. Definition

1. The essential feature of this disorder is preoccupation with the fear of having, or the belief that one has, a serious disease, based on the person's interpretation of physical signs or sensations as evidence of physical illness. A thorough physical evaluation does not support the diagnosis of any physical disorder that can account for the physical signs or sensations or for the person's unwarranted interpretation of them, although a coexisting physical disorder may be present. The unwarranted fear or belief of having a disease persists despite medical reassurance, but is not of delusional intensity, in that the person can acknowledge the possibility that he or she may be exaggerating the extent of the feared disease or that there may be no disease at all (*DSM*-III-R).
2. The term derives from the term for the subcostal abdominal region, the hypochondrium, which at one time was believed to be the seat or the origin of the disorder.
3. It is now presumed to be of psychogenic origin.
4. The hypochondriac is painfully aware of sensations that most people ignore. In general, he or she exaggerates the intensity and importance of the sensations.
5. The hypochondriac's somatic preoccupation precludes any concern with underlying feelings or conflicts.
6. The hypochondriacal patient may interpret normal functions (such as peristalsis or heartbeat) or minor symptoms (for example, tension headache or a mild viral infection) as evidence of serious disease.

B. Prevalence

This disorder is much more commonly seen in general medical practice than it is in psychiatric practice, because the patients are focused on physical symptoms and are resistant to the interpretation of any of their symptoms being of psychogenic origin.

C. Symptoms
1. Awareness and exaggeration of physical sensations that most others disregard.
2. Sometimes the somatic preoccupation is really an obsessional symptom, representing displacement of anxiety onto the body itself.
3. Anxiety, depression, and compulsive personality traits are commonly associated with hypochondriasis.
4. Sometimes the hypochondriacal symptoms are vague; at other times, they are organ-centered.
5. Physical findings are absent.

D. Psychopathology

1. It should be kept in mind that this diagnosis has had a number of different clinical meanings in the past.
2. Many show obsessive-compulsive traits and/or narcissistic traits. (They are often egocentric and excessively concerned with themselves and their bodies.)
3. In general, hypochondriasis is considered a reaction to any kind of conflictual situation. Thus, it might be considered a reaction to sexual conflict, to repressed hostility, to disappointment, to failure, and so forth.

E. Course and prognosis
1. The course is usually a chronic one. The patient may take to bed and adopt an invalid life-style, or
2. The course may be intermittent.

F. Treatment
1. No specific treatment has been very effective.
2. Psychotherapy has had only limited value; the best results have been obtained when treatment is begun early.
3. When hypochondriasis is suspected, careful physical and laboratory examinations should be made to rule out any underlying physical disease. It is important to remember that a hypochondriacal person can develop a serious physical disease.
4. Medications of various kinds have been prescribed for symptomatic relief, including antianxiety agents for anxiety symptoms, antidepressants for any depressive features, and so forth. Drugs often have only temporary effects.
5. Perhaps the best treatment program is a generally supportive one, in which a sympathetic physician listens and does not challenge the patient's symptoms. Such a relationship can best be offered by an internist or a general practitioner, with psychiatric consultation and advice available.
6. Whatever physician does treat the hypochondriac must recognize that "cure" is probably not a viable goal and accept "containment" as a more appropriate treatment goal.
7. Environmental modification is occasionally helpful.

G. Examples
1. Dr. Samuel Johnson was a hypochondriac.
2. In Molière's (1622–1673) play *The Hypochondriac,* Argan is a hypochondriac who gauges his health by the number of purges and clysters (enemas) he has had the previous month and who enjoys the attention of two physicians and an apothecary. His desire is to have a physician in the family to attend him at all times.

VII. **Somatization disorder**
A. Definition

1. The essential features of this disorder are recurrent and multiple somatic complaints, of several years' duration, for which medical attention has been sought, but that apparently are not due to any physical disorder. The disorder begins before the age of thirty and has a chronic but fluctuating course (*DSM*-III-R).
2. It is a new diagnostic term coined for *DSM*-III, but is based primarily on Briquet's syndrome (refers to the condition of hysteria as described by French psychiatrist Paul Briquet in his monumental treatise of 1859).

B. Prevalence

From .2 percent to 2 percent among females

C. Symptoms

1. Complaints invariably involve the following organ systems or types of symptoms: conversion or pseudoneurologic symptoms, gastrointestinal discomfort, female reproductive difficulty, psychosexual problems, and cardiopulmonary symptoms.
2. It is a chronic polysymptomatic disorder.
3. A screening list of seven symptoms (from a list totaling thirty-five items as the diagnostic criteria of the disorder) has been found highly specific for somatization disorder: shortness of breath, dysmenorrhea, burning sensation in the sexual organs or rectum, lump in the throat (difficulty in swallowing), amnesia, vomiting, and painful extremities.
4. The diagnostic criteria indicate that at least thirteen symptoms are necessary to make the diagnosis.
5. Often it is difficult to determine when the illness started or why the patient sought medical examination.
6. The conversion symptoms suggest neurological damage and are sometimes called pseudoneurological or grand hysterical symptoms.
7. Virtually everyone experiences many somatic symptoms, but we do not complain of them and rarely report them to a physician when we are examined because we interpret the physician's questions as referring to "significant" symptoms.

D. Associated features

1. Anxiety and depression are extremely common. It may be the depression for which the individual seeks psychiatric treatment.
2. Hallucinations are also reported, usually hearing one's name called (however, reality testing is intact).
3. Histrionic personality disorder and, more rarely, antisocial personality disorder often are also present (*DSM*-III-R).

4. Patients with this disorder have a propensity to abuse substances and to engage in impulsive behavior, as, for example, overdoses.
E. Onset and course
1. It begins in the teens or twenties (prior to the age of thirty).
2. It is rare in males.
3. The course is chronic but fluctuating.
4. Patients often have many medical examinations, are often admitted to hospitals for evaluation, and are frequently subjected to unnecessary surgery.
5. The patients' lives are often dominated by their symptoms, and they often lead lives as chaotic and complicated as their medical history.
6. They go from physician to physician.
7. They tend to overmedicate or become drug abusers.
F. Etiologic explanations for somatization disorders
The possibilities are nearly endless and include:
1. The specific cause is unknown.
2. The cause is presumed to be psychological, and assumptions are based on the usual presumed kinds of psychogenic factors.
3. There is increased incidence among family members, but there is not conclusive evidence of a genetic basis.
4. The somatizing person may be alexithymic (that is, unable to use emotional words to describe his or her feelings).
5. Social, political, religious, and economic issues place a premium on somatic diagnosis in preference to stigmatizing psychiatric diagnoses.
6. Many patients continue to emphasize their somatic complaints because the physician has made a symptomatic diagnosis such as nervous stomach, insomnia, or spastic colitis, not realizing that such symptoms can be physiological concomitants of psychiatric disorders.
G. Case example

A forty-six-year-old married woman presented herself at a hospital with a twenty-year history of multiple physical complaints, especially abdominal pain, dating back fifteen years. Asked her reason for seeking hospitalization, she immediately recited a long list of physicians, hospitals, and clinics she had visited, underscoring her dissatisfaction with all of them. She was very dramatic in her presentation. Although sexual themes appeared to underlie her symptomatology and behavior, she focused entirely on her physical symptoms, especially those referable to her abdomen. She reported that she had suffered for fifteen years and had continually sought medical care, and she stated, with a sort of glee, that all attempts had failed. Some of her physical symptoms were described in such a way that they seemed self-induced. For example, she said, "I was bleeding from the vagina, but I didn't pick at any specific place." In addition to seeing many internists, gastroenterologists, surgeons, gynecologists, and other specialists, she had seen several psychiatrists, who had attempted psychotherapy and psychotropic medication. A number of neurological examinations by excellent neurologists had been negative. A laparoscopy had been essentially negative. All medication had been unsuccessful.

On psychiatric examination, she was overly dramatic and superficial. She rambled on about her symptoms and tried to control the interview. She focused entirely on her physical symptoms, although there was a strong underlying sexual connotation.

After three or four weeks in the hospital, after attempts with various kinds of medication, psychotherapy, and joint therapy with her husband had failed, she left in an angry mood and proceeded to another hospital in a nearby city.

H. Treatment
   1. There is no standard effective treatment.
   2. Psychotherapy is usually recommended, although patients often can't link up psychological factors with their physical symptoms.
   3. Most patients end up refusing psychotherapy, so it is really the nonpsychiatric physician who often is the only one who might offer a helpful relationship to the troubled patient. To be helpful to such a patient, the physician must be comfortable accepting "incurable" complaints and have as a primary goal preventing the patient from "doctor shopping," without introducing *iatrogenic* factors (disorders unwittingly precipitated, aggravated, or induced by the physician's attitude, examination comments, or treatment).

VIII. **Somatoform pain disorder**
   A. Definition
      1. The essential feature of this disorder is preoccupation with pain in the absence of adequate physical findings to account for the pain or its intensity (*DSM*-III-R).
      2. As in conversion disorder, psychological factors are etiologically involved.
         a) When there is a clear temporal relationship between an environmental stimulus that is apparently related to a psychological conflict or need and the initiation or exacerbation of the pain.
         b) Or the pain permits the individual to avoid some activity that is noxious to him or her, or to get support from the environment that otherwise might not be forthcoming.
         c) Or in some cases, there may be no direct evidence of an etiological role for psychological factors (*DSM*-III-R).

3. Often the pain enables the patient to effect some secondary gain.

B. Associated features
  1. It may be accompanied by other localized sensory or motor function changes, such as paresthesia and muscle spasm.
  2. The afflicted person frequently visits physicians to obtain relief despite medical reassurance (doctor shopping), uses analgesics to excess without relief of the pain, requests surgery, and assumes an invalid role.
  3. The individual usually refuses to consider the role of psychological factors in the pain.
  4. In some cases, the pain has symbolic significance, such as pain mimicking angina in an individual whose father died from heart disease. A past history of conversion symptoms is common.
  5. Histrionic personality traits are seldom present, nor is *la belle indifference,* though concern about the pain symptom is usually less intense than its stated severity. Symptoms of depression are frequent (*DSM*-III-R).

C. Prevalence
  The prevalence of this disorder is not known, but is probably common in general medical practice, and such patients are probably usually seen by internists or general physicians rather than psychiatrists, because the patient focuses on the somatic aspects of his or her complaint. In addition, such a person is often extremely resistive of accepting even obvious emotional factors and hence refuses psychiatric consultation. Such persons are said to be alexithymic (persons who define their emotions only in terms of somatic sensations or in behavioral reactions rather than relating them to accompanying thoughts).

D. Concept of chronic pain
  1. According to Whittington (1985), the present-day conception of chronic pain is based on a biopsychosocial model—pain is viewed as a form of abnormal illness behavior influenced by a wide range of biological, psychological, and social factors. This broader conceptualization of chronic pain has emerged from social psychology, neurochemistry, learning theory, and psychophysiology.
  2. Some speak of the "sick role" behavior to account for the disparity between the pain/disability and the detectable disease.
  3. Since most chronic pain sufferers are emotionally disturbed, it has often been assumed that the emotional disturbance caused the chronic pain. When this emotional disturbance is depression, the pain has been interpreted as a "depressive

equivalent." (In part this is supported by the observation that antidepressants sometimes improve chronic pain.)

4. Characteristics of chronic pain patients (Whittington 1985)
   a) Generally they have started work at an early age and were dutiful, compliant, subassertive, and industrious in their work career before the injury.
   b) Their world view is essentially moralistic.
   c) They are not psychologically minded or especially insightful.
   d) They frequently feel alienated from the dominant political, social, and economic system.
   e) They do not have good verbal skills (alexithymia). It should be kept in mind, however, that individuals with poor language skills and poor ability to manipulate symbols are most often relegated to a life of menial labor and because of this are more likely to experience an industrial accident with a consequent injury to cause chronic pain. (The above are all characteristics of the pain patient *before* the pain begins.)

5. After the underlying injury, a very complex social system is brought into play including the patient and his or her immediate family, employers, physicians, co-workers, insurers and their agents, attorneys, judges, and workers' compensation referees.

6. In treatment they are dependent but noncompliant, are passive and have a sense of entitlement, are often very bitter and utilize projection extensively, and many are clinically paranoid by the time they enter a treatment program. Generally they are abusive of medications and of alcohol and show depressed affect. They are self-defeating.

E. The International Association for the Study of Pain (IASP) has promulgated a system of five axes as a nontheoretical comprehensive scheme for classifying pain in patients: (1) region, (2) system, (3) temporal characteristics, (4) intensity, and (5) etiology.

F. Treatment
   1. Treatment of such disorders is extremely difficult.
   2. Any psychiatric treatment must necessarily be based on adequate physical, neurological, and laboratory examinations, to rule out the evidence of physical disease. These are also a prerequisite to establishing the patient's trust in the physician's assurances about the patient's physical state.
   3. Supportive psychotherapy is probably the most useful approach in the treatment of this condition.

4. The judicious prescription of antianxiety agents and other psychotropic drugs, including tricyclics, for the appropriate symptoms is also often necessary.
5. The physician should be prepared to offer the patient an ongoing treatment plan.
6. Many patients with this disorder are referred to pain programs or pain clinics. These tend to have an eclectic approach and help the patient try to live with his or her difficulty rather than seeking relief through medications or surgery. Pain programs differ considerably in their patient selection and treatment modality. Most of the treatment focuses on rehabilitation rather than on cure, with emphasis on coping with rather than curing the pain.
7. However, it should be remembered that there are chronic pain sufferers who have not responded to the usual pain program, and some of these can only be maintained by the judicious prescription of appropriate analgesics and muscle relaxants.

## IX. Undifferentiated somatoform disorder
A. Definition
1. In this disorder there is either a single circumscribed symptom, such as difficulty in swallowing (globus hystericus), or more commonly, multiple physical complaints, such as fatigue, loss of appetite, and gastrointestinal problems. These symptoms are not explainable on the basis of demonstrable organic findings or known pathophysiologic mechanisms and are apparently linked to psychological factors (*DSM*-III-R).
2. Disorders in this category do not meet the full symptom picture of somatization disorder.

## X. Somatoform disorder not otherwise specified
A. Definition
Disorders with somatoform symptoms that do not meet the criteria for any specific somatoform disorder or adjustment disorder with physical complaints—for example: 1. an illness involving nonpsychotic hypochondriacal symptoms of less than six months' duration, or 2. an illness involving non-stress-related physical complaints of less than six months' duration. (*DSM*-III-R).

# References

American Psychiatric Association. *Diagnostic and Statistical Manual of Mental Disorders*. 3d ed., rev. Washington, D.C.: APA, 1987.

Blackwell, D., J. R. Galbraith, and D. S. Dahl. "Chronic Pain Management." *Hospital and Community Psychiatry* 35, no. 10 (October 1985): 99–107.

deLeon, J., et al. "Dysmorphophobia: Body Disorder or Delusional Disorder, Somatic Subtype?" *Comprehensive Psychiatry* 30, no. 6

(November/ December 1989): 457–72.

Ford, C. V. "The Somatizing Disorders." *Psychosomatics* (May 1986): 327.

Goldman, H. H. *Review of General Psychiatry*. Los Altos, Calif.: Lange Medical Publications, 1988.

Portenoy, R. K., and K. M. Foley. "Chronic Use of Opioid Analgesics in Nonmalignant Pain, Report of 38 Cases." *Pain* 25 (1986): 171–86.

Whittington, H. G. "The Biopsychosocial Model Applied to Chronic Pain." *Journal of Operational Psychiatry* 16, no. 2 (1985): 1–8.

# 13 Dissociative Disorders (or Hysterical Neuroses, Dissociative Type)

Not the power to remember,
But its very opposite,
The power to forget,
Is a necessary condition for our existence.

**Shalom Asch, *The Nazarene* (1939)**

## I. Introduction

In the *DSM*-II classification of mental disorders, psychogenic amnesia and multiple personality were categorized as hysterical neuroses, dissociative type. They are now classified as dissociative disorders, which also include depersonalization disorder (formerly termed depersonalization neurosis), defined as a disorder in which the person has feelings of unreality, altered personality, or altered identity and might deny his or her own existence along with that of his environment.

Thus, the characteristic that is common to all the dissociative disorders is a constellation of recent mental events that is out of the patient's awareness but is capable, under certain conditions, of being brought into consciousness.

## II. Definition

A. The essential feature of these disorders is a disturbance or alteration in the normally integrative functions of identity, memory, or consciousness. The disturbance or alteration may be sudden or gradual, and transient or chronic. If it occurs primarily in identity, the person's customary identity is temporarily forgotten, and a new identity may be assumed or imposed (as in multiple personality disorder), or the customary feeling of one's own reality is lost and is replaced by a feeling of unreality (as in depersonalization disorder). If the disturbance occurs primarily in memory, important personal events cannot be recalled (as in psychogenic amnesia and psychogenic fugue) (*DSM*-III-R).

B. Depersonalization disorder has been included in the dissociative disorders because the feeling of one's own reality, an important component of identity, is lost. Some, however, question this inclusion because disturbance in memory is absent (*DSM*-III-R).

C. Although sleepwalking disorder (somnambulism) has the essential feature of a dissociative disorder, it is now classified as a sleep disorder.

## III. Psychopathology

A. Essentially, these disorders reflect the mechanism of dissociation—that is, the unconscious detachment of certain behavior or aspects of personality from the normal or usual patterns of an individual. The detached material then usually functions alone (compartmentalization).

B. It is a more massive type of forgetting than is seen in simple repression.

C. Patients with dissociative disorders (as well as conversion disorders) have a diathesis (inborn tendency) for dissociation.

D. The ego is protecting itself against something that is critically dangerous and defending itself against overwhelming anxiety that develops because of an emotional bind.

E. Although the dissociation is handicapping, it relieves the individual's anxiety.

F. Dissociation is also symbolic and may have more than one meaning to the patient.

G. Primary gain (relief of anxiety) and secondary gain (advantage that accrues to the patient by virtue of the disorder) are evident in this condition (as they are in conversion disorders).

H. The premorbid personality is said to be immature and egocentric and have experienced some type of episodic emotional disturbance early in life. Still others are said to be histrionic, schizoid, or passive.

## IV. Types

A. Multiple personality disorder
B. Psychogenic fugue
C. Psychogenic amnesia
D. Depersonalization disorder (or depersonalization neurosis)
E. Dissociative disorder not otherwise specified

## V. Multiple personality

A. Definition
The essential feature of this disorder is the existence within the person of two or more distinct personalities or personality states. Personality is here defined as a relatively enduring pattern of perceiving, relating to, and thinking about the environment and

one's self, which is exhibited in a wide range of important social and personal contexts. Personality states differ only in that the pattern is not exhibited in as wide a range of contexts. In classic cases, there are at least two fully developed personalities; in other cases, there may be only one distinct personality and one or more personality states. In classic cases, the personalities and personality states each have unique memories, behavior patterns, and social relationships; in other cases, there may be varying degrees of sharing of memories and commonalities in behavior or social relationships. In children and adolescents, classic cases with two or more fully developed personalities are not as common as they are in adults. In adults, the number of personalities or personality states in any one case varies from two to more than one hundred, with occasional cases of extreme complexity. Approximately one-half of recently reported cases have ten personalities or fewer, and half have more than ten (*DSM*-III-R).

B. Characteristics of multiple personality (Nemiah in Kaplan and Sadock 1989)
   1. At any given time, the patient is dominated by one of two or more distinct personalities (the behavior and attitude are determined by that personality).
   2. The transition from one personality to another is usually sudden and often dramatic.
   3. There is amnesia pairing each state for the existence of the other personality or personalities and for any events that occurred.
   4. Each personality is a fully integrated, highly complex set of associated memories with personal relationships, characteristic attitudes, and behavior patterns.
   5. Mental-status evaluation reveals no abnormalities other than the amnesia for periods of time.

C. Prevalence
   Although at one time considered to be rare, within the last decade, multiple personality disorder has been diagnosed, treated, and studied with increasing frequency. What distinguishes it from all other psychiatric syndromes is the ongoing coexistence of relatively consistent but alternating separate identities plus recurrent episodes of memory distortion, frank amnesia, or both (Kluft 1987).

D. Age at onset
   It almost invariably begins in childhood but does not come to clinical attention until much later. Child abuse and incest are very common during childhood (75 to 88 percent experience sexual abuse during childhood), but because many are reluctant

to volunteer this information, it must be elicited by specific inquiry. Probably the victims dealt with the accompanying pain and despair through the use of dissociation).

E. Sex ratio

The ratio of victims of multiple personality disorder has been reported at 9:1 predominance in females.

F. Associated feature

Many clinicians working with both multiple personality disorder and post-traumatic stress disorder have remarked on the similarity of the two conditions.

G. While dissociation is the major mechanism operating in this disorder, identification is also evident in the fashioning of the second personality.

H. Course: Unattended, it tends to become a chronic condition; however, some may achieve synthesis of the personality through prolonged psychotherapy.

## VI. Psychogenic fugue

A. Definition

The essential feature of this disorder is sudden, unexpected travel away from home or customary work locale with assumption of a new identity and an inability to recall one's previous identity. Perplexity and disorientation may occur. Following recovery, there is no recollection of events that took place during the fugue. The diagnosis is not made in the presence of an organic mental disorder (*DSM*-III-R).

B. Predisposing factors and course

Heavy alcohol use may predispose an individual to the development of the disorder. The fugue is usually of brief duration. Recovery is usually rapid and recurrences are rare.

C. Prevalence

It is apparently rare but more common in wartime or in the wake of a natural disaster.

D. Unlike the patient with psychogenic amnesia, the patient with fugue is unaware that he or she has forgotten anything.

E. Case example

J. R., a twenty-five-year-old soldier, was admitted to the prison ward of a military hospital, accused of desertion. His history revealed that he had served with distinction in combat and was twice wounded. Following his second wound, he was evacuated to the U.S. mainland for further treatment. After a brief period at one hospital, the medical staff decided he could be managed best at another hospital several hundred miles away and placed him on a train for that destination. The man never arrived at the second hospital. Six months later, he was discovered in another section of the country, living the life of a civilian under an assumed name. He was unable to identify himself correctly and could not account for his activities during the entire six-month period. His real identity was established only through his fingerprints.

## VII. Psychogenic amnesia

A. The essential feature of this disorder is sudden inability to recall important personal information, an inability not due to an organic mental disorder (*DSM*-III-R). If the person travels to another locale and assumes a new identity, the case is diagnosed as psychogenic fugue.

B. Unlike somnambulism, the person with psychogenic amnesia usually does not give any indication to others that there is anything wrong with him or her.

C. There are four types of disturbance in recall.

1. Localized (circumscribed) amnesia
   *Localized amnesia* is failure to recall all events during a circumscribed period of time, usually the first few hours following a profoundly disturbing event (this is the most common type).

2. Selective (systematized) amnesia
   *Selective amnesia* is failure to recall some, but not all, of the events occurring during a circumscribed period of time (somewhat less common).

3. Generalized amnesia
   *Generalized amnesia* is failure to recall the individual's entire life.

4. Continuous amnesia
   *Continuous amnesia* is failure to recall events subsequent to a specific time and up to, and including, the present. (Generalized and continuous amnesia are the least common types.)

D. During an ongoing amnesia episode, perplexity, disorientation, and purposeless wandering may occur (*DSM*-III-R).

E. Psychogenic amnesia is a pathological loss of memory.

1. This type of amnesia must be distinguished from the amnesias associated with organic brain damage and alcoholism.

2. It is more than a mere forgetting. Rather, it is an active "blotting out" of consciousness containing conflictual material.

3. It is most often a response to intense feelings such as terror, anger, or guilt.

4. Its onset is usually sudden, and it is of brief duration.

5. It is apparently rare and is usually seen in wartime or during natural disasters.

6. The individual is usually indifferent to the loss of memory (a similar indifference is found in conversion disorder).

F. Case example

Mrs. H., a forty-two-year-old housewife, entered the hospital complaining of several brief periods of memory loss. History revealed that the onset of the first episode coincided with her learning that her husband was going out with another woman. Subsequent episodes usually followed some incident in which she was reminded of the "other woman."

## VIII. Depersonalization disorder (depersonalization neurosis)
A. Definition
   1. The essential feature of this disorder is the occurrence of persistent or recurrent episodes of depersonalization sufficiently severe to cause marked distress. The diagnosis is not made when the symptom of depersonalization is secondary to any other disorder, such as panic disorder or agoraphobia without history of panic disorder (*DSM*-III-R).
   2. The symptom of depersonalization involves an alteration in the perception or experience of the self in which the usual sense of one's own reality is temporarily lost or changed. This is manifested by a feeling of detachment from and being an outside observer of one's mental processes or body, or of feeling like an automaton, or as if in a dream. Various types of sensory anesthesia and a sensation of not being in complete control of one's actions, including speech, are often present. All of these feelings are ego-dystonic, and the person maintains intact reality testing (*DSM*-III-R).
   3. It may be defined as a disorder of affect, in which the person has feelings of unreality, altered personality, or altered identity. Patients may deny their own existence or that of their environment.
   4. An essential feature is the frequent occurrence of prolonged episodes.
   5. Derealization is frequently present. (This is a feeling that the environment has changed.)
B. Depersonalization
   1. Depersonalization disorder is not to be confused with depersonalization, which occurs as a secondary finding in other disorders.
   2. Depersonalization as a secondary finding or symptom is not considered an illness or disorder.
   3. Brief episodes of depersonalization, without significant impairment, are a common symptom, said to occur in 30 to 70 percent of young adults.

4. Some common examples of depersonalization are hypnagogic hallucinations (the mental images that occur just before sleep) and hypnopompic hallucinations (images seen in dreams that persist on awakening). These are experienced by healthy people.

C. Types

Related to depersonalization disorder are the following:

1. Trance states and trancelike states

A *trance state* is a psychological stupor characterized by immobility and unresponsiveness to the environment. It usually has a sudden onset, and amnesia follows. A *trancelike state* is a similar experience, ordinarily induced in normal individuals by prolonged and unusual concentration on a task or object.

2. Feelings of unreality

a) *Feelings of unreality* are feelings that one is unreal.

b) *Feelings of derealization* are feelings that the environment has changed.

c) *Depersonalization* (see previous discussion) is a sense of estrangement from oneself.

3. *Déjà vu*

*Déjà vu* is a subjective sensation that an experience that is really happening for the first time occurred on a previous occasion. It is the obverse of depersonalization. Experienced by normal people, it also occurs in certain disorders, including psychotic disorders and in organic mental disorders.

4. Feelings of estrangement

*Feelings of estrangement* are a sense of detachment from people, the environment, or concepts. The term embraces paramnesia, distortion, or falsification of memory in which the individual confuses reality and fantasy.

5. Fascination, or fixation

*Fascination,* or *fixation,* is a trancelike state induced in individuals (e.g., pilots) who are compelled to focus on a given object for long periods of time.

6. Cosmic consciousness, or illumination

*Cosmic consciousness,* or *illumination,* is a fabulous sense of joy or well-being, sometimes produced by hallucinogenic drugs.

D. Etiology

1. The etiology remains obscure.

2. There is little agreement regarding the exact mechanism of depersonalization.

E. Prevalence
1. It is apparently very rare as a pure syndrome.
2. It usually occurs between the ages of fifteen and fifty.
F. Course and prognosis
1. The course and prognosis depend upon the patient's motivation to get well, his or her ego strength, the duration of the disorder, and the strength of the secondary gain.
2. The onset is usually in late adolescence or early adult life and generally has a chronic course with remissions and exacerbations.
3. Little is known about precipitating factors.
4. The symptoms of all the dissociative disorders usually increase when the patient is confronted with mounting anxiety.
5. In general, the immediate prognosis is good when the dissociative episode has an acute onset.
6. When there is a close relationship between some environmental factor and the onset, the prognosis is good if the person is removed from the threatening environment.
7. In some cases, the long-term prognosis is only fair.

IX. **Dissociative disorder not otherwise specified**
A. Definition
Disorders in which the predominant feature is a dissociative symptom that does not meet the criteria for a specific dissociative disorder.
B. Among the examples of this would be Ganser's syndrome: "the syndrome of approximate answers" to questions, commonly associated with other symptoms such as amnesia, disorientation, perceptual disturbances, fugue, and conversion symptoms. This was named for Sigbert J. M. Ganser, German psychiatrist (1853–1931). It is also called the "nonsense syndrome" or prison psychosis because it is often observed in prisoners who, it is believed, hope to be treated leniently by the court in view of their symptoms.

In *DSM*-III, Ganser's syndrome was listed as a factitious disorder with psychological symptoms.

X. **Course**
Characteristically, dissociative disorders have sudden onset and sudden termination.

XI. **Treatment**
A. Most of the dissociative disorders respond to psychotherapeutic intervention.
B. Often, especially in psychogenic amnesia, the therapist can gain access to the unconscious mental conflict after a few interviews, by permitting the patient to free-associate to dream material or

to any incidents that family or other informants may recall about the patient's locale or behavior.

C. Occasionally it may be necessary to interview the patient under intravenous Amytal to help him or her recount the amnesic material and retain these in consciousness after awakening.

D. The presence of a significant degree of secondary gain may make it difficult to remove the symptoms.

## References

American Psychiatric Association. *Diagnostic and Statistical Manual of Mental Disorders.* 3d. ed., rev. Washington, D.C.: APA, 1987.

Eaton, M. T., Jr., M. H. Peterson, and J. A. Davis. *Psychiatry.* 4th ed. Garden City, N.Y.: Medical Examination Publishing, 1981.

Kaplan, H. I., and B. J. Sadock, eds. *Comprehensive Textbook of Psychiatry/V.* 5th ed. Baltimore: Williams & Wilkins, 1989.

Kluft, R. P. "An Update on Multiple Personality Disorder." *Hospital and Community Psychiatry* 38 (April 1987): 363–73.

Kolb, L. C., and H. K. H. Brodie. *Modern Clinical Psychiatry.* 10th ed. Philadelphia: Saunders, 1982.

Nemiah, J. "Psychoneurotic Disorders." In *The New Harvard Guide to Psychiatry,* edited by A. M. Nicholi. Cambridge: Belknap Press, 1988.

# 14 Factitious Disorders

And thus I clothe my naked villany
With odd old ends stol'n forth of holy writt,
And seem a saint when most I play the devil.

**William Shakespeare, *King Richard III***

I. **Introduction**
   A. "Factitious" means not real, genuine, or natural. Factitious disorders are, therefore, characterized by physical or psychological symptoms that are intentionally produced or feigned. The sense of intentionally producing a symptom is subjective; it can only be inferred by an outside observer (*DSM*-III-R).
   B. Factitious disorders are distinguished from acts of malingering. In malingering, the "patient" also produces the symptoms intentionally, but it is for a goal that is obviously recognizable when the environmental circumstances are known.
   C. In contrast, in a factitious disorder there is no apparent goal other than to assume the patient role. A long history of seeking hospitalization suggests that some persons have made a career of patienthood.
   D. Thus, factitious disorders are distinguished from other abnormal illness-affirming states, such as malingering and hysterical conversion disorders.
   E. Abnormal illness-affirming states
      1. Malingering: Signs and symptoms of illness are consciously produced and consciously motivated.
      2. Hysterical conversion disorders (also including somatoform pain, hypochondriasis, and Briquet's syndrome): Signs and symptoms are unconsciously produced and unconsciously motivated.
      3. Factitious disorders: Signs and symptoms are consciously produced but unconsciously motivated.

II. **Types**
   Factitious disorders usually present with either
   A. Physical symptoms

B. Psychological symptoms
## III. Levels of disorder
A. Factitious illness can exist at three levels.
1. Factitious history (without support of physical evidence)
2. Simulation of signs of illness (for example, dropping blood in the urine)
3. Producing abnormal *pathophysiological states* (for example, a) using dicoumarol to modify the bleeding and clotting time, or b) injecting insulin to produce hypoglycemia, or c) injecting foreign substances such as saliva to produce abscesses)
## IV. Factitious disorder with physical symptoms
A. Definition

The essential feature is the intentional production of physical symptoms. The presentation may be total fabrication, as in complaints of acute abdominal pain in the absence of any such pain; self-inflicted, as in the production of abscesses by injection of saliva into the skin; an exaggeration or exacerbation of a preexisting physical condition, as in the acceptance of a penicillin injection despite a known history of anaphylactic reaction; or any combination or variation of these (*DSM*-III-R).

The best-studied form of this disorder has been called Münchhausen syndrome. In this chronic form of the disorder, the person's plausible presentation of factitious physical symptoms is associated with multiple hospitalizations. The name was suggested by Richard Asher in 1951 (named after Baron Münchhausen, a real character of the eighteenth century who wandered from city to city and from tavern to tavern telling tall tales). He thought this name was appropriate because the patients wandered from hospital to hospital ("hospital hoboes"), feigned acute medical or surgical illness, and gave false and fanciful information. This has also been called "hospital addiction," although it is doubtful that it is dynamically similar to addiction, and "peregrinating professional patients." Impostership (fabrications of attainments, positions, or worldly possessions) is common to this disorder. Once hospitalized, patients are rarely quiet or cooperative. The behavior is frequently described as truculent, evasive, and hostile; when confronted with the evidence of factitiousness, they sign out against advice.

B. Prevalence

The prevalence is unknown. Some believe that it is rare and that those who have the disorder are overreported, whereas others think the disorder is common but rarely recognized.

C. Symptoms

Common clinical pictures include severe right lower quadrant pain associated with nausea and vomiting, dizziness and blacking out, massive hemoptysis (the expectoration of blood from some part of the respiratory tract), generalized rashes and abscesses, fevers of undetermined origin, bleeding secondary to ingestion of anticoagulants, and "lupuslike" syndromes. Any organ system may be involved, and the symptoms are reflections of the person's medical sophistication and imagination.

D. Sex ratio

*DSM*-III-R reports the disorder as "apparently more common in males," but others say that it seems to occur equally in men and women.

E. Etiology

1. From a psychodynamic point of view, the patient seems to be seeking a repetitive relationship with a physician to reenact a maternal type of relationship.

2. The psychodynamic origin seems to lie in early childhood experiences, that is, emotional and/or physical deprivation.

3. Some have noted that their patients often have borderline personality traits (with developmental difficulty during the separation/individuation phase of childhood).

4. The history often includes a period of hospitalization during early childhood. The developmental history may reveal several themes.

   a) A sense of needing to be taken care of
   b) Masochism
   c) Mastery of an early trauma (thus using factitious illness as a means of mastering a relationship with a parental figure)

F. Treatment

1. Treatment is difficult. A nonpunitive attitude on the part of the treatment staff and gentle, nonjudgmental confrontation would seem appropriate. This would include psychiatric consultation as an attempt to develop a supportive relationship with the patient prior to confrontation.

2. Additionally, the staff who have had to deal with the factitiously disordered patient need an opportunity to ventilate their anger at having been deceived.

3. Psychotherapy by an experienced and skilled psychotherapist, with treatment aimed at improving the patient's autonomy and self-esteem while reducing the sense of helplessness, vulnerability, and anger.

4. The goal of treatment is not necessarily to effect a cure, rather it is a try to prevent further morbidity and surgery and avert further hospitalization.
G. Differential diagnosis: Since it is an example of abnormal illness-affirming behavior, it must be differentiated from other forms of illness-affirming behaviors.
   1. The chief consideration is true physical disorder.
   2. Somatoform disorder (symptoms are not intentionally produced).
   3. Malingering (the goal is usually apparent).
   4. Antisocial personality disorder (rarely associated with chronic hospitalization as a way of life).
H. Natural history of the disorder is not clear because very few patients have had careful psychiatric evaluation.
   1. Most have thought to have had a deprived early childhood or had hospitalizations during the first five years of life.
   2. Children who remain home from school feigning illness are at risk for this disorder.
   3. The onset of the disorder is usually in adolescence or early adult years (Eisendrath 1988).

## V. Factitious disorder with psychological symptoms
A. Definition
   1. The essential feature of this disorder is intentional production or feigning of psychological (often psychotic) symptoms suggestive of mental disorder. The person's goal is apparently to assume the "patient" role and is not otherwise understandable in light of the person's environmental circumstances (as is the case in malingering).
   2. It is sometimes called "nonsense syndrome" (Ganser's syndrome) or the syndrome of deviously relevant answers.
B. Associated features
   1. Giving the approximate answers or talking past the point (*Vorbeireden*) may be present.
   2. This disorder is almost always superimposed on a severe personality disorder (for example, borderline personality disorder). The person surreptitiously uses psychoactive substances to produce symptoms suggesting a nonorganic mental disorder (e.g., stimulants, hallucinogens, analgesics, hypnotics).
C. "The conspicuous features of this disorder consist of a childish, ludicrous performance of simple acts, the correct procedure for which is fully known by the patient" (Kolb and Brodie 1982).
D. Sex ratio
Apparently more common in males

E. Course

May be limited to a single, brief episode or may be chronic.

F. Differential diagnosis

1. Other mental disorders.

2. Little is known about the incidence of these disorders.

3. The etiology, psychodynamics, and treatment are probably similar for patients with chronic factitious disorder (with physical symptoms).

4. Studies suggest that patients with factitious psychological disorder have a poorer prognosis than they would if they had a true major mental disorder (Pope, Jones, and Jones 1982: "It appears that acting crazy may bode more ill than being crazy.")

VI. **Factitious disorder not otherwise specified**

A. According to *DSM*-III-R, this is a category for cases that cannot be classified in any other specific categories.

B. Factitious physical and factitious psychological symptoms, sometimes called atypical factitious disorder, can often present a primary care physician with mild intermittent physical problems such as factitious dermatitis.

C. There seems to be a large number of such patients who can maintain stable family relationships.

D. Psychodynamics are similar to those of patients with chronic factitious illness.

# References

American Psychiatric Association. *Diagnostic and Statistical Manual of Mental Disorders*. 3d ed., rev. Washington, D.C.: APA, 1987.

Eisendrath, S. J. "Factitious Illness: A Clarification." *Psychosomatics* (February 1988): 110–17.

Goldman, H. H. *Review of General Psychiatry*. Los Altos, Calif.: Lange Medical Publications, 1988.

Kolb, L. C., and H. K. H. Brodie. *Modern Clinical Psychiatry*. 10th ed. Philadelphia: Saunders, 1982.

Livingston, R. "Maternal Somatization Disorder, and Münchhausen Syndrome by Proxie." *Psychosomatics* (April 1987): 213–17.

Nadelson, T. "The Münchhausen Spectrum: Borderline Character Features." *General Hospital Psychiatry* 1, no. 11 (1979).

# 15 Consultation Liaison Issues/ Eating Disorders/AIDS

For so your doctors hold it very meet,
Seeing too much sadness hath congealed your blood,
And melancholy is the nurse of frenzy.

**William Shakespeare, *The Taming of the Shrew***

## I. Introduction

A. Consultation liaison psychiatry is a discipline that bridges psychiatry/psychology, and general medicine and other medical specialties. In this respect, it resembles the psychosomatic or psychophysiological approach.

In *DSM*-I (1952), the term *psychophysiologic autonomic and visceral disorders* was listed as a diagnostic group. It was a term substituted for psychosomatic disorders, since according to *DSM*-I the latter term seemed to point more toward a point of view, rather than a discipline of medicine, or medicine as a whole rather than certain specified conditions. The term referred to the visceral expression of affect and included the so-called organ neuroses (for example, gastric neuroses and cardiac neuroses).

In *DSM*-II (1968), psychophysiologic disorders were referred to as physical disorders of presumably psychogenic origin. They were characterized by physical symptoms involving a single organ system, usually under autonomic innervation (for example, psychophysiologic cardiovascular disorder, psychophysiologic respiratory disorder, psychophysiologic endocrine disorder, psychophysiologic gastric intestinal disorder, psychophysiologic genital-urinary disorder, psychophysiological musculoskeletal disorder, and hemic and lymphatic disorder).

B. In neither *DSM*-III (1980) or *DSM*-III-R (1987) is there a category labeled psychosomatic or psychophysiologic disorders. Instead there is a classification of psychological factors affecting physical condition. This category enables a clinician to note that psychological factors contribute to the initiation or exacerbation of a physical condition to which psychological factors are judged to be contributory. It can be used to describe disorders that in the past have been referred to as either "psychosomatic" or "psychophysiological." Common examples of physical conditions for which this category may be appropriate include, but are not limited to: obesity, tension headache, migraine headache, angina pectoris, painful menstruation, sacroiliac pain, neurodermatitis, acne, rheumatoid arthritis, asthma, tachycardia, arrhythmia, gastric ulcer, duodenal ulcer, cardiospasm, pylorospasm, nausea and vomiting, regional enteritis, ulcerative colitis, and frequency of micturition (*DSM*-III-R).

C. In the past, the term *psychosomatic* was used in a nosological or classificatory sense to refer to a group of disorders whose etiology, at least in part, was believed to be related to emotional factors. Subsequently, psychiatric nomenclature substituted the term *psychophysiological disorders* for *psychosomatic disorders*.

D. Presently, psychosomatic concepts and their application to patient care are viewed more as an approach or a movement rather than a special field of practice or medical inquiry.

E. The psychosomatic approach assumes that psychological and social factors are significant predispositions, onsets, and continuations of any illnesses. It can, in fact, be an approach to all patients rather than to just those who, in the past, had been considered to have traditional psychosomatic illnesses. More specifically, it is a *biopsychosocial approach*. (Some would say that the biopsychosocial approach is the successor to the psychosomatic approach!)

F. Modern consultation liaison psychiatry is based on the psychosomatic approach. Here, the psychiatrist is part of a medical team and directs attention to the intrapsychic forces within the patient, the ego defenses (adaptations to stress), life-style, and interpersonal relationships with the nurses and physicians. The psychiatrist directs attention to the special kinds of emotional problems an individual faces in the particular setting (e.g., intensive care unit, coronary care unit, renal dialysis) and also evaluates the family and social roles of the management of the patient.

G. While older theories were somewhat simplistic in their conceptions of psychosomatic approaches, with the advent of more research we are aware of the complexities of interacting biological, psychological, and social factors.

II. **Consultation liaison psychiatry**

A. Definition

The term *consultation liaison psychiatry* has been used in two ways:

1. The application of a specific body of knowledge and skills from psychiatry to patient care or physician education (J. L. Houpt).
2. A subspecialty in psychiatry that is concerned with clinical service, teaching, and research at the borderline of psychiatry and medicine (Lipowski 1986).
   a) The clinical service includes the provision of formal psychiatric consultation to other physicians and care-givers or liaisons with them to increase their awareness of psychosocial issues of patients.
   b) Teaching would include the instruction of medical students and other care-givers in the aspects of psychosocial medicine.
   c) Research includes studies by consultation liaison psychiatrists about psychosocial issues in relation to various physical illness and physical injury as well as abnormal illness behavior (for example, somatoform and factitious disorders).
B. Historical background
   Among the names of those who have attempted to integrate psychiatry and medicine are the following:
   1. Benjamin Rush (1745–1813). He was a physician and a signer of the Declaration of Independence. His *Medical Inquiries and Observations Upon Diseases of the Mind*, published in 1812, was the first American treatise on psychiatry. This is considered the first attempt to integrate psychiatry and medicine in clinical practice into the teaching of medical students. His holistic approach was a precursor of the modern psychosomatic movement.
   2. Adolf Meyer (1866–1950), founder of *psychobiology*, which was a comprehensive and holistic approach to the understanding of the individual. He became the director of the Henry Phipps Psychiatric Clinic of Johns Hopkins Hospital in the early twentieth century. This helped pave the way for the emergence of the psychosomatic approach and consultation liaison psychiatry.
   3. Subsequently, other psychiatrists were engaged in pioneering efforts that would advocate collaboration between psychiatrists and other physicians in teaching, clinical work, and research.
   4. Edward G. Billings is credited for founding the first formal division of consultation liaison psychiatry at the University of Colorado School of Medicine in 1934 (Lipowski 1986).

III. **The psychosomatic movement**
   A. Definitions

1. Earlier definitions equated psychosomatic medicine with specific disease or specific disease states (for example, essential hypertension, bronchial asthma, peptic ulcer, ulcerative colitis, rheumatoid arthritis, neurodermatitis, and hyperthyroidism). This definition has been superseded by the following.
2. Psychosomatic medicine has been used as a term that is interchangeable with consultation liaison psychiatry (Lipowski 1986).
3. Psychosomatic medicine most frequently refers to a particular theoretical approach to illness including the biopsychosocial model as described by George Engel.

B. Historical perspective
1. Specialists in this approach have seen the early origins of this approach in the writings of Hippocrates. Credit is also given to Francis Bacon, who spoke of "the sympathies and concordances between the mind and the body, which being mixed, cannot be properly assigned the sciences of either" (Schwab 1985).
2. Interest in this approach waxed and waned over the centuries, but "faded into obscurity during 1840–1920" (Schwab 1985).
3. The current era of interest in psychosomatic medicine dates back to Flanders Dunbar, M.D., whose book *Emotions and Bodily Changes* (1935) reviewed the literature dating back to the early part of the century and described certain personality traits (or types) that she correlated with a variety of physical conditions.
4. Although in the middle of this century, it appeared as if psychosomatic medicine might become a specialty within a short time, the movement later appeared fated for obscurity once again.
5. Currently, the psychosomatic movement seems to be in a phase of rapid development. "A number of cultural and intellectual processes favor its growth and importance. These include widespread public concern about stress, deleterious life-styles and the diseases of civilization, which many now agree, are psychosomatic" (Schwab 1985).
6. Thus, the psychosomatic concept seems to fit in very well with the current focus on the biopsychosocial model of health and illness.
7. In this chapter, we will discuss eating disorders and AIDS as conditions that seem to blend well into the matters discussed under consultation liaison psychiatry in the psychosomatic movement.

## IV. Eating disorders

A. Introduction

1. Most everyone is aware of the relationship between emotions and the gastrointestinal tract. It is thought by many that food is, very early on, associated with feelings of security, attention, and love. Various types of psychosomatic disturbances are associated with eating, digesting, and eliminating food.

2. In 1676, Morton described the characteristic triad—loss of appetite, amenorrhea, and extreme wasting without lassitude—in cases of "nervous consumption" or "prodigious abstinence."

3. About two hundred years later, Gull and Laseque labeled this condition anorexia nervosa.

4. Eating disorders, particularly anorexia nervosa and bulimia nervosa, have attracted the increasing attention of the general public and psychiatrists.

5. Despite the volume of recent research, etiology, pathology, and treatment remain largely unknown.

B. Classification

1. Eating disorders are characterized by gross disturbances in eating behavior.

2. Included in this group are: anorexia nervosa, bulimia nervosa, pica, and rumination disorder of infancy. Pica and rumination disorder are primarily found in young children and very likely not related to the other two. Anorexia nervosa and bulimia nervosa seem to be related and typically begin in adolescence or early adult life.

3. Obesity, which is probably many disorders, is *not* classified as an eating disorder in *DSM*-III-R.

C. Anorexia nervosa

1. Definition

The essential features are: refusal to maintain body weight over a minimal normal weight for age and height; intense fear of gaining weight or becoming fat, even though underweight; a distorted body image; and amenorrhea in females (*DSM*-III-R).

2. Description

a) Ninety-five percent are females. The typical anorectic is a white teenage female from a middle- or upper-class family, who plans to attend college.

b) It must be distinguished from other illnesses that are accompanied by weight loss, such as endocrine and other organic illnesses that produce malnutrition, loss of appetite, and loss of weight.

c) Clinical picture
   (1) Refusal to maintain body weight over the normal minimum for one's age and height.
   (2) Loss in weight of 15 percent; or, if under eighteen years of age, a 15 percent loss in weight when the gain in weight projected from pediatric growth charts is added. In the proposed tenth edition of the *International Classification of Diseases,* significant weight loss is defined as a body mass index (BMI) of 16 or less. BMI is defined as:

   BMI = **weight in kilograms**
   
   height in meters
   (3) Disturbance of body image and inability to perceive body size accurately.
   (4) Intense fear of becoming obese that does not diminish as weight is lost.
   (5) There is no known medical illness to account for the loss of weight.
   (6) Amenorrhea in females.
d) Anorexia is rare.
e) Essentially, the behavior of the person with this illness is governed by the desire to lose weight and the intense fear of gaining it. The behavior includes marked dietary limitation; abuse of laxatives or diuretics or both; and, sometimes, self-induced vomiting. (The last is a symptom of bulimia nervosa, which also may be present.)

3. Etiology
   The etiology of anorexia nervosa and bulimia nervosa, as with most psychiatric disorders, remains unknown.
   a) Many of these patients are described as "model" children, with perfectionistic tendencies and above-average achievement in school. (After the onset of anorexia nervosa, they become terrified of their lack of control and immobilized by their own perceived helplessness.)
   b) Two prominent features of this disorder are:
      (1) Distorted perception of their body image
      (2) Dread of not being in control
   c) Theories of etiology
      Several theoretical models have been offered to explain the etiology of these two disorders.
      (1) Psychodynamics
         (a) Early psychoanalytic interpretations regarded this as "fear of oral impregnation."
         (b) Many authors have assumed the psychodynamic factors contribute to the development of both of

these disorders. But few of these psychodynamic theories have actually attempted to relate anorexia to early childhood events.

(c) Abnormalities in the family (for example, as described by Hilda Bruch [1978]). However, almost all of the family studies have been uncontrolled, and it is difficult to establish if the abnormalities within the family were cause or effect.

(2) Biological

(a) Recent studies have indicated a variety of neuroendocrine abnormalities, but it is not clear whether these are related to the cause or merely effects of the cachectic state.

(b) Bulimia has been regarded as a convulsive disorder. This theory is based on the rationale that binge-eating episodes are stereotypic and automatic and there are a variety of electroencephalographic (EEG) changes.

(c) Recent studies have considered the possibility that anorexia nervosa and bulimia nervosa are related to bipolar and major depressive disorders (a high proportion of patients with these two disorders also have a mood disorder, and there is a high prevalence of mood disorder in the first degree relatives). There does seem to be a relationship between these eating disorders and mood disorders, but the relationship is not clear.

(3) Sociocultural

These are in response to society's recent emphasis on thinness, especially among women (sociocultural pressures at least seem to be a significant contributory influence).

4. Clinical course

a) Anorexia nervosa

(1) It usually begins in adolescent females (continues to lose weight even after she may have reached a normal weight).

(2) Becomes obsessed with food and weight.

(3) According to *DSM*-III-R, the most common course is a single episode with return to normal weight, but it is important to keep in mind that anorexia nervosa can be a lethal disease and the course may be "unremitting until death."

b) Bulimia nervosa
   (1) May follow an episode of anorexia nervosa or may begin on its own in late adolescence.
   (2) Binges usually involve high carbohydrate foods.
   (3) The binges vary from those in which a person vomits after eating any amount of food, to others in which bingeing and vomiting alternate with each other over protracted periods of time.
   (4) Preoccupation with food and body weight.
5. Psychiatric disorders associated with anorexia nervosa and bulimia nervosa
   a) Mood disorders (including bipolar and major depressive)
   b) Anxiety disorders (including panic disorder, agoraphobia, and obsessive-compulsive disorder)
   c) Substance abuse disorder (alcohol, amphetamines, and poly drug use)
   d) Impulse control disorders (for example, kleptomania)
6. Medical complications
   Many medical disorders can complicate these two conditions, which may be life threatening (as the consequences of cachexia, electrolyte imbalance, or acid base imbalance, etc.).
7. Prognosis
   a) The bouts will usually remit spontaneously.
   b) The full disorder is not common after the age of forty.
8. Treatment
   No specific treatment exists because the etiology of these disorders remains unknown and the needs of patients are far from uniform. Treatment should be pragmatic and designed to improve major areas of dysfunction (Hsu 1986).
   a) Hospitalization may be indicated to effectively assess the anorexia nervosa patient's condition and needs, and also to foster the development of a therapeutic alliance. In some instances it may be "lifesaving." It might also provide an opportunity to teach the patient how to eat properly. However, many patients can be treated in an outpatient setting. The best inpatient eating disorder units are usually eclectic in orientation. A certain percentage of people with this disorder remain refractory to repeated programs.
   b) Bulimia nervosa can usually be handled on an outpatient basis.
   c) Traditional psychoanalytic interpretative approaches are ineffective. However, psychotherapy has been found useful.
   d) Pharmacotherapy

(1) Certain psychotropic medications may enhance weight gain in the short term when used in conjunction with behavior or milieu therapy. (Included in these would be thorazine and tricyclic antidepressants.)

(2) Because of the coexistent depression commonly found in anorexia nervosa, many clinicians have used antidepressants, either tricyclics or MAOI drugs. (However, one must keep in mind the tyramine-free diet in the use of the latter.)

e) Outpatient therapy

The less emaciated, less severely ill patients who are not vomiting, purging, or suicidal may be treated as outpatients, using psychotherapy in an attempt to resolve underlying psychological problems.

f) Relapses

Although *DSM*-III-R indicates that a single episode of anorexia is the most common story, some authors feel relapses are common, especially within the first year.

g) Summary

The prevalence of anorexia nervosa has been increasing. Despite this fact, there has been no major breakthrough in treatment in recent years. However, it does seem that use of coercive treatments such as hyperalimentation and tube feeding are rarely necessary anymore.

D. Bulimia nervosa

1. Introduction

Although anorexia nervosa was described three hundred years ago, bulimia was not recognized until the 1950s.

2. Definition

The essential features are recurrent episodes of binge eating (rapid consumption of a large amount of food in a discrete period of time); a feeling of lack of control over eating behavior during the eating binges; self-induced vomiting, use of laxatives or diuretics, strict dieting or fasting, or vigorous exercise in order to prevent weight gain; and persistent overconcern with body shape and weight (*DSM*-III-R).

Amenorrhea is uncommon, and there usually is no weight loss.

3. Description

Bulimics view their bingeing behavior as pathological and dread their difficulty in controlling their eating. Their self-induced vomiting is usually common. Bingeing usually stops when the patient is discovered, falls asleep, induces vomiting, or develops abdominal pain. They are preoccupied with their appearance and body image. Some of the people with this disorder also have psychoactive substance abuse or dependence, most frequently involving alcohol, amphetamines, sedatives, or cocaine.

4. Clinical course
   This is usually a chronic disorder arising in the teens or twenties.
5. Etiology
   (a) The cause of bulimia nervosa is largely unknown. Some psychodynamic theories see bingeing as a gratification of sexual and aggressive wishes and vomiting as a symbolic "purging of the bad self." Descriptive and biological psychiatrists see it as having some relationship to depression.
   (b) See Etiology under Anorexia nervosa.
6. Treatment
   (a) See summary under Anorexia nervosa.

## V. AIDS (acquired immunodeficiency syndrome)—definition[1]

A. Acquired immunodeficiency syndrome (AIDS) is a late manifestation of infection by the human immunodeficiency virus (HIV), characterized by various opportunistic infections and Kaposi's sarcoma (KS). It represents the end stage of a gradual collapse of the "immune defense system."

B. AIDS is a disease that spreads through sexual intercourse and through the sharing of intravenous drug needles and syringes for the injection of illicit drugs.

C. Presently the U.S. population most likely to become infected with the AIDS virus are homosexual or bisexual men and male and female intravenous drug users. However, it is expected that heterosexual transmission will probably account for an increasing proportion of the infected (in Africa the spread is by heterosexual relations and neonatal transmissions).

## VI. Occurrence

A. More than 150,000 cases of AIDS have been reported in the United States, and more than half of these victims (mostly young, productive people) have died (*The Psychiatric Times,* March 1991).

B. It is an infection of worldwide scope with the highest occurrences in Africa, Western Europe, and the United States.

C. It has brought *fear* to many Americans in addition to the illness, disability, and death.

D. HIV (human immunodeficiency virus), the cause of AIDS and AIDS-related complex (ARC), has been recovered from many body fluids including blood, semen, vaginal secretions,

---

1. The authors are indebted to Gary R. Kravitz, M.D., for his contributions to the section on AIDS.

cerebrospinal fluid, and more rarely from saliva, tears, breast milk, and urine. Blood and semen have the highest viral concentrations.

## VII. Etiology and Pathogenesis

A. The cause of AIDS is the human immunodeficiency virus (HIV), which results in immune suppression that can lead to AIDS and AIDS-related complex (ARC).

B. HIV infects monocytes and helper-inducer (CD4) lymphocytes, the focal cell of the immune system, with resulting gradual depletion of these cells and progressive cellular immune deficiency.

C. Additionally, gastrointestinal, renal, cardiac, and central nervous system (CNS) disorders have been described in HIV-infected patients, which may be caused by opportunistic infections, malignancies, or directly by HIV.

D. Syndromes other than AIDS caused by HIV infections.
The clinical outcome of HIV infection includes a spectrum from chronic healthy carrier state to AIDS itself.

1. Acute HIV infection: Some people with primary HIV infection develop an acute nonspecific flu-like syndrome usually within three to six weeks after exposure. Common symptoms include fevers, rigors, arthralgia, myalgia, gastrointestinal symptoms, malaise, and often symptoms of lymphocytic (aseptic) meningitis, etc. Lymphadenopathy and skin rash may occur.

2. Asymptomatic HIV infection (a large percentage of HIV-infected individuals are clinically asymptomatic): The interval from HIV infection until the development of any clinical HIV-related illness may be as long as five to seven years or more.

3. Symptomatic HIV infection: Common constitutional symptoms include chronic diarrhea, malaise, weight loss, fatigue, fever, etc. (formerly called ARC).

4. Medical aspects of AIDS

   a) AIDS is a lethal illness with a one-year postdiagnosis mortality rate of about 60 percent.

   b) The two major disease categories are: (1) opportunistic infections, most commonly pneumocystis carinii pneumonia (PCP) and (2) Kaposi's sarcoma (KS).

   c) AIDS is a disease in which the body's immune system is progressively destroyed by the viral infection.

   d) AIDS can also attack the central nervous system and lead to AIDS dementia complex (with deterioration of memory, thought, judgment, and motor coordination), which is now believed to be caused directly by the HIV virus.

e) The average time from infection to development of full-blown AIDS is eight years. Many patients remain asymptomatic despite extremely low levels of CD4 lymphocytes, but most, if not all, will eventually develop AIDS.

5. Transmission of HIV can result from unprotected sexual intercourse, sharing of contaminated needles, and maternal-fetal transmission from HIV-positive mothers.

## VIII. Psychiatric aspects of AIDS

A. Psychiatric symptoms usually develop after the diagnosis of AIDS or ARC.

B. After the diagnosis is made, patient reactions are usually characterized by disbelief and denial followed by depression (with fearful uncertainty, hopelessness, and suicidal ideations) and anxiety (including panic attacks and insomnia).

C. Feelings of anger are common and directed toward ineffective medical care and the perception of public discrimination.

D. Neuropsychiatric deficits are frequently the result of CNS complications.

1. AIDS dementia complex (ADC) is characterized by deterioration in thought, memory, judgment, and motor coordination.

Postmortem findings indicate that 70 to 90 percent of AIDS victims have gross or microscopic evidence of CNS disease attributable to HIV, other infections, or neoplasms.

## IX. Treatment

A. The medical treatment of AIDS is not discussed in this outline. There is no cure for the illness and no known vaccine to protect people against it, but intensive investigation continues.

B. AZT is helpful but is not a cure. It can retard development of HIV dementia and improve cognitive functions in patients with established HIV dementia.

C. DDC (an experimental antiretroviral drug) is currently being investigated. Combination therapy for HIV infection is seen by some as the wave of the future.

## X. Psychiatric Treatment

A. Includes treatment of anxiety or depression in the same manner as they would be treated elsewhere, keeping in mind the limits AIDS may place on a treatment program.

B. Patient management should also include dissemination of the most recent updates on AIDS.

# References

American Psychiatric Association.
*Diagnostic and Statistical Manual of
Mental Disorders*. 3d ed., rev.
Washington, D.C.: APA, 1987.

Bruch, H. *The Golden Cage: The Enigma
of Anorexia Nervosa*. Cambridge,
Mass.: Harvard University Press,
1978.

Davison, G. C., and J. M. Neale.
*Abnormal Psychology*. New York:
Wiley, 1990.

Faulstich, M. E. "Psychiatric Aspects of
AIDS." *American Journal of
Psychiatry* 144–5 (May 1987): 551ff.

Hsu, L. K. G. "The Treatment of
Anorexia Nervosa." *American
Journal of Psychiatry* 143 (May
1986): 5.

Kaplan, H. I., and B. J. Sadock, eds.
*Comprehensive Textbook of
Psychiatry/V*. 5th ed. Baltimore:
Williams & Wilkins, 1989.

Lipowski, Z. J. "Consultation-Liaison
Psychiatry: The First Half Century."
*General Hospital Psychiatry* 8
(1986): 305–15.

Maxmen, J. S. *Essential Psychopathology*.
New York: Norton, 1986.

Schwab, J. J. "Psychosomatic Medicine:
Its Past and Present."
*Psychosomatics* 26, period 7 (July
1985).

*The Psychiatric Times* 8, no. 3 (March
1991).

# 16 Personality Disorders

There is something in the character of every man which cannot be altered:
It is the skeleton of his character. Trying to change it is like trying to train
sheep to pull a car.

G. C. Lichtenberg, *Reflections* (1799)

I. **Definition**

Personality traits are enduring patterns of perceiving, relating to,
and thinking about the environment and oneself, and are exhibited
in a wide range of important social and personal contexts. It is only
when personality traits are inflexible and maladaptive and cause
either significant functional impairment or subjective distress that
they constitute personality disorders. The manifestations of personality disorders are often recognizable by adolescence or earlier and
continue throughout most of adult life, although they often become
less obvious in middle or old age (*DSM*-III-R).

II. **Personality development**

A. Definition: There are very likely as many definitions of personality as there are authorities who have written about it. No single definition of personality exists.

B. Personality is defined by Campbell as follows: the characteristic,
and to some extent predictable, behavior-response patterns that
each person consciously or unconsciously evolves as his or her
life-style. The personality represents a compromise between
inner drives and needs and the inner (conscious) and external
(reality) controls that limit or regulate their expression. The personality functions to maintain a stable, reciprocal relationship
between the person and the environment; it is thus a composite
of the ego defenses, the autoplastic and the alloplastic maneu-
vers that are automatically and customarily employed to maintain intrapsychic stability.[1]

C. The American Psychiatric Association's *Psychiatric Glossary*
defines personality as "The characteristic way in which a person

1. R. J. Campbell, *Psychiatric Dictionary*, 5th ed. (New York: Oxford University Press, 1989).

thinks, feels, and behaves; the ingrained pattern of behavior that each person evolves, both consciously and unconsciously, as the style of life or way of being in adapting to the environment."[2]

D. More simply stated, personality is the sum total of a person's internal and external patterns of adjustment to life. Although there may be some variation in a person's behavior, the individual's adjustment is generally in a state of equilibrium because he or she has accumulated a repertoire of problem-solving techniques during growth and development. Personality reflects those coping mechanisms and ego defenses that one uses to maintain emotional equilibrium. (See chapter 6.) It also reflects the compromise that one has made among the pressures from instinctual drives, the environment, and the superego.

Thus, personality usually reflects the individual's techniques of getting along with other people and results from early developmental factors, including the influences of society, culture, and child-rearing patterns. Certain well-developed personality traits such as compulsiveness, narcissism, or dependency may be so minimal that they do not interfere with the individual's functioning.

III. **Characteristics of personality disorder**

A. Individuals with personality disorders do not develop symptoms that bother them. In psychoanalytic terminology, they have a *character neurosis* (in which impulses and ideas are acceptable to the ego as consonant and compatible with its principles) rather than a *symptom neurosis* (in which the stimuli from any source are rejected by the ego or are prevented from reaching the ego for consideration).

B. The personality disorder is characterized by its lifelong nature and the person's repetitive, maladaptive, and often self-defeating behavior (rather than discomfort or physical and psychological symptoms).

C. The disorders usually begin in childhood or adolescence and persist throughout most of adult life.

D. People with personality disorders are usually anxiety-free except when they are confronted with environmental stress.

E. Because problems are expressed in a maladaptive form of living rather than in symptoms, it is rare for character-disordered individuals to seek help at their own initiative. In general, such people tolerate stress poorly. If they are confronted by minor stresses, they are apt to become anxious; if confronted by moderate stresses, they may develop transient psychotic reactions.

---

2. American Psychiatric Association, "Personality Disorders," in *A Psychiatric Glossary,* 6th ed. (Washington, D.C.: APA, 1988), 137–64.

F. It should be remembered that many of the difficulties people have adjusting to the world may be due to social stress or disarrangement rather than to disordered character.

G. When the occupation or environment accepts or rewards the individual's behavior, such personality patterns may be compatible with success and satisfaction. For example, a narcissistic person might be very successful in the entertainment world.

H. Some evidence suggests that individuals with personality disorders are at greatest risks for other psychiatric disorders.

## IV. Etiological factors

A. Although the concept of personality disorders has a long history, at this point, little is known about causality and pathogenesis. Although little research has been published on personality disorders (exception: borderline personality and antisocial personality) in recent years, it seems likely that personality disorders are common.

B. Among the possible etiological factors are:
1. Genetic predisposition
2. Childhood experiences that have fostered deviant behavior:
   a) Being rewarded for "acting-out" behavior (such as temper tantrums or hostile-aggressive behavior)
   b) Being encouraged when overly conforming and being discouraged when creative
   c) Circumstances in which normal behavior is not allowed to develop—for example, having a rigid, unreasonable parent who adamantly refuses to accept any reason for nonconformity
3. Identification with parents or other authority figures who have similar deviancies

## V. Types of personality disorders

A. The personality disorders are grouped into three clusters
1. Cluster A (previously referred to as odd or eccentric). This group includes paranoid, schizoid, and schizotypal personality disorders.
2. Cluster B (previously described as dramatic, emotional, or erratic). This group includes antisocial, borderline, histrionic, and narcissistic personality disorders.
3. Cluster C (previously described as anxious or fearful). This group includes avoidant, dependent, obsessive-compulsive, and passive-aggressive personality disorders.

B. Included under this classification are
1. Paranoid personality disorder
2. Schizoid personality disorder
3. Schizotypal personality disorder
4. Antisocial personality disorder

5. Borderline personality disorder
6. Histrionic personality disorder
7. Narcissistic personality disorder
8. Avoidant personality disorder
9. Dependent personality disorder
10. Obsessive-compulsive personality disorder
11. Passive-aggressive personality disorder

C. In the new multiaxial classification of *DSM*-III-R, these disorders are listed under Axis II. This axis includes specific developmental disorders of children and adolescents. This axis allows for the inclusion of diagnostic entities that are usually not given consideration when the usually more florid Axis I disorder is under treatment (e.g., major depressive disorder, substance use disorder, etc.). Such a classification assumes that the attention to more than one clinical parameter of the disorder will "provide greater specificity and objectivity and a firmer basis for identifying subtypes."

D. The definitions of the personality disorders discussed in the rest of this chapter are based on the descriptions in *DSM*-III-R.

## VI. Paranoid personality disorder

A. Definition
1. The essential feature of this disorder is pervasive and unwarranted tendency, beginning by early adulthood and present in a variety of contexts, to interpret the actions of people as deliberately demeaning or threatening, as indicated by at least *four* of the following (*DSM*-III-R):
   a) Expects, without sufficient basis to be exploited or harmed by others
   b) Questions, without justification, the loyalty or trustworthiness of friends or associates
   c) Reads hidden demeaning or threatening meanings into benign remarks or events (e.g., suspects that a neighbor put out trash early to annoy him)
   d) Bears grudges or is unforgiving of insults or slights
   e) Is reluctant to confide in others because of unwarranted fear that the information will be used against him or her
   f) Is easily slighted, quick to react with anger, or to counterattack
   g) Questions, without justification, fidelity of spouse or sexual partner (*DSM*-III-R)
2. Does not meet the criteria for schizophrenia or delusional disorder.

B. Prevalence
1. People with this disorder rarely come to clinical attention, so its prevalence is not really known.

2. Substantially, all the psychiatric classification systems promulgated in the last two hundred years have noted some types of paranoid disorders. Paranoid disorders are poorly understood.
C. Associated features
1. Persons with paranoid personalities rarely seek psychiatric treatment on their own.
2. The disorder is more common in men.
3. Most paranoid people avoid intimacy.
4. Such a person may be "litigious, moralistic, and a collector of injustices" (Kaplan and Sadock 1989).
5. Paranoid patients often "personalize" fortuitous or coincidental events.
6. Impairment tends to be minimal because people with this personality disorder realize that it is wise to keep their unusual ideas to themselves.
D. Etiology
1. The specific causes of this disorder are unknown.
2. Abuse or early deprivation, coupled with genetic predisposition, may lead to the development of paranoid personality.
E. Treatment
1. In an effort to build a trusting therapeutic relationship, the therapist should include the patient in decision making.
2. Psychotropic medications may be helpful, including neuroleptics (such as phenothiazines, etc.), or tricyclic antidepressants or MAO inhibitors for fearfulness, anxieties, or depression.
3. Group therapy may be difficult because it might provoke the paranoid person's sensitivity.
4. "Not a single report of successful treatment has ever been recorded" (Freeman and Gunderson 1989).
F. Case example

J. H., a thirty-eight-year-old married man, was referred to the court's psychiatric consultant for evaluation after he had pleaded guilty to a charge of assault growing out of a complaint filed by his wife, whom he had beaten up one evening in a bar.

He admitted to one previous court appearance for leaving the scene of an accident and also admitted to being jailed overnight once for drunkenness. In an interview, he admitted to having beaten his wife once previously, but said that he only slapped her with his open hand. He admitted to arguing with his wife but claimed the arguments were not too different from those most married couples have.

His wife reported that he carried a chip on his shoulder most of the time and felt that people owed him something. She indicated that he was "very suspicious" of her friends and that he would not talk to them. He constantly suspected that his wife was unfaithful and was unable to place any trust and confidence in physicians even though, by neglecting to do so, he had impaired his health. His Minnesota Multiphasic Personality Inventory profile was consistent with a diagnosis of paranoid personality. He seemed to be the sort of person who could keep his paranoid feelings under control as long as he did not drink. When he drank, his suspicions and projected feelings were enhanced, and he acted on them.

## VII. Schizoid personality disorder
A. Definition
1. The essential feature of this disorder is a pervasive pattern of indifference to social relationships and a restricted range of emotional experience and expression, beginning by early adulthood and present in a variety of contexts, as indicated by at least *four* of the following (*DSM*-III-R):
   a) Neither desires nor enjoys close relationships, including being part of a family
   b) Almost always chooses solitary activities
   c) Rarely if ever claims or appears to experience strong emotions such as anger or joy
   d) Indicates little if any desire to have sexual experiences with another person (age being taken into account)
   e) Is indifferent to the praise or indifference of others
   f) Has no close friends or confidants (or only one) other than first-degree relatives
   g) Displays constricted affect, e.g., is aloof, cold, rarely reciprocates gestures or facial expressions such as smiles or nods (*DSM*-III-R)
2. Also known as *introverted personality*
B. Occurrence not exclusively during the course of schizophrenia or delusional disorder (*DSM*-III-R)
C. Associated features
People with this disorder are often unable to express their aggressiveness or hostility. They lack social skills.
D. Prevalence
1. The prevalence in clinical settings is low.
2. The term *schizoid* was originally coined by Eugene Bleuler (he described schizoid as "shut-in").
3. In *DSM*-III, the term *schizoid* was divided into:
   a) Schizotypal
   b) Schizoid
   c) Avoidant
E. Impairment
Socialization is severely restricted, and occupational functioning may be impaired.
F. Etiology
1. The role of genetic predisposition is not known.

2. May have an emotionally deprived childhood.
G. Treatment
   1. The therapist should try to establish a psychodynamically oriented relationship in which support and advice can comfortably be accepted (attempt to develop trust).
   2. Psychotropic medications may be useful (neuroleptics if psychotic-like features appear, antidepressant medications if depressive or anxious symptoms, and benzodiazepines if fearfulness or anxiety develop).
H. Case example

C. N., a twenty-five-year-old single woman, was referred to the court's psychiatric consultant for evaluation after she had been arrested in the lobby of a downtown hotel for drunkenness. Aside from her drunken state, no behavioral disturbance had brought her to the attention of the authorities. She had never been arrested previously.

During the interview, she was very quiet. Most of the information obtained from her was through a question-and-answer approach. She responded to direct questions but volunteered very little about herself. She had a somewhat disheveled appearance and wore an unusual amount of cheap jewelry. Although she was a college graduate, she was working as a cocktail waitress in one of the local country clubs. She readily admitted to having a drinking problem and estimated that about twice a month she drank to the point of blacking out. Most of her drinking was done alone, although some of it was in the company of other waitresses. She did not seem to be very introspective or reflective. When asked to give her opinion of herself, she said that she never thought much about herself. She admitted to being very passive and said that she felt easily led. The probation officer who had investigated her reported that she was a very shy, withdrawn person, sadly lacking in self-confidence.

## VIII. Schizotypal personality disorder
A. Definition
   The essential feature of this disorder is a pervasive pattern of peculiarities of ideation, appearance, and behavior and deficits in interpersonal relatedness, beginning by early adulthood and present in a variety of contexts, as indicated by at least *five* of the following (*DSM*-III-R):
   1. Ideas of reference (excluding delusions or reference)
   2. Excessive social anxiety, e.g., extreme discomfort in social situations involving unfamiliar people
   3. Odd beliefs or magical thinking influencing behavior and inconsistent with subcultural norms, e.g., superstitiousness, belief in clairvoyance, telepathy, or "sixth sense," "others can feel my feelings" (in children and adolescents, bizarre fantasies or preoccupations)

4. Unusual perceptual experiences, e.g., illusions, sensing the presence of a force or person not actually present (e.g., "I felt as if my dead mother were in the room with me.")
5. Odd or eccentric behavior or appearance, e.g., unkempt, unusual mannerisms, talks to self
6. No close friends or confidants (or only one) other than first-degree relatives
7. Odd speech (without loosening of association or incoherence)—for example, speech that is impoverished, digressive, vague, or inappropriately abstract
8. Inappropriate or constricted affect, e.g., silly, aloof, rarely reciprocates gestures or facial expressions, such as smiles or nods
9. Suspiciousness or paranoid ideation

B. Occurrence
Not exclusively during the course of schizophrenia or a pervasive developmental disorder (*DSM*-III-R)

C. Associated features
During periods of extreme stress, such individuals may experience transient psychotic episodes.

D. Prevalence
According to *DSM*-III-R, approximately 3 percent of the population has this disorder.

E. Impairment
Social or occupational function is commonly impaired.

F. Family
There is some evidence that people with this disorder are more common in the first-degree biologic relatives of schizophrenics.

G. Etiology
Schizotypal personality disorder is genetically related to schizophrenia, if we consider twin, family, and adoption studies (Goldman 1988).

H. Treatment
1. Psychodynamic attempts to establish helping relationships in which support and advice are accepted.
2. Because of the severe dysfunction in such patients, social and vocational rehabilitation are central parts of the treatment (Freeman and Gunderson 1989).
3. Medications depending upon clinical symptoms (for example, low-dose neuroleptics for illusions, ideas of reference, psychoticism, etc.).

## IX. Antisocial personality disorder

A. Definition
The essential feature of this disorder is a pattern of irresponsible and antisocial behavior beginning in childhood or early

adolescence and continuing into adulthood. For this diagnosis to be given, the person must be at least eighteen years of age and have a history of conduct disorder before the age of fifteen.

B. Prevalence
   1. Recent estimates indicate a prevalence of about 3 percent of American men and less than 1 percent of American women.
   2. It is more common in lower socioeconomic groups with backgrounds of rejection, deprivation, neglect, and abuse.
   3. Predisposing factors are attention-deficit hyperactivity disorder and conduct disorder during prepuberty years.
   4. The fathers of those affected often have the same disorder.

C. Symptoms, according to *DSM*-III-R criteria
   1. Current age at least eighteen
   2. Evidence of conduct disorder before the age of fifteen—at least three of the following: truancy; running away from home overnight; frequent initiation of physical fights; the use of a weapon in more than one fight; forced someone into sexual activity; physical cruelty to animals; physical cruelty to other people; deliberate destruction of other's property; deliberate engagement in fire setting; lying; stealing (with and without confrontation of the victim)
   3. Irresponsible and antisocial behavior after the age of fifteen—at least four of the following:
      a) Inability to sustain consistent work behavior (significant unemployment, repeated absences from work unexplained by illness in self and family, abandonment of several jobs without realistic plans for others)
      b) Failure to conform to social norms with respect to lawful behavior
      c) Irritability and aggressiveness as indicated by repeated physical fights or assaults
      d) Repeated failures to honor financial obligations
      e) Failure to plan ahead or impulsivity as indicated by one or both of the following: traveling from place to place without a prearranged job or clear goal and lack of a fixed address for a month or more
      f) No regard for the truth
      g) Reckless regard for his or her own or others' personal safety
      h) If a parent, lacks the ability to function as a responsible parent (inattention to a child's basic needs)
      i) Inability to sustain a totally monogamous relationship for more than one year
      j) Lacks remorse

4. Generalizations

Antisocial personalities persistently violate the laws, customs, and mores of the community in which they live. They show a lifelong pattern of acting-out behavior (disordered behavior) rather than the subjective discomfort.

D. Etiology

1. The causes of antisocial personality disorder are not clearly understood.

2. Family history

a) A history of antisocial personality disorder is often found in the fathers of both males and females with the disorder.

b) Findings in twin studies and adoption studies support the hypothesis of a genetic component.

3. Multiple causation

Recent studies indicate that both genetic and environmental influences are important (*DSM*-III-R).

4. Organic

At present there is no evidence that organic brain damage contributes to antisocial personality disorder. In the past, some cases of antisocial behavior have been precipitated by brain damage, for example, by severe head trauma or encephalitis. Although the behavior may be classified as antisocial, technically such individuals are not usually considered antisocial personalities, but are more properly diagnosed as having organic mental disorders.

5. Psychosocial

Some authorities consider psychological and social factors to be chiefly responsible for the development of antisocial personality disorder.

a) Social factors

(1) The antisocial personality comes largely from the lower socioeconomic groups. There is a high rate of delinquency in the slum areas of larger urban communities.

(2) Living according to the pleasure principle without regard for the reality principle is in part determined by social factors as well as by parental relationships.

(3) The families and environment from which antisocial persons come have high rates of broken homes, alcoholism, and antisocial behavior.

b) Psychological factors

(1) Johnson and Szurek (1952) describe the "superego lacunae" that developed in antisocial personalities

as a result of unconscious fostering of such behavior by the parents during the developmental years.

   (2) Antisocial personality disorder has been correlated with maternal deprivation in a child's first five years of life.

   (3) Some studies report that the mothers of children who develop this disorder show a lack of consistent discipline, lack of affection, and increased incidence of alcoholism and impulsiveness.

E. Psychopathology

1. The essential defect in antisocial personalities involves their character structure (hence, this disturbance is sometimes called a *character disorder* or *character neurosis*).

2. Like infants, antisocial personalities give direct expression to their impulses. They are seemingly incapable of adapting their urges to the demands of society and unable to postpone immediate gratification of their desires.

3. They defy, or come into conflict with, authority, and they lack sensitivity to other people's feelings.

4. Since they are dominated by unsocialized drives, they have difficulty in their relationships with others. Although intellectually they recognize that their acts are illegal or unethical, they seem uninfluenced by such knowledge.

5. They might be considered emotionally deficient. They are egocentric, selfish, make excessive demands, and are unable to view their own behavior objectively. They are usually free of anxiety, remorse, or guilt.

6. From the foregoing, it becomes apparent that the antisocial person has a poorly developed conscience (defective superego).

   a) Conscience is largely dependent upon relationships with parents or parent substitutes. One's value system is usually developed through one's relationships with parents (largely by identification) and is based on affection and trust.

   b) In antisocial persons, the identification process is faulty. Either they are unable to evolve a value system through the normal process of identification or they develop pathological types of identification.

      (1) *Hostile identification* is internalization of undesirable personality traits of parents or authority figures.

      (2) *Identification with the aggressor* is internalization of the characteristics of a frustrated or feared parent or parent substitute.

c) We often find a history of difficulty with parents or authority figures from the earliest years.

d) This history seems related to parental attitudes that are commonly unreasonable, neglectful, cruel, hypocritical, or inconsistent (e.g., vacillating or unpredictable). The child has difficulty attaching him- or herself to either parent as an example to follow or as a source of security because there has been a lack of mutual affection, tenderness, or trust.

e) Because of this detachment from parents and parent figures, the behavior of antisocial personalities develops no sense of direction (i.e., they are uninfluenced by any concepts of right and wrong).

f) Some authorities feel that in a sense, their willful, unsocialized behavior is a seeking for attention, affection, and acceptance.

F. Historical note

1. C. J. Prichard in the early nineteenth century described "moral insanity" (insanity primarily related to moral functioning).

2. Robert Koch, also in the nineteenth century, suggested the term *constitutional psychopathic insanity* (to describe chronic liars, swindlers, etc., who were thought to have some genetic defect in their inhibitory apparatus).

3. The term *sociopathy* (sociopathic personality) was introduced by L. N. Robins in her book *Deviant Children Grown Up: A Sociological and Psychiatric Study of Sociopathic Personality* (1966).

4. Hervey Cleckley, in his book *The Mask of Sanity* (first written in 1941 with editions through 1964), described the psychopathic personality and referred to it as semantic disorder.

G. Treatment

1. Persons with this disorder are usually poorly motivated for treatment. This is especially true because they often lack trust.

2. Peer pressure, described by Maxwell Jones in "The Concept of Therapeutic Community," (*American Journal of Psychiatry* 112 (1956): 647–50) in structured or confined settings may encourage change.

3. Family therapy may be helpful if the family dynamics are such that they encourage the antisocial person to "act out."

4. Trials of medication have given inconsistent results.

H. Case report

Bob, the eighteen-year-old son of well-to-do parents, was brought to the hospital for psychiatric examination upon the order of a judge. One night four weeks earlier, the patient had, in the company of three other boys, entered a cemetery, tipped over several gravestones, and mutilated a monument.

When Bob first entered grade school, he had some minor difficulties. He performed below his intellectual capacity and frequently did things that the other children considered "daring," such as letting the air out of automobile tires. At nine, he began to smoke, not just experimentally, like some of the other boys, but often and somewhat defiantly.

He first came into difficulty with the law at the age of eleven when he stole two cigarette lighters and a wristwatch from a jewelry store. Following this, he was sent to a military boarding school upon the advice of the judge and the family physician. Two months after he entered the new school, he broke into the school store, stole candy and cigarettes, and ran away to a nearby city. He was found two days later in a hotel room by himself. He was returned to his home and completed the school year at the local school.

At thirteen, he and two other boys stole a large amount of gasoline from a nearby storage plant. This was used in a "jalopy" purchased for the patient by his father. At first, he denied the theft but, when confronted with irrefutable proof, admitted his guilt; however, he was unable to give any reason for wanting the gasoline. From the age of thirteen until seventeen, he was frequently involved in minor delinquencies but always escaped punishment because of his family's position in the community and because his father always made restitution. At seventeen, he began drinking beer and shortly was getting "high" regularly.

Bob was the older of two brothers but was reared as an only child because his infant brother died when Bob was four. After this, the parents overindulged him. At five, he fell from a horse, following which he had a few convulsions. He was examined at a well-known clinic and placed on anticonvulsants. After a few weeks of this treatment, he quit taking the medications. He says he has never been really close to anyone and has never felt toward his parents as other youngsters do. Although the parents verbally disapproved of his behavior, they encouraged it in subtle ways—for example, increasing his already overly generous allowance after he was caught stealing from a hardware store.

At no time has he ever shown any guilt for his delinquent and antisocial behavior, and he always seems free of anxiety. His case illustrates some of the typical aspects of the antisocial personality disorder.

## X. Borderline personality disorder
### A. Definition
The essential feature of this disorder is a pervasive pattern of instability of self-image, interpersonal relationships, and mood, beginning by early adulthood and present in a variety of contexts, as indicated by at least *five* of the following (*DSM*-III-R):

1. A pattern of unstable and intense interpersonal relationships characterized by alternating between extremes of overidealization and devaluation

2. Impulsiveness in at least two areas that are potentially self-damaging, e.g., spending, sex, substance use, shoplifting, reckless driving, binge eating (does not include suicidal or self-mutilating behavior, covered in 5 below)
3. Affective instability: Marked shifts from baseline mood to depression, irritability, or anxiety, usually lasting a few hours and only rarely more than a few days
4. Inappropriate, intense anger or lack of control of anger, e.g., frequent displays of temper, constant anger, recurrent physical fights
5. Recurrent suicidal threats, gestures, or behavior, or self-mutilating behavior
6. Marked and persistent identity disturbance manifested by uncertainty about at least *two* of the following: self-image, sexual orientation, long-term goals or career choice, type of friends desired, preferred values
7. Chronic feelings of emptiness or boredom
8. Frantic efforts to avoid real or imagined abandonment (*DSM*-III-R)

B. Historical notes
1. "Borderline" has had different meanings over the past century. Among the previous labels were: *ambulatory schizophrenia, latent schizophrenia, preschizophrenia, schizophrenic character, abortive schizophrenia, pseudoneurotic schizophrenia,* and so forth.
   The *DSM*-III-R definition is classified as an Axis II disorder rather than an Axis I and represents an amalgam of the Kernberg (1967) and Gunderson (1975) "items."

C. Prevalence
It is apparently common and more frequently diagnosed in females.

D. Associated features
1. Features of other personality disorders such as narcissistic, histrionic, schizotypal, and antisocial are commonly present.
2. An Axis I diagnosis is fairly common as well (e.g., depression).

E. Typical clinical picture.
1. The borderline personality patient is stormy, unstable, over-anxious, anger-prone, impulsive, and destructive of self or others (Stone 1990).
2. The suicide rate is as high as that observed in the major psychoses (ibid).

F. Etiology and psychopathology
1. Early formulations of borderline psychopathology were based on the ego-psychological model of psychoanalysis;

thus, the borderlines were viewed as having weak ego structures that remained intact and able to cope with reality when reality was structured and consistent but that could be easily flooded by primary process thinking (largely unconscious psychological expressions of underlying basic drives that follow the pleasure principle) when external structure was lacking or internal pressures had upset the ego's precarious equilibrium (thus, such diagnostic terms as *borderline psychosis, borderline schizophrenia, ambulatory schizophrenia, preschizophrenia*).

More recent formulations have been influenced by object relations theory (the psychoanalytic description of the internalization of interpersonal relations and the organizing effects of internalized human object relationships on the structure of psyche), leading to the concept of borderline disorganization.

2. Most causal theories have been based on cases treated with psychodynamically oriented therapy. Most of the theoretical formulations have been psychoanalytic in orientation.

   a) Masterson (1972) sees the borderline personality in adolescence as characterized by a persistent symbiosis with parental figures. There is a predominance of negative feelings that are shared by parent and child, which persists and yet binds the two together by mutual guilty and bad feelings.

   b) Kernberg (1975) suggests that early pathological object relations are internalized and maintained by the use of primitive defense mechanisms that healthier people give up in normal development. These psychotic-like defensive operations are denial, projection, splitting, and projective identification (see chapter 6). Further, Kernberg sees the person with borderline personality disorder as categorizing people as all good (nurturant) and all bad (hateful). He relates this to the patient's early stages of psychosexual development, in which the mother figure is experienced in two contradictory ways (good and bad).

      Thus Kernberg hypothesized that the arrest in normal psychological development, with failure to integrate ambivalent feelings, originally arose against the primary caretaker but later occurred in other close relationships as well.

3. Mahler (1971) and Masterson (1972) have hypothesized that this disorder results after a disturbance occurring in children between sixteen and twenty-five months of age

during the rapprochement phase of separation and individuation. In this phase, the child practices independent behavior and returns to the primary caretaker for approval, admiration, and emotional "refueling." The critical, rejecting parent or the suffocating, smothering parent interferes with optimal progression of attachment-separation sequences.

4. Although most authorities regard etiology as largely psychodynamic some feel there is a genetic role, and Kernberg (1975) and Klein (1977) have suggested that patients with borderline personality have a "constitutionally based" inability to regulate effects, especially anger. There may also be a relationship between borderline personality and depressive illness.

5. This is the most written about personality disorder in the psychiatric literature. The hope is that this will lead to findings leading to better treatment, better definition, and stable outcome.

6. Recent studies indicate a high prevalence of physical and sexual abuse in patients ultimately diagnosed as having borderline personality disorder (Goodwin 1990).

G. Course and prognosis
   1. In the past, short-term follow-up studies have suggested that borderline patients do not change much.
   2. Recent evidence suggests that the long-term prognosis of this condition is relatively good with gradual improvement (provided the patient does not commit suicide or succumb to alcohol abuse).

H. Treatment
   1. Psychotherapy
      In the past, there were two viewpoints about treatment approaches to borderline personality disorder.
      a) Attempts at long-term psychotherapy for borderline personality disorder are fraught with anguish and hostility for both the patient and the therapist. Regression is a repeated problem.
         (1) A modified psychoanalytic approach was considered helpful and aimed at the resolution of the underlying psychopathology. Such treatment often required special ongoing support systems.
         (2) In supportive reality-oriented therapy the patient was offered a limited psychotherapeutic relationship, but the therapist expected to be indefinitely available. The goal in this treatment was gradual social adjustment. (Such an approach may include some behavioral approaches as well.)

2. Recent strategies are based chiefly on cognitive behavioral techniques of support, education and construction of alternatives. (Patients are asked to make a commitment to diminishing self-destructive behaviors and are supported in their efforts to do so. They are educated about the maladaptive nature of such behaviors.) (Linehan 1987)
3. Psychotropic medication
   a) Antipsychotic drugs may be useful during brief psychotic periods, and lower doses may be indicated for anger, hostility and suspiciousness, paranoid thinking, and so forth.
   b) Carbamazepine may increase impulsivity.
   c) Tricyclic antidepressants may be helpful during periods of depression, and monoamine oxidase inhibitors may also be helpful in improving mood (caution: dietary restrictions).
   d) Those who have bipolar traits might benefit from lithium.
4. Some authorities suggest the use of pharmacotherapy together with psychotherapy in the context of an ongoing supportive relationship with the therapist.
5. Treating borderline patients is a challenge, and the therapist must be continually on the alert for countertransference issues.

I. Case example

A sixteen-year-old white female was admitted to a residential treatment center upon referral of a psychiatrist who had treated her in an acute adolescent hospital for approximately six months. In his referral note, he reported that she was unable to function in her chaotic home situation. In addition to this, she was depressed in the hospital and had made suicidal gestures—specifically, cutting herself with fragments of glass and drinking bottles of cologne. In addition, he reported that she was showing academic underachievement, truancy, poor peer relationships, and had frequent headaches and temper outbursts.

Evaluation at the residential treatment center revealed that her manifest symptoms had begun to surface about a year and a half earlier, following a move from one part of the country to another. About this time, she became truant and engaged in activities that kept her four other siblings in constant turmoil. In addition, her peer relationships at school deteriorated, and she showed bellicosity toward her teachers. She even became physically assaultive of others in her school. There was evidence of a great deal of intense ambivalence, on her part, surrounding her mother and her relative degree of separation from and closeness to her mother. (The mother had had a series of men living with her, and about six months before the girl was admitted to the residential treatment center, her stepfather entered into a sexual relationship with her, of which the mother was unaware until just before the girl's hospitalization.) Shortly before her initial hospitalization, she had run away from home for a two-week period and suddenly reappeared in the police station to report that she had been physically abused by her mother and raped by her stepfather. After the parents were cleared of these accusations by an investigation, she was placed in a crisis home and then admitted to the local hospital.

From assessment performed at the residential center, it was learned that she had developed an ever-increasing degree of separation anxiety as a result of her impaired separation-individuation process. The periods of acting out seemed to be correlated with the imminent separation from her mother, and the speculation was that her sexual involvement with her stepfather was perhaps a search for a lost nurturant mother. Her identification seemed confused. She seemed to lack a consistent role model.

Her treatment plan, which included intense individual psychoanalytic therapy, lasted for approximately two and a half years. She made good progress in therapy and was able to surrender unstable relationships that were patterned after her mother; she also was able to express vulnerability instead of covering it up. In treatment, she showed a great deal of splitting and projective identification.

## XI. Histrionic personality disorder

A. Definition

The essential feature of this disorder is a pervasive pattern of excessive emotionality and attention seeking, beginning by early adulthood and present in a variety of contexts, as indicated by at least *four* of the following (*DSM*-III-R):

1. Constantly seeks or demands reassurance, approval, or praise
2. Is inappropriately sexually seductive in appearance or behavior
3. Is overly concerned with physical attractiveness
4. Expresses emotion with inappropriate exaggeration, e.g., embraces casual acquaintances with excessive ardor, experiences uncomfortable sobbing on minor sentimental occasions, has temper tantrums
5. Is uncomfortable in situations in which he or she is not the center of attention
6. Displays rapidly shifting and shallow expression of emotions
7. Is self-centered, actions being directed toward obtaining immediate satisfaction; has no tolerance for the frustration of delaying gratification
8. Has a style of speech that is excessively impressionistic and lacking in detail, e.g., when asked to describe mother, can be no more specific than, "She was a beautiful person." (*DSM*-III-R)

B. People with this disorder constantly seek or demand reassurance, approval, or praise from others and are uncomfortable in situations in which they are not the center of attention. They characteristically display rapidly shifting and shallow expression of emotions. Their behavior is overly reactive and intensely expressed; minor stimuli give rise to emotional excitability. Emotions are often expressed with inappropriate exaggeration; for example, the person may appear much more sad, angry, or delighted than would seem to be warranted. People with this disorder tend to be very self-centered, with little or no tolerance for the frustration of delayed gratification. Their actions are directed to obtaining immediate satisfaction.

C. These people are typically attractive and seductive, often to the point of looking flamboyant and acting inappropriately. They are typically overly concerned with physical attractiveness. In addition, their style of speech tends to be expressionistic and lacking in detail. For example, a person may describe his vacation as "just fantastic" without being able to be more specific.

D. Prevalence
*DSM*-III-R notes that the disorder is "apparently common" and diagnosed "much more frequently in females," in part because of the sex class and its description.

E. Associated features (*DSM*-III-R)
People with this disorder are lively and dramatic and are always drawing attention to themselves. They are prone to exaggeration in their interpersonal relations and often act out a role such as that of "victim" or "princess" without being aware of it. They crave novelty, stimulation, and excitement and quickly become bored with normal routine. Others frequently perceive them as superficially charming and appealing but lacking genuineness. They are often quick to form friendships, but once a relationship is established, can be egocentric and inconsiderate. They may constantly demand reassurance because of feelings of helplessness and dependency. Their actions are often inconsistent and may be misinterpreted by others.

In relationships they attempt to control the opposite sex or to enter into a dependent relationship. Flights into romantic fantasy are common. The actual quality of their sexual relationships is variable. Some are promiscuous; others, naive and sexually unresponsive; and still others, apparently normal in their sexual adjustment.

Usually these people show little interest in intellectual achievement and careful, analytic thinking, but they are often creative and imaginative.

People with this disorder tend to be impressionable and easily influenced by others or by fads. They are apt to be overly trusting of others and suggestible, and to show an initially positive response to any strong authority figure who, they think, can provide a magical solution for their problems. Though they adopt convictions strongly and readily, their judgment is not firmly rooted, and they often play hunches.

Frequent complaints of poor health, such as weakness or headaches, or subjective feelings of depersonalization may be present. During periods of extreme stress, people with this disorder may experience transient psychotic symptoms, but they are generally of insufficient severity or duration to warrant an additional diagnosis.

F. Symptoms

In addition to the symptoms listed under Definition, the patient often displays *"la belle indifference."* Women with this disorder may be coquettish, and men with the disorder may play the "Don Juan" role.

G. Case example

Scarlett O'Hara, the heroine of Margaret Mitchell's *Gone with the Wind,* seems to be a histrionic personality type. At the end of the novel, after she is rejected by Rhett Butler, she can't think of letting him go and thinks, "I won't think of it now—I'll go home to Tara tomorrow—I'll think of it all tomorrow at Tara. I can stand it then. Tomorrow, I'll think of some way to get him back. After all, tomorrow is another day."

## XII. Narcissistic personality disorder

A. Definition

The essential feature of this disorder is a pervasive pattern of grandiosity (in fantasy or behavior), hypersensitivity to the evaluation of others, and lack of empathy that begins by early adulthood and is present in a variety of contexts, as indicated by at least *five* of the following (*DSM*-III-R):

1. Reacts to criticism with feelings of rage, shame, or humiliation (even if not expressed)
2. Is interpersonally exploitive: Takes advantage of others to achieve his or her own ends
3. Has a grandiose sense of self-importance, e.g., exaggerates achievements and talents, expects to be noticed as "special" without appropriate achievements
4. Believes that his or her problems are unique and can be understood only by other special people
5. Preoccupied with fantasies of unlimited success, power, brilliance, beauty, or ideal love
6. Has a sense of entitlement: Unreasonable expectation of especially favorable treatment, e.g., assumes that he or she does not have to wait in line when others must do so
7. Requires constant attention and admiration, e.g., keeps fishing for compliments

8. Lack of empathy: Inability to recognize and experience how others feel, e.g., annoyance and surprise when a friend who is seriously ill cancels a date

9. Is preoccupied with feelings of envy (*DSM*-III-R)

B. Prevalence

It seems to be more common recently than in the past, although this may be due to recent clinical interest in this disorder.

C. Associated features

Histrionic, borderline, and antisocial personality characteristics are frequently found in association with this disorder. Depressed mood is common.

D. Clinical notes

1. The concept of narcissism was first described by Freud when he wrote about the psychosis of Schraeber.

2. The concept of borderline personality and narcissistic personality became widely popular in psychiatric literature after the appearance of the book by Otto Kernberg, *Borderline Conditions and Pathological Narcissism* (1975).

3. Although borderline and narcissistic personality disorders were originally regarded as discrete entities, they are now regarded by some as part of a continuum.

4. Much attention has been focused on the subject of narcissism not only in the psychiatric literature but also in the popular press. (For example, Tom Wolfe has labeled the 1970s as "the me decade.")

5. Renewed interest in narcissism has been fostered by the works of Otto Kernberg and Heinz Kohut.

a) Kohut believes that the diagnosis of narcissistic personality disorder can be established only by observing a spontaneously developing transference relationship in a trial analysis. He differentiates a narcissistic personality disorder from the borderline states.

b) Kernberg's description of the narcissistic personality agrees in general with the *DSM*-III-R proposed classification and regards the defensive organization of narcissistic patients as quite similar to that of borderline patients.

6. Margaret Mahler postulates a sequence of three "phases" of infantile development, directed ultimately toward the child's attainment of a sense of separateness from the mother.

a) Absolute autism—the period of William James's "blooming, buzzing, confusion"—occupies the first postnatal month and is characterized by the operation of basic life-sustaining reflex activities, and responses are essentially devoid of mental representation. During this period the infant's kaleidoscope world is organized around a "primitive good-bad" dichotomy of perceptions in accordance with the pleasure principle, which dictates that whatever reduces it is "good tension" and whatever increases or fails to reduce it is "bad."

b) Symbiosis, the second through the sixth postnatal month. During this phase the infant's "good-bad" perceptual dichotomy undergoes organization in relation to the figure or person of the mother.

c) The separation-individuation process. The child's sense of separateness from the world about him. This is divided into four phases:

   (1) Differentiation
   (2) Practicing
   (3) Rapprochement
   (4) Consolidation
       (See chapter 2.)

E. Treatment

  1. Dynamically oriented individual psychotherapy or psychoanalysis are the recommended treatments for patients with this disorder.

  2. Inpatient treatment may be necessary if the patient develops a severe depression or some other Axis I disorder.

  3. Group therapy (although narcissistic personalities often avoid this).

F. Case example

J. C., a thirty-two-year-old corporate junior executive, was initially seen in consultation, jointly with his wife, because of marital distress. This was his second marriage, and the couple had two children in elementary school. His wife complained that he was extremely self-centered and was always cool and distant with her. He was also remote from the children, but expected them to accomplish much to enhance his own name.

At work, he prided himself on his ruthless decisiveness in dealing with subordinates who might show signs of incompetency. About his superiors, he privately acknowledged that he would "play on their sympathy and compassionate feelings" to enhance his corporate position. He also confided that he had numerous brief extramarital affairs, and on a few occasions had homosexual encounters. A handsome man, he prided himself on his sexual technique and his ability to be able to enjoy both sexes.

In discussing his work relationships, it became clear that he had no loyalty to any colleague or company policy and felt that he would leave to establish his own business to "run things my own way." He had had some strong disagreements with some of his superiors about his own practices, which were at odds with the ethics of the company.

It was believed that part of his own motivation for seeking joint consultation was that he felt a divorce would cost him more financially and hinder his business plans. He felt that he could reduce the financial cost by superficially complying with his wife's wishes.

He abruptly announced his plans to terminate the counseling, and did so.

## XIII. Avoidant personality disorder
### A. Definition
The essential feature of this disorder is a pervasive pattern of social discomfort, fear of negative evaluation, and timidity, beginning by early adulthood and present in a variety of contexts, as indicated by at least *four* of the following (*DSM*-III-R):
1. Is easily hurt by criticism or disapproval
2. Has no close friends or confidants (or only one) other than first-degree relatives
3. Is unwilling to get involved with people unless certain of being liked
4. Avoids social or occupational activities that involve significant interpersonal contact, e.g., refuses a promotion that will increase social demands
5. Is reticent in social situations because of the fear of saying something inappropriate or foolish, or of being unable to answer a question
6. Fears being embarrassed by blushing, crying, or showing signs of anxiety in front of other people
7. Exaggerates the potential difficulties, physical dangers, or risks involved in doing something ordinarily outside of his or her usual routine, e.g., may cancel social plans because she anticipates being exhausted by the effort of getting there (*DSM*-III-R)

### B. Prevalence
According to *DSM*-III-R, it is currently apparently common; it is a new term in *DSM*-III-R.

### C. Associated features
1. Depression, anxiety, and anger at oneself for failing to develop social relations are commonly experienced. Specific phobias may also be present (*DSM*-III-R).
2. Unlike people with schizoid personality disorders who are socially isolated but have no desire for social relationships, those with avoidant personality disorder yearn for affection and acceptance.

### D. Treatment
A variety of psychotherapeutic interventions may be beneficial:

1. Psychodynamically oriented psychotherapy with interpretation seeking to alleviate fearfulness relative to unconscious conflicts.
2. Behavioral approach: Assertiveness and social skills training to increase the patient's confidence and, also, desensitization/exposure techniques.
3. Cognitive techniques may be helpful in eliminating and removing pathological assumptions that erode the patient's self-confidence.
4. Group therapy
5. Antianxiety medications, including benzodiazepines and/or buspar, may be helpful in removing the initial anxiety.

E. Case example

A twenty-nine-year-old single white male consulted a psychiatrist with complaints of loneliness and lack of friends.

He had grown up in a small community in a resort area and attended college for approximately two years, with a goal toward entering forestry. However, he never did complete college and worked in resort areas in the West until he entered the marines, where he served honorably for four years. He did not feel lonely during his military service because, "There always seemed to be people around me." His parents were divorced when the patient was about nine years of age. His father was absent from the home a lot because of his employment. The patient felt that he did not have a close relationship with his mother and had "negative" feelings toward his father. He was not close to his sister, who was two years older, nor to his brother, who was four years younger.

In discussing his personality, he reported that he felt there was "something wrong with me." He saw himself as self-centered and wanting friends but unable to make them. "I just can't make friends," he said. He was a weekend drinker and at such times went out to bars to play pool or stayed at home to watch television. He did not speak with any of the residents of his apartment building, and although he was able to converse some with fellow employees, he still said, "I'm kind of a stranger to them." He also realized that he did something to "keep people away from me."

Despite the fact that he had an isolated life, he did express an underlying yearning for affection and acceptance and was seeking help in how he might learn to relate to others.

## XIV. Dependent personality disorder
A. Definition
The essential feature of this disorder is a pervasive pattern of dependent and submissive behavior beginning by early adulthood and present in a variety of contexts, as indicated by at least *five* of the following (*DSM*-III-R):
1. Is unable to make everyday decisions without an excessive amount of advice or reassurance from others

2. Allows others to make most of his or her important decisions, e.g., where to live, what job to take
3. Agrees with people even when he or she believes they are wrong, because of fear of being rejected
4. Has difficulty initiating projects or doing things on his or her own
5. Volunteers to do things that are unpleasant or demeaning in order to get other people to like him or her
6. Feels uncomfortable or helpless when alone, or goes to great lengths to avoid being alone
7. Feels devastated or helpless when close relationships end
8. Is frequently preoccupied with fears of being abandoned
9. Is easily hurt by criticism or disapproval (*DSM*-III-R)

B. Associated features
   1. Commonly another personality disorder is present (e.g., histrionic, schizotypal, narcissistic, or avoidant personality disorder. Anxiety and depression are common.).
   2. People with this disorder invariably lack self-confidence.

C. Prevalence and sex ratio
   This disorder is apparently common and is diagnosed more frequently in women.

D. Predisposing factors
   Chronic physical illness or separation anxiety disorder may predispose to the development of this disorder.

E. Treatment
   1. Patients with this disorder often originally present for treatment when independent functioning or some degree of autonomy is required of them.
   2. In treating such patients, the therapist must keep in mind the patient's desire to transfer the responsibility to the therapist (this can pose countertransference problems for the therapist as well as transference problems for the patient).
   3. Behavioral and cognitive therapies have all reported some success.
   4. Group therapy presents opportunities to encourage autonomy in the patient.
   5. Medications and inpatient treatment are usually not indicated.

XV. **Obsessive-compulsive personality disorder**
   A. The essential feature of this disorder is a pervasive pattern of perfectionism and inflexibility, beginning by early adulthood and present in a variety of contexts, as indicated by at least *five* of the following (*DSM*-III-R):

1. Perfectionism that interferes with task completion, e.g., inability to complete a project because overly strict standards are not met
2. Preoccupation with details, rules, lists, order, organization, or schedules to the extent that the major point of the activity is lost
3. Unreasonable insistence that others submit to exactly his or her way of doing things, or unreasonable reluctance to allow others to do things because of the conviction that they will not do them correctly
4. Excessive devotion to work and productivity to the exclusion of leisure activities and friendships (not accounted for by obvious economic necessity)
5. Indecisiveness: Decision making is either avoided, postponed, or protracted, e.g., the person cannot get assignments done on time because of ruminating about priorities (do not include if indecisiveness is due to excessive need for advice or reassurance from others)
6. Overconscientiousness, scrupulousness, and inflexibility about matters of morality, ethics, or values (not accounted for by cultural or religious identification)
7. Restricted expression of affection
8. Lack of generosity in giving time, money, or gifts when no personal gain is likely to result
9. Inability to discard worn-out or worthless objects even when they have no sentimental value (*DSM*-III-R)

B. Prevalence and sex ratio
This disorder seems to be common and is more frequently diagnosed in males.

C. Associated features
Often people with this disorder lack confidence and are dependent. Typically, they are pessimistic about the future and have no realization that their behavior is responsible for their difficulty.

D. Complications
Obsessive-compulsive disorder, hypochondriasis, major depression, and dysthymia may be complications. Many of the features of obsessive-compulsive personality disorder are apparently present in people who develop myocardial infarction, particularly those with overlapping "Type A" personality traits of time urgency, hostility-aggressiveness, and exaggerated competitiveness (*DSM*-III-R).

E. Etiology
1. The person who possesses such traits is referred to as an *anankastic personality* or *anal character* (such an individual

needs to feel in control of him- or herself and the environment).

2. According to psychoanalytic theory, such anal qualities develop in the infant during the period of toilet training (the anal phase of infantile sexuality).

3. According to Erikson, disturbance in this stage of development characterized by the issues of autonomy versus shame and self-doubt predisposes to the development of obsessive-compulsive personality disorder.

4. The compulsive personality probably has encountered excessive discipline during the developmental years.

5. Family life is characterized by constrained emotions, and members are often criticized and socially ostracized if they express anger.

6. According to learning theory, obsessions are conditioned responses to anxiety, and compulsions are behavioral patterns that reduce the anxiety.

F. Course and prognosis
This is variable and not predictable. As noted earlier, persons with compulsive personality traits do well in positions demanding accurate, deductive, or detailed work. People such as this are rigid and are usually vulnerable to unexpected changes. Such personalities may also develop frank obsessions and compulsions and are susceptible to major depressive disorders, especially those of late onset.

G. Treatment

1. Unlike persons with the other personality disorders, compulsive personalities often are aware of their discomfort and are more apt to voluntarily seek treatment. However, treatment of obsessive-compulsive personalities is not easy and may be protracted. Focus should be on feelings rather than thoughts and on clarification of the defenses of intellectualization and displacement of hostility.

2. Dynamically oriented psychotherapy is the treatment of first choice for the obsessive-compulsive disorder.

3. In contrast, behavioral and pharmacological approaches are advocated for treating circumscribed rituals and obsessions as seen in obsessive-compulsive disorders.

4. Psychotropic medication: Clomipramine (Anafranil) is effective in treating many who have rituals of obsessive thinking. Fluoxetine (Prozac) is also effective in some.

## XVI. Passive-aggressive personality disorder

A. Definition
The essential feature of this disorder is a pervasive pattern of passive resistance to demands for adequate social and occupational

performance, beginning by early adulthood and present in a variety of contexts, as indicated by at least *five* of the following (*DSM*-III-R):

1. Procrastinates, i.e., puts off things that need to be done so that the deadlines are not met
2. Becomes sulky, irritable, or argumentative when asked to do something he or she does not want to do
3. Seems to work deliberately slowly to do a bad job on tasks that he or she really does not want to do
4. Protests, without justification, that others make unreasonable demands of him or her
5. Avoids obligations by claiming to have "forgotten"
6. Believes that he or she is doing a much better job than others think he or she is doing
7. Resents useful suggestions from others concerning how he or she could be more productive
8. Obstructs the efforts of others by failing to do his or her share of the work
9. Unreasonably criticizes or scorns people in positions of authority (*DSM*-III-R)

B. Prevalence and sex ratio

Unknown. Oppositional defiant disorder in childhood or adolescence apparently predisposes to the development of this disorder.

C. Associated features

Often people with this disorder are dependent and lack self-confidence. Typically, they are pessimistic about the future, but have no realization that their behavior is responsible for their difficulties (*DSM*-III-R).

D. Etiology

1. Prospective studies of this disorder are lacking.
2. A reasonable hypothesis seems to be that the person with a passive-aggressive personality is one whose parents were both assertive and aggressive in their relationships with him or her, yet blocked the expression of normal assertiveness and aggressiveness in the child and reluctantly met his or her dependency needs. As a consequence, the child learns to retroflex his or her anger and at first glance appears polite and undemanding, but overtly punishes the oppressor with inefficiency. (He or she adopts the style of pseudopoliteness, hiding resentment, which then can only be covertly expressed.)
3. The name of this disorder is based on the assumption that such people are passively expressing covert aggression.
4. This is a concept arising from military psychiatry during World War II.

E. Treatment
1. Insight-oriented psychotherapy, involving examination of the patient's covert expression of hostility, with a goal of gradually converting passive-aggressive behavior to more successful behavior, has been helpful.
2. Supportive psychotherapy seems to be the more practical approach. The therapist must repeatedly confront such individuals with the consequences of their behavior.
3. Psychotropic medication is indicated on those rare occasions where severe anxiety or severe depression can bring on symptoms.

## XVII. Personality disorders needing further study

*DSM*-III-R, Appendix A, lists proposed diagnostic categories needing study. Three diagnoses are included. These are late luteal phase dysphoric disorder, sadistic personality disorder, and self-defeating personality disorder.

A. Late luteal phase dysphoric disorder (reprinted from *DSM*-III-R).
1. Definition
   a) The essential feature of late luteal phase dysphoric disorder is a pattern of clinically significant emotional and behavioral symptoms that occur during the last week of the luteal phase and remit within a few days after the onset of the follicular phase. In most females these symptoms occur in the week before, and remit within a few days after, the onset of menses.
   b) The diagnosis is given only if the symptoms are sufficiently severe and cause marked impairment in social or occupational functioning and have occurred during the majority of the menstrual cycles of the past year.
   c) The diagnosis should not be made if the person is experiencing only a late luteal phase exacerbation of another disorder such as major depression, panic disorder, dysthymia, or a personality disorder.
2. Symptoms
   Among the most commonly experienced symptoms are marked affective lability (sudden episodes of tearfulness, sadness, or irritability); persistent feelings of irritability, anger, or tension (feeling "on edge"); and feelings of depression and self-deprecating thoughts. Also common are decreased interest in usual activities, fatigability and loss of energy, a subjective sense of difficulty in concentrating, changes in appetite, cravings for specific foods (especially carbohydrates), and sleep disturbance. Other physical symptoms, such as breast tenderness or swelling, headaches,

joint or muscle pain, a sensation of "bloating," and weight gain, may also be present.
3. Associated features
Some studies suggest that there may be a higher frequency of depressive disorder in females with this disorder.
4. Females seeking treatment generally report that this condition worsens with age.
5. Prevalence
Unknown.

B. Sadistic personality disorder (reprinted from *DSM*-III-R)
1. Definition
The essential feature of this disorder is a pervasive pattern of cruel, demeaning, and aggressive behavior directed toward other people, beginning by early adulthood. The sadistic behavior is often evident both in social relationships (particularly with family members) and at work (with subordinates), but seldom is displayed in contacts with people in positions of authority or higher status.
a) Many people with this disorder use physical violence or cruelty to establish dominance in interpersonal relationships. Other people with this disorder are never physically violent, although in many cases they are fascinated by violence, weapons, martial arts, injury, or torture.
b) A variety of behaviors reflect the basic lack of respect or empathy for others (e.g., humiliation or demeaning; such a person often gets others to do what he or she wants by frightening them with tactics ranging from intimidation by hostile glances to terror through threats of violence).
c) Often people with this disorder seem to be amused or enjoy psychological or physical suffering of others (including animals).
2. Associated features
Almost invariably the sadistic behavior is ego-syntonic, and the person rarely comes to clinical attention unless this has been mandated by the courts. Often these people victimize others who suffer from self-defeating personality disorder. Frequently many features of narcissistic and antisocial personality disorder are present.
3. Predisposing factors
People with this disorder have been physically, sexually, or psychologically abused as children or have been reared in a family in which there was abuse of a spouse.

4. Prevalence

It is rarely seen in clinical settings but is not uncommon in forensic settings.

5. Sex ratio

It is far more common in males.

6. Differential diagnosis

Sexual sadism, in this sadistic behavior, is for the purpose of sexual arousal.

C. Self-defeating personality disorder (reprinted from *DSM*-III-R)

1. Definition

The essential feature of this disorder is a pervasive pattern of self-defeating behavior, beginning by early adulthood and present in a variety of contexts. The person may often avoid or undermine pleasurable experiences, be drawn to situations or relationships in which he or she will suffer, and prevent others from helping him or her. The diagnosis is not made if the self-defeating behaviors occur only in situations in which the person is responding to or anticipating being physically, sexually, or psychologically abused. Similarly, the diagnosis is not made if the self-defeating behaviors occur only when the person is depressed.

a) The disorder has been called masochistic personality disorder, but the name of the category has been changed to avoid the historic association of the term *masochistic* with older psychoanalytic views of female sexuality and the implication that a person with the disorder derives unconscious pleasure from suffering. A variety of theories—psychoanalytic, cognitive, and social learning—have been offered to explain the origins of this pattern.

b) The person repeatedly enters into relationships with persons or places him- or herself in situations that are self-defeating and have painful consequences even when better options are clearly available.

c) Reasonable offers of assistance from others are rejected.

d) The person's reaction to positive personal events, such as graduation, a job promotion or raise, or any form of praise or encouragement from others, may be depression or feelings of guilt.

e) Characteristically, people with this disorder act in such a way as to cause others to be angry or to reject them.

f) Opportunities for pleasure may be repeatedly avoided.

g) The person reports a number of situations in which he or she had the opportunity to accomplish a task crucial to his or her personal success, but despite having the capacity to complete the task, failed to do so.

      h) People who consistently treat the person well are often experienced as boring or uninteresting.

      i) The person frequently attempts to do things for others that require excessive self-sacrifice, even though these sacrifices are unsolicited by the intended recipients.

2. Associated features

Other personality disorders are common, particularly borderline, dependent, passive-aggressive, obsessive-compulsive, and avoidant personality disorders.

3. Complications

Dysthymia and major depressive episodes are common complications.

4. Predisposing factors

Physical, sexual, or psychological abuse as a child, or having been reared in a family in which there was abuse of a spouse may predispose.

5. Prevalence

Initial studies suggest that this disorder may be one of the more common personality disorders in clinical samples.

6. Sex ratio

3:2 to 2:1 females to males.

## XVIII. Treatment of personality disorders

A. Treatment of the personality disorders is very difficult because the patients usually lack any fundamental motivation for change.

B. The positive rewards of their behavior overbalance the socially incurred ill-feeling that may result.

C. When they do seek treatment, it is often likely to be

1. Because of anxiety developing secondarily in response to the social repercussions of their behavior

2. At the insistence of another person (a parent, spouse, or employer)

3. Because of the slowly developing awareness of an unsatisfactory life-style

D. Intensive psychoanalytically oriented psychotherapy is useful in narcissistic personality disorders and borderline personality disorders.

E. In individual therapy, the therapist may focus on the individual's maladaptive behavior rather than on a discussion of his or her inner life.

F. The therapist's negative countertransference feelings must be dealt with in many of these disorders; recognizing feelings of resentment is an important cornerstone in developing an appropriate management strategy that will create a favorable therapeutic alliance to help facilitate change.

G. Such persons often need a different model with whom to identify and from whom to obtain reliable information about their emotional impact on others. In general, the therapist must remain flexible and be prepared to take an active role in the treatment process if necessary.

H. In general, the therapist should focus on the behavior rather than trying to deal with the "reasons" for it.

I. Limit setting and structure are also important in treating many disorders.

# References

American Psychiatric Association. *Diagnostic and Statistical Manual of Mental Disorders.* 3d ed., rev. Washington, D.C.: APA, 1987.

Cleckley, H. *The Mask of Sanity.* 4th ed. St. Louis: Mosby, 1964.

Frances, A., ed. "Personality Disorders." *Psychiatric Annals* 19, no. 3 (March 1989): 120–57.

Freeman, P. S., and J. G. Gunderson. "Treatment of Personality Disorders." *Psychiatric Annals* 19, no. 3 (1989): 147–53.

Goldman, H. H., ed. *Review of General Psychiatry.* 2d ed. Norwalk, Conn.: Appleton & Lange, 1988.

Gunderson, J. G. "Pharmacotherapy for Patients with Personality Disorder." *Archive of General Psychiatry* 43 (July 1986): 698–700.

Jacobsberg, L. B., et al. "Symptoms of the Schizotypal Personality Disorder." *American Journal of Psychiatry* 143, no. 10 (October 1986): 1222–27.

Johnson, A. M., and S. A. Szurek. "The Genesis of Antisocial Acting Out in Children and Adults." *Psychoanalytic Quarterly* 21 (1952): 323–43.

Kaplan, H. I., and B. J. Sadock, eds. *Comprehensive Textbook of Psychiatry/V.* 5th ed. Baltimore: Williams & Wilkins, 1989.

Kernberg, O. *Borderline Conditions and Pathological Narcissism.* New York: Aronson, 1975.

Kolb, L. C., and H. K. H. Brodie. *Modern Clinical Psychiatry.* 19th ed. Philadelphia: Saunders, 1982.

Masterson, J. *Treatment of the Borderline Adolescent: A Developmental Approach.* New York: Wiley-Interscience, 1972.

Nicholai, A. M., Jr., ed. *The New Harvard Guide to Modern Psychiatry.* Cambridge: Belknap Press, 1988.

Perry, J. C., et al. "Passive-Aggressive Personality Disorder." *Journal of Nervous and Mental Diseases* 170, no. 3 (1982): 164–73.

Rinsley, D. B. "Developmental Etiology of Borderline and Narcissistic Disorders." *Bulletin of the Menninger Clinic* 44, no. 2 (1980): 127–34.

Stone, M. H., ed. "Borderline Personality Disorder." *Psychiatric Annals* 20, no. 1 (January 1990): 8–10.

Wong, N. "Borderline and Narcissistic Disorders: A Selected Overview." *Bulletin of the Menninger Clinic* 44, no. 2 (1980): 101–26.

# 17  Disorders of Impulse Control

In order to do certain crazy things, it is necessary to behave like a coachman who has let go of the reins and fallen asleep.

**Jules Renard, *Journal* (November 1888)**

## I. Introduction
A. Not all antisocial behavior is identified with persons diagnosed as having antisocial personality disorders.
B. Excluded from the antisocial personality disorders are a residual group of disorders characterized by the irresistible, repetitious expression of a *single* pleasurable impulse.
C. This antisocial behavior may be the expression of any type of impulse. From a psychodynamic point of view this specific symptom often seems to have a symbolic significance as related to the patient's life history.
D. In these disorders, the superego is usually well developed and is only defective to the extent that it permits acting out of one type of antisocial behavior.
E. In the past, these disorders were called impulse-ridden states, or impulse neuroses. In the current nomenclature (*DSM*-III-R), they are called disorders of impulse control.

## II. Definition
The essential features of disorders of impulse control are:
A. Failure to resist an impulse, drive, or temptation to perform some act that is harmful to the person or others. There may or may not be conscious resistance to the impulse. The act may or may not be premeditated or planned.
B. An increasing sense of tension or arousal before committing the act.
C. An experience of either pleasure, gratification, or release at the time of committing the act. The act is ego-syntonic (acceptable to the ego) in that it is consonant with the immediate conscious wish of the individual. Immediately following the act there may or may not be genuine regret, self-reproach, or guilt (*DSM*-III-R).

### III. Types
  A. Intermittent explosive disorder
  B. Kleptomania
  C. Pathological gambling
  D. Pyromania
  E. Trichotillomania
  F. Impulse control disorder not otherwise classified; this includes atypical, idiosyncratic, nonspecific irresistible impulses including spending sprees or buying binges, compulsive buying, and dromomania (an abnormal impulse to travel, also known as vagabond neurosis).
  G. At one time, substance use disorders (including alcoholism) and the paraphilias were considered disorders of impulse control. Under the present nomenclature these disorders are classified separately.
### IV. General psychodynamic considerations
  A. From the psychoanalytic point of view, these disorders could be considered as resulting from the temporary loss of control of the reality principle (with the loss of ego control, thus allowing the individual to express a pleasurable drive).
  B. Psychodynamically, the expression of the impulse represents an attempt to relieve underlying anxiety, depression, guilt, or other painful affects (and, secondarily, to provide distorted satisfaction of underlying instinctual drives).
  C. Some have stressed the oral fixation of such people (in the psychoanalytical model).
  D. The impulsive (ego-syntonic) character of the disorders distinguishes it from compulsive (ego-dystonic) and ego-alien drives. (This is not always easy to verify clinically.)
  E. Some believe that the tension-relieving aspect of the impulse expression is not goal directed and that the underlying need is for the relief of pain rather than for the production of pleasure.
  F. It must be kept in mind that certain organic factors, such as cerebral atrophy, alcohol, or drugs, may permit release of underlying impulses.
### V. Intermittent explosive disorder
  A. Definition
   The essential features of this disorder are discrete episodes of loss of control of aggressive impulses, resulting in serious assaultive acts or destruction of property. The degree of aggressiveness expressed during the episodes is grossly out of proportion to any precipitating psychosocial stressors. There are no signs of generalized impulsivity or aggressiveness between the episodes.
   The person may describe the episodes as "spells" or "attacks." The symptoms are said to appear within minutes or

hours and, regardless of duration, remit almost as quickly. Genuine regret or self-reproach about the consequences of the action and the inability to control the aggressive impulse may follow each episode.

Other disorders that are sometimes associated with loss of control of aggressive impulses must be ruled out before the diagnosis can be made. These include psychotic disorders, organic personality syndrome, antisocial or borderline personality disorder, conduct disorder, or intoxication with a psychoactive substance (*DSM*-III-R).

This category has been retained in *DSM*-III-R despite the fact that many doubt the existence of a clinical syndrome characterized by episodic loss of control that is not symptomatic of one of the disorders that must be ruled out before the diagnosis of intermittent explosive disorder can be made.

B. Prevalence

The disorder apparently is very rare.

C. Sex ratio

It is apparently more common in males.

D. Differential diagnosis (see previous paragraph)

E. Etiology

In addition to the factors listed under General psychodynamic considerations, some authorities suggest that neurophysiological factors may play a role in the disorder.

F. Case example

A twenty-two-year-old married man was referred to the court psychiatric consultant for evaluation after he had pleaded guilty to a charge of simple assault, growing out of an incident in which he was verbally and physically abusive to his wife. He was on probation at the time of the offense for a similar disorderly conduct offense committed nine months earlier.

At the interview, he was cooperative and pleasant but did not spontaneously volunteer much about himself. He was quiet, nonverbal, and not at all reflective. In discussing his difficulty he said, "Basically it's temper," which had been an issue in his marriage for the preceding three years. He said that the difficulty was that his temper began during the time that he was in the service for two years following his eighteenth birthday. "It just seemed to come on by itself." It had its onset shortly before he was sent overseas to Vietnam, where he served as an infantry rifleman and was wounded.

The kind of subsequent anger that included the physical and verbal abuse of his wife occurred about every six months. At such times he usually would awaken angry and, as a consequence, would overreact throughout the entire day.

Mental status evaluation revealed him to be free of anxiety and depression. He didn't think that there was anything wrong with his mind, and he denied delusions, hallucinations, and other types of perceptual distortions. He denied any thinking disturbance. He thought that it was sometimes hard for him to trust others.

It was the consultant's opinion that this man had an explosive personality. Since the outbursts seemed to develop chiefly in relationships with his wife, it was suggested that they both be referred for marriage counseling if the wife planned to remain in the marriage.

## VI. Kleptomania

A. Definition
1. The essential feature of this disorder is a recurrent failure to resist impulses to steal objects not needed for personal use or their monetary value; the objects taken are either given away, discarded, returned surreptitiously, or kept and hidden. Almost invariably the person has enough money to pay for the stolen objects. The person experiences an increasing sense of tension immediately before committing the act and intense gratification or relief while committing it. Although the theft does not occur when immediate arrest is probable (e.g., in full view of a police officer), it is not preplanned, and the chances of apprehension are not fully taken into account. The stealing is done without long-term planning and without assistance from or collaboration with others. Further, there is no association between the stealing and anger or vengeance (*DSM*-III-R).
2. The diagnosis is not made if stealing is due to conduct disorder or antisocial personality disorder.
3. True kleptomania is rare.
B. Associated features
The kleptomaniac may exhibit depression, anxiety, and guilt over the possibility of apprehension.
C. Sex ratio
The majority of the individuals apprehended for shoplifting are female, but only a small portion of these have kleptomania.
D. Etiology
1. It was once considered a monomania.
2. Currently viewed as a behavioral manifestation of underlying conflict.
3. Most dynamic theories center on stealing as an attempt to obtain nourishment, self-esteem, and love or as a sexual equivalent.
E. Prognosis
The course is recurrent. The recurrences tend to occur in times of stress (separation, loss, or termination of significant relationships).

F. Treatment
  1. Individual (insight-oriented) psychotherapy is indicated in those individuals who feel guilt and shame and are motivated to change.
  2. Behavioral therapy (including desensitization, aversive conditioning, etc.) has been successful in some cases.
G. Case example

A twenty-seven-year-old married man, who had just formed his own small business, consulted a psychiatrist about difficulties in his relationship with his wife and the hostile feelings he had toward his hypercritical father. He expressed a great deal of anger and negativism toward both parents, but especially toward the father, who was unreasonable, paranoid, and insensitive.

In discussing his past history, he reported that he had a habit of stealing small items from the shops he visited for business or personal reasons. These items were almost never of any use to him and usually were inexpensive. He saved all of them and kept them in drawers in his workshop at home. No one knew of his stealing habit—not even his wife, who was irritated by what he described to her as his "impulse buying."

At first he reported no associated feelings with the stealing incidents, but later in therapy, he recalled that he felt anxious before and at the time of the thefts—and remorseful afterward. He could not relate these incidents to any psychological determinant, but he suspected it had something to do with his rebellious feelings toward his father. He terminated therapy a few months later, when he left the city. At that time, he still did not know the reasons for his stealing.

(Note in the previous case example: It was not the impulsive stealing that led to his seeking psychiatric treatment. The history of kleptomania was only incidentally reported in the therapeutic process.)

## VII. Pathological gambling
  A. Definition
  The essential features of this disorder are a chronic and progressive failure to resist impulses to gamble, and gambling behavior that compromises, disrupts, or damages personal, family, or vocational pursuits. The gambling preoccupation, urge, and activity increase during periods of stress. Problems that arise as a result of the gambling lead to an intensification of the gambling behavior. Characteristic problems include extensive indebtedness and consequent default on debts and other financial responsibilities, disrupted family relationships, inattention to work, and financially motivated illegal activities to pay for gambling (*DSM*-III-R).
  B. Associated features
  1. Generally, people with pathological gambling disorder have the attitude that money causes and is also the solution to all their problems. As the gambling increases, the person is

usually forced to lie in order to obtain money and to continue gambling. There is no serious attempt to budget or save money. When borrowing resources are strained, antisocial behavior in order to obtain money is likely (*DSM*-III-R).

2. The gambler usually appears overconfident, energetic, easily bored, and is a "big spender"; but at other times he or she may show signs of personal stress, anxiety, and depression.

C. Etiology
1. *DSM*-III-R considers the following to be predisposing factors: inappropriate parental discipline (absent, inconsistency, or harshness); exposure to gambling activities as an adolescent; high family value placed on material and financial symbols; and a lack of family emphasis on saving, planning, and budgeting.
2. Some psychoanalysts have regarded it as related to conflicts about masturbation.
3. Others have seen it as an Oedipal conflict.
4. Some have considered it to be associated to some neurophysiological dysfunction (e.g., epilepsy, subcortical lesions, minimal brain dysfunction).
5. The prevailing view is that pathological gambling is an expression of unconscious conflicts (regarding guilt based on unconscious need to lose).

D. Prognosis
It is considered a chronic cyclic disorder.

E. Treatment
Various modalities have been tried.
1. Individual psychotherapy.
2. Group therapy.
3. Peer support, such as Gamblers Anonymous (based on the AA model).
4. Treatment can usually begin when significant people in the gambler's life help him or her see that the gambler's behavior is a problem.
5. There are inpatient facilities that specialize in the treatment of compulsive gambling.

F. Case example

Mrs. J. P., the fifty-two-year-old wife of a social agency executive, was referred for psychiatric treatment because of her "addiction to bingo." Her gambling had its onset after she learned of the tragic death of her thirty-year-old scientist son. Her irresistible urge to gamble (and lose) at bingo seemed to represent an equivalent of depression.

Repeated efforts at outpatient psychotherapy and hospital treatment were to little avail. She wrote worthless checks, stole, and went into debt to continue her habit. Ultimately, her husband divorced her. Unfortunately, there was no follow-up beyond that point.

## VIII. Pyromania

A. Definition

The essential features of this disorder are deliberate and purposeful (rather than accidental) fire setting on more than one occasion; tension or affective arousal prior to setting the fires; and intense pleasure, gratification, or relief when setting the fires or witnessing or participating in their aftermath. In addition, there is fascination with, interest in, curiosity about, or attraction to fire and its situational context or associated characteristics (e.g., uses, consequences, exposure to fires). The fire setting is not done for monetary gain, as an expression of sociopolitical ideology, to conceal criminal activity, to express anger or vengeance, to improve one's living circumstances, or in response to a delusion or hallucination.

Although the fire setting results from a failure to resist an impulse, there may be considerable advance preparation for starting the fire, and the person may leave obvious clues. People with the disorder are often recognized as regular "watchers" at fires in their neighborhoods, frequently set off false alarms, and show interest in firefighting paraphernalia. Their fascination with fire leads some to seek employment or volunteer work in firefighting. They may be indifferent to the consequences of the fire for life or property, or they may get satisfaction from the resulting destruction (*DSM*-III-R).

B. Age of onset

Usually in childhood. There is usually a history of lifelong fascination with fires and the firefighting scene (including firefighters, firefighting equipment, etc.)

C. Sex ratio

It is more common in men; with women it is often associated with low IQ. Some reports indicate that pyromania in females is associated with petty theft and promiscuity.

D. Etiology

1. It is regarded as a symptom of underlying psychological conflicts.
2. Recent authorities have noted coincidental learning disabilities and brain dysfunction.
3. Psychoanalytic literature generally focuses on three major issues:
   a) An association of fire setting and sexual gratification
   b) Concerns about feelings of inferiority, impotence, and annihilation
   c) Conscious hostility toward parent figure

4. Lewis and Yarnell (1951) in a monograph reported that the fire setter has a craving for power and prestige, and setting the fire is an exercise in power.

E. Treatment

1. Treatment is difficult because of denial.
2. Behavioral therapy approaches have had some success.
3. Treatment with children has been more encouraging and the afflicted ones have been responsive to group and family therapy.
4. Most of the individuals with this disorder have been sent to treatment through the court system.

F. Case example

An eighteen-year-old married man was arrested for having set a number of fires in the city. In discussing the setting of the fires, he indicated that he got a ''thrill'' or a ''feeling of excitement'' as he watched the fires. In addition, he experienced some sexual gratification from setting the fires. He would set the fires in an area in which he could witness them from his home, and he and his wife would become sexually excited and have sexual intercourse while observing the blaze.

Apart from the particular offense that brought him to the attention of the law, there was evidence that he had had adjustment difficulties for many years. Obesity, for example, had been a problem with him for a long time, and he gave a history of an arrest four years earlier for an assault on a two and one-half year old boy. He felt that he turned to homosexuality at that point because he was not able to date in high school. He denied that he had had any homosexual feelings since he had been married in March of the previous year.

From clinical examination, there was no evidence that he was psychotic. In a general way, he indicated that he probably knew right from wrong and that at the time he set the first fire he knew it was wrong, but after that the rightness or wrongness of his behavior in setting additional fires did not enter his head—''It was just something I needed.'' There was also evidence that setting the fires relieved sexual, aggressive, and anxious feelings. At the time of psychiatric examination in the county jail, he was still experiencing strong desires to set fires.

G. The pyromaniac must be distinguished from the arsonist.

## IX. Trichotillomania

A. Definition

1. The essential feature of this disorder is a recurrent failure to resist impulses to pull out one's own hair. The diagnosis is not made when hair pulling is associated with a preexisting inflammation of the skin or is in response to a delusion or hallucination.
2. Specific patterns and rituals involving the plucking of the hair and its dispositions are common: trichophagy or mouthing of the hair may follow the plucking.

3. Unlike in alopecia areata, regrowth of the hair is without pigmentary change, and a scalp biopsy will uncover signs of the traumatic nature of the disorder: catagen hairs, absence of inflammation and scarring, the presence of keratin plugs, and dilated follicular infundibula. Characteristic histopathologic changes in the hair follicle, known as trichomalacia, are demonstrated by biopsy and help to distinguish the condition from other causes of alopecia (*DSM*-III-R).
4. It is usually a lifelong habit pattern beginning in childhood (between the ages of four and ten).

B. Associated features: long-standing denial of the disorder is commonly encountered. Other acts of self-mutilation may be present (head banging, nail biting, scratching, gnawing, excoriation, etc.).

C. Age of onset
It usually begins in childhood (between the ages of four and ten) and is usually a lifelong habit pattern.

D. Predisposing factors
1. Although the disorder is regarded as "multidetermined," onset has been linked to stressful situations in more than one-quarter of the cases.
2. Disturbances in mother-child relationships, fear of being left alone, and recent object loss are often cited as critical factors in the genesis of the condition. Psychoactive substance abuse may contribute to the development of this disorder.

E. Prevalence
No information. It is more common in people with mental retardation and possibly with schizophrenia or borderline personality disorder.

F. Differential diagnosis
1. It must be differentiated from other kinds of alopecia (e.g., alopecia areata is a disorder with which it is often confused).
2. All other types of psychiatric disorders that have alopecia as a symptom.

## X. Impulse control disorders not otherwise specified
A. Introduction
1. This comprises the rarely occurring impulse control disorders that nonetheless have conformed to the trilogy of symptoms found in the identified impulse control disorders.
2. In the past they have been considered to be "monomanias" and include dromomania and hair cutting and braid snipping.

B. Treatment

Although these conditions are rare, they are usually thought to be responsive to insight-oriented psychotherapy.

XI. **Summary of impulse control disorders**

Impulse control disorders are disorders of behavior that result from the inability to resist an impulse, drive, or temptation, which is characterized by mounting tension before the commission of the act and feelings of relief and gratification when the act has been committed. All of the behaviors mentioned in this chapter are ego-syntonic when the act is committed.

## References

American Psychiatric Association. *Diagnostic and Statistical Manual of Mental Disorders.* 3d ed., rev. Washington, D.C.: APA, 1987.

Goldman, H. H. *Review of General Psychiatry.* Los Altos, Calif.: Lange Medical Publications, 1988.

Kaplan, H. I., and B. J. Sadock, eds. *Comprehensive Textbook of Psychiatry/V.* 5th ed. Baltimore: Williams & Wilkins, 1989.

Lewis, N. D. C., and H. Yarnell. "Pathological Fire Setting (Pyromania)." *Nervous and Mental Diseases,* Monograph 82, no. 8 (1951).

# 18 Sexual Disorders

If venereal delight and the power of propagating the species were permitted only to the virtuous, it would make the world very good.

**James Boswell, *London Journal* (March 26, 1763)**

## I. Definition

In *DSM*-III-R the sexual disorders are divided into two groups: the paraphilias, characterized by arousal and response to sexual objects or situations that are not part of normative arousal-activity patterns and that in varying degrees may interfere with the capacity for reciprocal, affectionate sexual activity; and sexual dysfunctions, characterized by inhibitions in sexual desire or the psychophysiologic changes that characterize the sexual response cycle. Other sexual disorders is a residual class for disorders in sexual functioning that are not classifiable in any of the specific categories.

## II. Background

A. Historical notes

1. In previous classifications paraphilias have been called sexual perversions or sexual deviations.
2. Sexual deviations have been practiced throughout history and by all races.
3. Sexual deviancy includes any sexual behavior that is at variance with more or less culturally accepted norms.
4. To be considered deviant, either the quality or the object of the sexual drive must be deemed abnormal.
5. Some authorities speak of "sexual variants" rather than "sexual deviancies."
6. For centuries, deviations of sexual preference were regarded as offenses against the laws of religion. Generally, our concepts of sexual normalcy and deviancy are related to the values of our society. Since these values change, concepts and definitions of sexual deviance also change.
7. The first systematic studies of paraphilias began about one hundred years ago. In 1886 Richard von Krafft-Ebbing

published *Psychopathia Sexualis*. Subsequent studies by Henry Havelock Ellis (1859–1939) and others followed.

8. Among others who wrote about sexual abnormalities were Sigmund Freud, who saw the causes "in the failures of development processes."
9. Most of the publications on paraphilias are in the psychoanalytic tradition, but they have not been as successful at modifying or explaining the behaviors.
10. The deviant is usually one who has difficulty achieving normal or satisfactory sexual relations with a mature human partner. Thus, according to Marmor (1978), the deviant practices represent alternative ways of attempting to achieve sexual gratification.

B. Previous classification

In *DSM*-III, published in 1980, the psychosexual disorders were divided into four groups:

1. Gender identity disorders
2. Paraphilias
3. Psychosexual dysfunctions
4. Other psychosexual disorders (which included ego-dystonic homosexuality)

The current classification in *DSM*-III-R is divided into two groups: paraphilias and sexual dysfunctions. There is also a residual class of other sexual disorders for disorders in sexual functioning that are not classifiable in any of the other categories. (This last group includes a place for "persistent and marked distress about one's sexual orientation.")

C. Gender identity disorders including transsexualism are listed in *DSM*-III-R under Disorders Usually First Evident in Infancy, Childhood, or Adolescence. In this outline, these disorders will be listed and described in this chapter on sexual disorders.

D. Etiology

There is no universal or unifying theory of etiology (Adson 1992).

III. **Types**

A. Paraphilias
1. Exhibitionism
2. Fetishism
3. Frotteurism
4. Pedophilia
5. Sexual masochism
6. Sexual sadism
7. Transvestic fetishism
8. Voyeurism
9. Paraphilia not otherwise specified

B. Sexual dysfunctions

The essential feature of this subclass is inhibition in the appetitive or psychophysiologic changes that characterize the complete sexual response cycle. It includes:

1. Sexual desire disorders
    a) Hypoactive sexual desire disorder
    b) Sexual aversion disorder
2. Sexual arousal disorders
    a) Female sexual arousal disorder
    b) Male erectile disorder
3. Orgasm disorders
    a) Inhibited female orgasm
    b) Inhibited male orgasm
    c) Premature ejaculation
4. Sexual pain disorders
    a) Dyspareunia
    b) Vaginismus
5. Sexual dysfunction not otherwise specified

C. Other sexual disorders

Sexual disorders that are not classifiable in any of the previous categories include nonparaphilic sexual addiction and "persistent and marked distress about one's sexual orientation."

IV. **Gender identity disorders**

Our maleness or femaleness (gender identity) is deeply ingrained from earliest childhood, and regardless of the stresses encountered throughout life, most people are certain of their gender.

However, some—more commonly men—feel deeply within themselves from earliest childhood that they are of the opposite sex.

A. Definition

The essential feature of the disorders included in this subclass is an incongruence between assigned sex (i.e., the sex that is recorded on the birth certificate) and gender identity.

1. Gender *identity* can be defined as one's sense of femininity or masculinity, or, according to Campbell (1989), it is "the inner conviction that one is either male, female, ambivalent, or neutral."
2. Gender *role,* according to Campbell, is "the behavior and appearance that one presents in terms of what the culture considers to be 'masculine' or 'feminine.' " One might also consider this to be the individual's perception of his or her social role as being either masculine or feminine. While gender identity is usually established and fixed early in life, gender role evolves over a period of time.

3. Gender identity is the private experience of gender role, and gender role is the public expression of gender identity (*DSM*-III).

B. Transsexualism

1. Definition

The essential features of this disorder are a persistent discomfort and a sense of inappropriateness about one's assigned sex in a person who has reached puberty. In addition, there is persistent preoccupation, for at least two years, with getting rid of one's primary and secondary sex characteristics and acquiring the sex characteristics of the other sex. Therefore, the diagnosis is not made if the disturbance is limited to brief periods of stress. Invariably there is the wish to live as a member of the other sex. In the rare cases in which physical intersexuality or a genetic abnormality is present, such a condition should be noted on Axis III.

People with this disorder usually complain that they are uncomfortable wearing the clothes of their assigned sex and therefore dress in clothes of the other sex. Often they engage in activities that in our culture tend to be associated with the other sex. These people often find their genitals repugnant, which may lead to persistent requests for sex reassignment by hormonal and surgical means (*DSM*-III-R).

2. Types

*DSM*-III-R types (subdivided according to the history of sexual orientation)

a) Asexual—the person denies ever having had strong sexual feelings.

b) Homosexual—object choice has been the same anatomic sex.

c) Heterosexual—the individual claims to have had an active heterosexual life.

3. Etiology

a) There is a history of gender identity problems as a child.

b) Some consider that all types of transsexual disorders stem from unresolved separation anxiety during the early stages of infantile development.

c) In primary male transsexuals, some believe that the father is distant and passive and the mother is a woman with strong bisexual aspects in her personality.

d) In female transsexuals, fragmentary evidence suggests that the female child's mother was unavailable for mothering (but not necessarily physically absent). This seems to set up a process in which the female child tries to restore her mother.

e) No biological factors have been reported in either male or female transsexualism.

f) Transsexuals are sometimes called "gender dysphoric."

4. Course

Chronic. The long-term prognosis of combined psychiatric, hormonal, and surgical sex-reassignment treatment is not well known (*DSM*-III-R).

5. Treatment

a) Psychiatric treatment of this disorder has been disappointing.

b) Psychotherapy has been unsuccessful.

c) Aversive therapy has also been unsuccessful.

d) Whether behavior therapy will be of help in the future is unknown.

e) Sex transformation, or reconstructive surgery, has been used for a carefully screened group of patients. Persons with psychotic or borderline behavior, a criminal record, or gross sexual disturbances have been excluded. Although such surgery does not always relieve symptoms (e.g., depression), the patients seem to have done well postoperatively. Some authorities state that in the absence of long-term follow-up studies, the outcome remains controversial.

6. Case example

A twenty-four-year-old, single, genetic male was admitted to the hospital for transsexual surgery. He had been born in a small town in southern Minnesota and had an unusually healthy life.

He stated that from his earliest memories he had regarded himself as a girl and that throughout his life he had never felt differently. Some of his earliest memories were of dressing up in the clothes of his sister, who was two years older. He was interested exclusively in dolls, little girls' games, and playing with girls. He did not like playing with boys or engaging in their games. He was also interested in dolls and cooking and, in high school, baton twirling. He said that he was always accepted "as a girl" by the girls in the small town in which he grew up.

By the end of grade school, he was taunted by boys for his feminine ways. It was during his midteens, while coming across descriptions of a famous case of transsexuality, that it began to dawn upon him that he might be a transsexual.

He denied any overt sexual experiences of any type except for a few anal sexual experiences. He was afraid of having relationships with a male "because he would quickly find out about me." He had never attempted sexual relations with a genetic female—"this would disgust me." He masturbated frequently and in his fantasies played the role of a woman, lying on his back and accepting the penis from his imaginary male lover. About four and one-half years earlier, he had begun to take estrogens and dress and live like a woman. During this time, there was substantial breast development, his male genitalia became "smaller," and he became unable to have erections. He felt disgust for his penis and testicles, never felt them, and kept them constantly tucked between his legs. He also enrolled in a school for beauticians, where he met his first fellow transsexual. About two years before admission to the hospital, he had had his breasts injected with liquid silicone to make them "more solid."

He was a natural blond and had never had much trouble with excessive bodily and facial hair. He had a "peaches-and-cream" complexion, and a depilatory used about every ten days controlled the relatively small amount of facial fuzz. In the hospital, a one-stage transsexual operation was performed.[1]

C. Gender identity disorder of adolescence or adulthood, nontranssexual type (GIDAANT)
   1. Definition
      The essential features of this disorder are a persistent or recurrent discomfort and sense of inappropriateness about one's assigned sex, and persistent or recurrent cross-dressing in the role of the other sex, either in fantasy or in actuality, in a person who has reached puberty. This disorder differs from transvestic fetishism in that the cross-dressing is not for the purpose of sexual excitement; it differs from transsexualism in that there is no persistent preoccupation (for at least two years) with getting rid of one's primary and secondary sex characteristics and acquiring the sex characteristics of the other sex (*DSM*-III-R).
   2. Age at onset and course
      Age at onset and course are both variable, but in most cases before puberty there was a history of some or all of the features of gender identity disorder of childhood.
   3. Sex ratio
      More common in males.
D. Gender identity disorder not otherwise specified
   This is a class for gender identity disorders that are not classifiable elsewhere. For example: children with persistent cross-dressing without the other criteria for gender identity disorder of childhood; adults with transient stress-related cross-dressing behavior, etc.

V. **Exhibitionism**
   A. Definition
      1. The essential feature of this disorder is recurrent, intense sexual urges and sexually arousing fantasies, of at least six

---

1. Courtesy of the late Donald W. Hastings, M.D., University of Minnesota Hospitals.

months' duration, involving the exposure of one's genitals to a stranger. The person has acted on these urges or is markedly distressed by them. Sometimes the person masturbates while exposing himself (or fantasizing exposing himself).

If the person acts on these urges, there is no attempt at further sexual activity with the stranger, and therefore people with this disorder are usually not physically dangerous to the victim (*DSM*-III-R).

2. The act is preceded by a feeling of mounting tension and accompanied by intense excitement and exhilaration.
3. The term is sometimes used in the popular sense to describe somebody who is "showing off."
4. Some believe it is related to voyeurism.
5. The exhibitionist is sometimes referred to as a "flasher."

B. Prevalence
1. Exhibitionistic play among children is common and is not considered a deviancy.
2. It is one of the more common deviations among adults.
3. It is nearly always a deviation of males. Females usually do not derive erotic satisfaction from exhibiting their genitalia, but derive more pleasure from displaying other parts of their bodies.
4. The exhibitionist often returns repeatedly to the same scene to expose himself. As a consequence, he is frequently arrested.
5. In senile men, it may be a symptom of impaired judgment and poor impulse control.

C. Etiology
1. Psychodynamically, the exhibitionist seems to be seeking reassurance for his underlying castration anxiety.
2. The exposure may thus be an attempt to seek reassurance by
   a) Having another person react to the sight of his genitalia
   b) Having other persons show fear of him
   c) Showing the female what he wishes she could show him, thus reassuring himself that she also has a penis.
3. Some say that exhibitionists suffer from sexual impotence or premature ejaculation and deep-seated feelings of masculine inadequacy.

D. Prognosis
1. The prognosis depends upon the exhibitionist's desire for change.
2. It is also related to the severity of the deviancy.

3. The deviancy usually ceases with aging—at least, few arrests are made in the older age group.

E. Case example

G. J., a thirty-six-year-old married man, was referred to the court's psychiatric consultant for evaluation after he had pleaded guilty to a charge of exposing himself to a woman in the downtown area. His history indicated that he had begun exposing himself several months earlier and, although he could not give any conscious reason for the behavior, it was interesting to note that he had become impotent shortly before he experienced the first urge to expose himself.

Although he indicated that he was worried about his impotence, he had not yet summoned up enough courage to discuss the matter with his personal physician. He seemed to have no understanding that his impotence might be psychogenic and that this might have some relationship to his exhibitionism. Mental-status examination did not reveal any thinking disorder or any major personality disturbance.

## VI. Fetishism
A. Definition
1. The essential feature of this disorder is recurrent, intense sexual urges and sexually arousing fantasies, of at least six months' duration, involving the use of nonliving objects (fetishes). The person has acted on these urges or is markedly distressed by them (*DSM*-III-R).
2. Begins in adolescence and occurs almost exclusively in heterosexual males (but a small percentage are homosexual).
3. Common fetish objects are bras, women's undergarments, stockings, shoes, boots, or other wearing apparel, or nongenital body parts.
4. The person with the fetishism frequently masturbates while holding, rubbing, or smelling the fetish object, or may ask his sexual partner to wear the object during sexual encounters.
5. The fetish is used as the masturbatory object; thus, it is clearly a symbolic substitute for the female, rather than the male, genitals.
6. Preoccupation with certain parts of the female body (e.g., breasts, buttocks, legs, hips) is called *partialism* (classified as Paraphilia Not Otherwise Specified in *DSM*-III-R).
7. Fetishism shades into normal sexual behavior.
B. Prevalence
1. Fetishism seems to be peculiar to men.
2. Kinsey believed that there was a relationship between sadomasochistic behavior and fetishism.
3. No figures are available on its prevalence.
4. Sometimes a fetishist is arrested for stealing an article of female clothing, especially undergarments (''fetish theft'').

5. Once established, the disorder tends to be chronic.
C. Etiology
1. Freud attributed fetishism to the castration anxiety originating in early childhood.
    a) The fetish represents a symbolic "female penis" and reassures the male that the female also has a penis, thus allaying castration anxiety.
    b) Such theories are of dubious value because castration anxiety is seen as a cause of many disorders that are not sexual deviations.
2. Like many homosexuals, fetishists do not achieve a healthy identification with their fathers, who, according to Marmor (1978), have usually been distant, absent, or rejecting.
D. Treatment
1. As in other sexual deviations, motivation to change is critical.
2. Psychotherapy is focused on the patient's basic feelings of masculine inadequacy and heterosexual inhibition.
3. Group psychotherapy may be helpful.
4. Behavioral therapy has been tried.
5. Marmor believes that a combination of dynamic and behavioral techniques may ultimately prove the most effective therapy.
E. Case example

A twenty-eight-year-old married man was referred to the court's psychiatric consultant after he had been arrested for touching an eighteen-year-old girl on the buttocks on two occasions on a downtown street. He admitted that he had touched between thirty to fifty girls, usually between fourteen and twenty-one years old, on the buttocks, breasts, or genitalia. He rarely touched the same girl twice. In addition, he admitted that on three or four occasions he had made obscene propositions to the girls. He said the incidents usually occurred on his way to work or on his way home in the evening and were most apt to occur when his wife was menstruating and unavailable for sexual relationships. In all instances he denied having an erection or an orgasm, but he did describe a feeling of "excitement," which he compared to the experience he had in other situations, such as shooting deer. He denied other kinds of sexual problems, claiming that he got along well with his wife.

During the interview, he behaved very much like a schizoid person, showing a rather blunted affect and a lack of verbal spontaneity. He said that on many occasions in the past, he had vowed to himself to give up his deviancy but had always found it difficult to stop.

He was recommended for probationary supervision with the stipulation that he attend a psychiatric clinic.

## VII. Frotteurism
A. Definition

The essential feature of this disorder is recurrent, intense sexual urges and sexually arousing fantasies, of at least six months' duration, involving touching and rubbing against a nonconsenting person (*DSM*-III-R).

The person has acted on these urges or is markedly distressed by them.

  B. Prevalence
    1. Usually a male deviation
    2. Is usually committed in crowded places

## VIII. Pedophilia

  A. Definition

The essential feature of this disorder is recurrent, intense sexual urges and sexually arousing fantasies, of at least six months' duration, involving sexual activity with a prepubescent child. The person has acted on these urges or is markedly distressed by them (*DSM*-III-R).

  B. This may be exclusively heterosexual or exclusively homosexual, but heterosexually oriented pedophiles are twice as common as homosexually oriented ones.

  C. The person may limit his activities to his own children, stepchildren, or relatives, or may victimize children outside his family.

  D. Prevalence

This paraphilia is the most likely to engender feelings of contempt or disgust in people.

    1. The disorder usually begins in adolescence.
    2. Prevalence is most difficult to estimate, although it is most common in adult males.
    3. This is the most common paraphilia that comes to the attention of the law.
    4. Heterosexual offenses are more common than homosexual ones.
    5. The popular belief that homosexuals tend to be child molesters seems to be a myth.
    6. Mostly, the behavior is genital petting. Most pedophiles do not resort to force or aggression.
    7. The course is usually chronic, especially in those attracted to boys.

  E. Etiology
    1. Most pedophiles are mild-mannered men who have profound feelings of masculine inadequacy and a fear of being castrated by mature women. They are frequently sexually impotent. As a result, they expect rejection and failure in any attempts at adult heterosexual relationships.
    2. On the other hand, the male pedophile is often said to be masochistic.

3. Many of the men feel that their penis is small; hence, children are seen as less threatening or less challenging.
4. Although no single family constellation is identifiable, a large percentage of pedophiles seem to come from unhappy home situations and to have had a poor relationship with the father.
5. Incest, although not classified as a perversion, is superficially related to pedophilia because of the frequent selections of an immature sexual child as a sexual object.

F. Types

Men who approach children sexually can be divided into the following groups:
1. Occasionally, males who are under the influence of alcohol
2. Males who are responding to a special situation
3. Pedophiles
4. Mentally retarded persons
5. Sociopathic types
6. Disorganized schizophrenics
7. Men with organic brain disease (senile dementia)

G. Other types

Some have divided pedophiles into two groups:
1. Adolescent
   An adolescent group who have sexual intercourse with girls who are only a few years younger and are often at an age when sexual behavior would be permissible in some societies
2. A second group of older men who deliberately choose a child as a sexual partner

H. Case example

Mr. I. H., a thirty-six-year-old single man, was referred to the court's psychiatric consultant after he had pleaded guilty to drunkenness when he was found picking up a three-year-old boy and walking away with him. History revealed that he had been arrested on several occasions and had appeared in court three times. Seven years earlier, he had been picked up by police for questioning after there had been complaints in a neighborhood about his frequent appearances there when there were small children around. He was released. About five years earlier, he had been arrested for drunkenness and held in jail overnight. A few months later, he was arrested for disturbing the peace. On that occasion, he had picked up a three-year-old boy but claimed that he did nothing to him. About four years earlier, he was arrested on a charge of indecent assault after picking up a four-year-old girl. He said that he was so drunk at the time that he could not remember exactly what happened.

During the interview, he was quiet but frank in discussing his problem and his previous court appearances. There were certain schizoid qualities to his behavior. Although he admitted that he had a problem, he was not certain it was sexual. He felt that his basic attraction to children was toward those who were in need of care or attention. Mental-status examination did not reveal any signs of a disturbance in thinking or perception. He was committed to a state hospital under the sexual psychopathic law.

IX. **Sexual masochism**

Named for Leopold Sacher-Masoch (1836–1905)

A. Definition

The essential feature of this disorder is recurrent, intense sexual urges and sexually arousing fantasies, of at least six months' duration, involving the act (real, not simulated) of being humiliated, beaten, bound, or otherwise made to suffer. The person has acted on these urges or is markedly distressed by them (*DSM-III-R*).

1. *Flagellation* (erotic whipping) is one example of masochism.

2. *Moral masochism* is the seeking of humiliation and failure rather than physical pain.

3. *Hypoxyphilia,* sexual arousal by oxygen deprivation, is a particularly dangerous form of masochism.

4. *Infantilism* is sometimes used to describe a desire to be treated as a helpless infant and clothed in diapers.

5. Some men with this disorder also have fetishism, transvestic fetishism, or sexual sadism.

6. At times masochists may permit dangerous forms of assault to be performed on them.

B. Prevalence

1. Elements of mild masochism are common. Masochistic fantasies are experienced by nearly everyone.

2. The actual prevalence of this disorder is not known.

3. Masochistic fantasies are likely to begin in childhood, but masochistic activities with partners commonly begin in early adulthood.

4. The disorder is usually chronic.

C. Etiology

1. Again, castration anxiety is the psychoanalytic explanation for both moral and physical masochism.

2. Some think the origins may lie in a child's identification with someone being punished while at the same time experiencing sexual pleasure.

D. Treatment

1. Treatment should be aimed at the underlying feelings of inadequacy.

2. Aversive therapies have been tried.

3. Perhaps a combination of dynamic psychotherapy and some behavioral therapy would offer the best prospect for resolution.

## X. Sexual sadism

Named for the Marquis de Sade (1774–1814), who inflicted extreme cruelty on women for sexual purposes.

A. Definition

The essential feature of this disorder is recurrent, intense sexual urges and sexually arousing fantasies, of at least six months' duration, involving acts (real, not simulated) in which the psychological or physical suffering (including humiliation) of the victim is sexually exciting. The person has acted on these urges or is markedly distressed by them.

1. Some people with this disorder are bothered by their sadistic fantasies, which may be invoked during sexual activity but not otherwise acted upon.
2. Others act on their sadistic sexual urges with a consenting partner who willingly suffers pain and humiliation. Still others act on their sadistic sexual urges with nonconsenting victims.
3. In all of these cases, it is the suffering of the victim that is sexually arousing (*DSM*-III-R).
4. Rape is an extreme form of sadism.
5. Beating, whipping, and tying are common forms of sadistic behavior. "Lust murders" are extreme examples of sadism.
6. Repeated sadistic behavior is usually performed with a person who is a masochist or with a prostitute who is paid.

B. Prevalence

1. Mildly sadistic trends are common in all males.
2. The exact prevalence is not known.
3. Sadism also refers to other acts of excessive cruelty not related to sexuality, such as beating of children.
4. Extreme sadism is usually a psychotic symptom.
5. Sadistic fantasies are apt to begin in childhood, but the onset of sadistic activities is common in early adulthood.

C. Etiology

According to psychoanalytic theory, underlying castration anxiety is the cause of this type of behavior also.

D. Case example

Mr. Creakle, the cruel headmaster of Salem House in Charles Dickens's *David Copperfield:* "He [Creakle] then showed me the cane, and asked me what I thought of that, for a tooth? Was it a sharp tooth, hey? Was it a double tooth, hey? Had it a deep prong, hey? Did it bite, hey? At every question, he gave me a fleshy cut with it that made me writhe; so I was very soon made free of Salem House—and was very soon in tears also.''

## XI. Sado-masochism
A. Definition
1. The occurrence of sadism and masochism in the same person. These two deviancies often occur together, and Freud regarded masochism as sadism turned inward.
2. The two conditions are sometimes included under the term *algolagnia*. Thus, *active algolagnia* is sadism, and *passive algolagnia* is masochism.
3. Sadism and masochism often represent the active and passive poles of the subjugation-humiliation axis.
B. Case example

A thirty-seven-year-old man, separated from his wife, was referred for psychiatric consultation by the attorney who was defending him in a suit filed by a woman who accused him of tying her up and beating her.

He reported that he had been aware of sado-masochistic feelings from about the age of eighteen, although he recalled pleasurable responses to being tied up by another boy at the age of eleven, when they played cowboy and Indian. Since his marriage at twenty-one, he had gone out with a number of women. He would derive sexual pleasure from either tying up a woman or being tied up by her. He usually terminated the relationship with sexual intercourse. He said he found that women liked to be treated roughly. For the preceding five years, he had had intermittent sexual impotence.

## XII. Transvestic fetishism
A. Definition
The essential feature of this disorder is recurrent, intense sexual urges and sexually arousing fantasies, of at least six months' duration, involving cross-dressing. The person has acted on these urges or is markedly distressed by them. Usually the person keeps a collection of women's clothes that he intermittently uses to cross-dress when alone. While cross-dressed, he usually masturbates and imagines other males being attracted to him as a woman in his female attire.
1. This disorder has been described only in heterosexual males. The diagnosis is not made in cases in which the disturbance has evolved into gender identity disorder of adolescence or adulthood, nontranssexual type, or transsexualism.
2. Transvestic phenomena range from occasional solitary wearing of female clothes to extensive involvement in a transvestic subculture.

3. Transvestism is to be distinguished from transsexualism. Transvestites, unlike transsexuals, accept their biological gender and get excited by cross-dressing.

B. Prevalence
   1. Cross-dressing occurs on a continuum from a single guilt-laden dressing to ego-syntonic membership in a transvestite subculture.
   2. Children sometimes dress up in the garb of the opposite sex. According to the folklore of people with this condition, "petticoat punishment," the punishment of humiliating a boy by dressing him in the clothes of a girl, is common in the history of those who later develop this disorder (*DSM*-III-R). Some transvestites recall incidents in which the boy was considered "cute" when wearing female attire.
   3. Transvestism is almost always found in heterosexual males. In our culture, dressing in the clothes of the opposite sex is considered less deviant in females.

C. Etiology
   In addition to what has been said previously about the etiology of sexual deviancy:
   1. The confusion about sexual identification may date from the earliest years in the lives of such individuals.
   2. The parents may have preferred a child of the opposite sex.
   3. There may have been envy of the opposite sex role.
   4. It is thought that the male transvestite reacts to his castration anxiety by identifying with the phallic woman. The mothers of such patients are often reported as being seductive.
   5. Some authorities consider that transvestism is a refuge from the responsibility of being a male (that is, female clothing may have a *meaning* for transvestites that goes beyond sexual arousal).

D. Prognosis
   The prognosis is questionable; transvestites are reluctant to surrender their deviancy because the syndrome is pleasurable (ego-syntonic). Motivation for change usually results from external pressures.

E. Treatment
   Because of the reluctance of transvestites to alter their behavior, treatment has been discouraging. In recent years there have been attempts at aversive behavioral therapy, using electroshocks or emetics.

F. Case example

R. U., a twenty-one-year-old married man, was referred to the court's psychiatric consultant after he had pleaded guilty to a disorderly conduct charge growing out of his arrest in a fitting room of the dress department of a department store while he was dressed in women's clothing.

Upon examination by the police physician, it was discovered that he was completely dressed in women's clothing, including a padded brassiere and women's hose. He admitted that he had dressed in women's clothing on a previous occasion, about two weeks earlier. He felt his problem was a climax to a rather deep-seated sexual problem and reported that he received a thrill upon entering the women's fitting room in the department store, as he had, previously, when he entered the women's washroom of a downtown theater. Just wearing the clothing stimulated him sexually. He seemed to be immature and naive but did not show other evidences of sociopathic behavior. He was placed under probationary supervision and referred to a psychiatric clinic.

## XIII. Voyeurism

A. The essential feature of this disorder is recurrent, intense sexual urges and sexually arousing fantasies, of at least six months' duration, involving the act of observing unsuspecting people, usually strangers, who are either naked, in the process of disrobing, or engaging in sexual activity. The person has acted on these urges or is markedly distressed by them.

The act of looking ("peeping") is for the purpose of achieving sexual excitement, and no sexual activity with the person is sought. Orgasm, usually produced by masturbation, may occur during the voyeuristic activity, or later in response to the memory of what the person has witnessed. Often these people enjoy the fantasy of having a sexual experience with the observed person, but in reality this does not occur. In its severe form, peeping constitutes the exclusive form of sexual activity (DSM-III-R).

1. A voyeur is known as a "peeping Tom."
2. Voyeurism is considered "the flip side of exhibitionism."

B. Prevalence

1. Sexual curiosity is universal, and voyeuristic tendencies are widespread in the male population, as indicated by the extent to which nude or nearly nude women are used in the various communications media.
2. It is normal to be excited by the sight of a love object.
3. It is probably a common deviancy, although the extent is not known because voyeurs are quiet and unobtrusive and, hence, rarely caught.

4. The onset of this disorder is usually in adolescence, and the course is usually chronic.
C. Etiology
1. Voyeuristic urges are universal; it is the inability to keep them within socially accepted limits that poses problems.
2. The psychoanalytic explanation is centered on feelings of castration anxiety; the deviation provides reassurance.
3. Some authorities view this deviation as an attempt to re-create exciting and pleasurable childhood experiences with the mother.
4. Some say a voyeur has been exposed, in an aggressive way, to the nudity of his mother.
D. Prognosis
1. This depends upon the voyeur's desire for change.
2. It is also related to the severity of the deviancy.
3. Although this is usually a harmless paraphilia, there are cases that can proceed from looking to touching, and later to seizing and assault.
E. Treatment
1. The voyeur rarely seeks help voluntarily.
2. Treatment is an attempt to help the person deal with underlying feelings of inadequacy.
3. Some patients say they suffer from impotence and premature ejaculation.
F. Case example

A twenty-three-year-old married man was examined by the court's psychiatric consultant after he had pleaded guilty to a charge of window peeping.
He stated that he began his voyeuristic activities in his first year of college. He estimated that he peeped in windows about once every three or four months. In that period of time, he had been picked up by the police on two occasions but formally charged only once. He was a mild-mannered, frank, and open individual who was basically shy and retiring but could verbalize easily about his problem. He denied any other types of sexually deviant behavior and denied that he had ever been aggressive in any sexual or asocial way. He came from an upper-middle-class family and had an austere father who was emotionally remote from him. He described his mother as a seductive person who had never allowed him to have a warm relationship with his father.
Arrangements were made for him to be seen in a psychiatric clinic.

## XIV. Paraphilia not otherwise specified
A. Telephone scatologia
1. *Telephone scatologia* (*lewdness*) is sexual gratification derived usually by men who telephone women, make obscene

remarks, and suggest that the women meet them and engage in sexual activity.

2. The man is usually apprehended when the woman agrees to meet him where the police can arrest him.

3. Case example

E. L., a twenty-year-old single male, was referred to the court's psychiatric consultant for evaluation after he had been arrested for making obscene phone calls to a sixteen-year-old girl over a six-month period. He would make such comments as, "Do you still have your cherry?" Or, "I want to put my fingers in your hairy cunt." Or, "If you don't let me fuck you, I will force you to fuck me." He admitted that he became sexually excited and on a couple of occasions masturbated when he made these phone calls.

During the interview, he seemed uneasy and defensive and was not very revealing of himself. There was a certain strangeness about his behavior. He was evasive when questioned about his thought processes, although he denied any psychotic mentation, delusions, hallucinations, or other types of perceptual distortions. The MMPI profile suggested depression, passive dependency, and homosexual impulses.

He was recommended for probationary supervision, with the stipulation that he be seen for further evaluation at the local mental health center to see if he could participate in any meaningful kind of treatment.

B. Necrophilia is the deriving of sexual gratification from corpses. This is an extremely rare paraphilia.

C. Partialism (exclusive focus on parts of the body)

D. Zoophilia (also called *bestiality*)

1. Definition: The essential feature is the use of animals as a repeatedly preferred or exclusive method of achieving sexual excitement. The animal may be the object of intercourse or may be trained to sexually excite the human partner by licking or rubbing. Usually the preferred animal is one with which the individual had contact during childhood, such as a household pet or farm animal. The animal is preferred no matter what other forms of sexual outlet are available (*DSM*-III).

2. Prevalence

a) It is rare, even though sexual relations with animals are relatively common.

b) Zoophilia is most commonly found in adolescents and usually involves a household pet or farm animal.

c) It is said to be more common in people who live in rural areas or are socially isolated.

d) The disorder is apparently rare in other circumstances.

e) Such patients are often schizoid, mentally retarded, or psychotic.

3. Case example
   In the following clinical vignette, the patient does not satisfy the current true criteria for zoophilia but does indicate zoophilic interests.

   Mrs. J. W., a thirty-year-old married woman, came for psychiatric treatment because of depressive symptoms. These were in part a result of a somewhat estranged relationship with her husband, who, although attentive, was not sexually interested in her. During the course of her hospitalization, she became profoundly depressed when her pet dog died. At that point she revealed that on a number of occasions she had engaged in sexual relations with the dog.

   E. Coprophilia
      1. *Coprophilia* is a pathological sexual interest in excretions. It includes the desire to defecate on a partner or to be defecated upon. Coprophagia (ingestation of feces) may follow.
   F. *Klismaphila* is the love of enemas and a dependence on their use for sexual arousal.
   G. *Urophilia* is a pathologic love for, or interest in, urine.
   H. Sexual urethran is erotic arousal through stimulation of the urethra (primarily a female paraphilia).

XV. **Prognosis for paraphiliacs**
   A. In general, the prognosis for paraphiliacs depends upon the severity and the chronicity of the deviation. When the paraphilia is well developed and firmly fixed, and there is lack of desire for change, the prognosis is extremely poor.
   B. The best prognosis seems to exist when there is a relationship between the deviant behavior and some precipitating environmental stress, and for younger deviants (especially adolescents).
   C. Since the symptom is pleasurable (ego-syntonic), it is often difficult to treat, especially since deviants seldom seek psychiatric treatment on their own.
   D. Some personality types are commonly found with the paraphiliacs. For example: perverse polymorphous sexuality (sexual behavior that includes many different forms, expressing both adult and infantile tendencies, both normal and abnormal trends). It is commonly found in patients with borderline personality organization. Also, paraphilias that involve overt cruelty to others are often found in patients who have antisocial personality disorders.

XVI. **Treatment of paraphiliacs**
   A. There is no ideal treatment.
   B. Psychotherapy is a long, drawn-out, tedious process with sometimes doubtful results. For those who are uncomfortable, anxious, or depressed (an indication that they cannot accept their deviance), psychotherapy is more promising. Such treatment is

usually insight oriented. Such a therapeutic approach affords the opportunity to trace the onset of the disorder and hopefully eliminate it.

C. Behavioral therapy has been tried with some reported success.

D. Because their behaviors and desires are ego-syntonic, paraphiliacs seldom seek treatment and are most often encountered in the legal system as "sex offenders." A new discipline of sex offender assessment and treatment has emerged (Adson 1992).

E. Perhaps setting goals for treatment would be helpful, as, for example, whether or not the patient wants merely to control his symptoms or surrender his disorder, or whether or not he wishes to make a better adaptation to his paraphilia.

F. Psychotropic medications, including antipsychotic drugs, may be helpful in those paraphilias that are acutely or dangerously compulsive.

G. Antiandrogens (e.g., cyproterone acetate and Depo-Provera) in selected cases have been reported to decrease hypersexual behavior.

## XVII. Homosexuality

A. The American Psychiatric Association has officially taken the position that homosexuality does not constitute a psychiatric disorder.

B. Homosexuality is not listed in *DSM*-III-R.

C. *DSM*-I listed homosexuality as a sexual deviation, and this was considered a type of sociopathic personality disturbance.

D. In *DSM*-II—until 1973—it was also considered one of the sexual deviations. In 1973, however, the term *homosexuality* was dropped, and the term *sexual orientation disturbance* was substituted to apply to gay men and women who were "disturbed by, in conflict with or wanted to change their sexual orientation."

E. *DSM*-III listed *ego-dystonic homosexuality,* for a person who was homosexually aroused but found this arousal to be a persistent source of distress and wanted to become heterosexual.

F. *DSM*-III-R does not specifically mention homosexuality as a disorder. Rather, in a category of Sexual Disorder Category Not Otherwise Specified, there is given an example of "persistence and marked distress about one's sexual orientation" without specifying a *particular* orientation. This could technically allow for the possibility of ego-dystonic heterosexuality.

## XVIII. Sexual dysfunctions

Focus in this section is on a range of problems that represent inhibitions in the normal sexual response cycle.

A. Definition

1. The essential feature of this subclass is inhibition in the appetitive or psychophysiologic changes that characterize the

complete sexual response cycle. Ordinarily this diagnostic category will be applied only when the disturbance is a major part of the clinical picture, even though it may not be part of the chief complaint. The diagnosis is not made if the sexual dysfunction is attributed entirely to organic factors, such as a physical disorder or a medication, or if it is due to another Axis I mental disorder (*DSM*-III-R).

2. The complete sexual response cycle as described by Masters and Johnson (1966, 1970) and Kaplan (1974) can be divided into the following phases (*DSM*-III-R):

   a) *Appetitive*. This consists of fantasies about sexual activity and a desire to have sexual activity.

   b) *Excitement*. This consists of a subjective sense of sexual pleasure and accompanying physiologic changes. The major changes in the male consist of penile tumescence, leading to erection, and the appearance of Cowper's gland secretion. The major changes in the female consist of vasocongestion in the pelvis, vaginal lubrication, and swelling of the external genitalia. Other changes include development of the orgasmic platform, that is, narrowing of the outer third of the vagina by increased pubococcygeal muscle tension and vasocongestion; vasocongestion of the labia minora; breast tumescence; and lengthening and widening of the inner two-thirds of the vagina.

   c) *Orgasm*. This consists of a peaking of sexual pleasure, with release of sexual tension and rhythmic contraction of the perineal muscles and pelvic reproductive organs. In the male there is the sensation of ejaculatory inevitability, which is followed by emission of semen, caused by contractions of the prostate, seminal vesicles, and urethra. In the female there are contractions, not always subjectively experienced as such, of the wall of the outer third of the vagina. In both the male and the female there is often generalized muscular tension or contractions, such as involuntary pelvic thrusting.

   d) *Resolution*. This consists of a sense of general relaxation, well-being, and muscular relaxation. During this phase, males are physiologically refractory to further erection and orgasm for a period of time. In contrast, women may be able to respond to additional stimulation almost immediately.

3. Inhibitions may occur during one or more of these four phases of the response cycle.
4. Sexual avoidance (phobic) is not really a psychosexual problem. Many are preoccupied with their sexual performance.

B. Prevalence

This is not really known, but most of these dysfunctions are believed to be common, especially in their milder forms.

C. Types of sexual dysfunctions
   1. Sexual desire disorders
      a) Hypoactive sexual desire disorder: persistently or recurrently deficient or absent sexual fantasies and desire for sexual activity.
      b) Sexual aversion disorder: persistent or recurrent extreme aversion to, and avoidance of, all or almost all, genital sexual contact with a sexual partner.
   2. Sexual arousal disorders
      a) Female sexual arousal disorder: (1) persistent or recurrent partial or complete failure to attain or maintain the lubrication-swelling response of sexual excitement until completion of the sexual activity; (2) persistent or recurrent lack of a subjective sense of sexual excitement and pleasure in a female during sexual activity.
      b) Male erectile disorder: persistent or recurrent partial or complete failure in a male to attain or maintain erection until completion of the sexual activity.
   3. Orgasm disorders
      a) Inhibited female orgasm: persistent or recurrent delay in, or absence of, orgasm in a female following a normal sexual excitement phase during sexual activity that the clinician judges to be adequate in focus, intensity, and duration.
      b) Inhibited male orgasm: persistent or recurrent delay in, or absence of, orgasm in a male following a normal heterosexual excitement phase during sexual activity that the clinician, taking into account the person's age, judges to be adequate in focus, intensity, and duration.
      c) Premature ejaculation: persistent or recurrent ejaculation with minimal sexual stimulation or before, upon, or shortly after penetration and before the person wishes it.
   4. Sexual pain disorders
      a) Dyspareunia: recurrent or persistent genital pain in either a male or female before, during, or after sexual intercourse.

b) Vaginismus: recurrent or persistent involuntary spasm of the musculature of the outer third of the vagina that interferes with coitus.

D. Course

The course is variable. All of the dysfunctions may be acquired or lifelong. Most commonly have their onset in early adult life.

E. Etiology

Most of the information on causality is based on studies from uncontrolled case studies and thus must be viewed with caution. It is assumed that physiological factors have been ruled out.

1. Predisposing factors

There is a slight correlation between certain personality traits and the presence of certain psychosexual dysfunctions.

a) Histrionic characteristics in females are frequently associated with inhibited sexual excitement and inhibited orgasm.

b) Compulsive traits in males are frequently associated with inhibited sexual desires and inhibited sexual excitement.

c) Anxiety appears to predispose to the development of premature ejaculation.

d) Any negative attitude toward sexuality (from internal conflicts, rigid subcultural values, or particular experiences) seems to predispose to psychosexual dysfunction.

2. Masters and Johnson (1966, 1970) emphasize the importance of performance fears and the assuming of a spectator role in which a sexual participant may be distracted from the natural reception of sexual stimulation or expression of sexual responsiveness.

3. Psychodynamic theory regards sexual dysfunctions as having their roots in early developmental conflict.

4. Women's sexual responsiveness, more than men's, tends to depend on feelings of tenderness, intimacy, affection, and security. Any factors that interfere with these underlying feelings may also impair the woman's ability to be sexually responsive.

5. A frequent problem in the woman's impaired sexual response is the male's premature ejaculation (some say premature ejaculation in men is disappearing).

6. Perhaps even more common is some disturbance in the total relationship with the partner.

7. Primary male impotence usually indicates serious underlying psychopathology. Such men usually come from backgrounds of sexual repression.

8. Men with secondary impotence are usually responding to some situational factor (e.g., excessive indulgence in alcohol, occupational or economic tensions, depression).
9. Testosterone is the libido hormone in both sexes.

F. Treatment
1. Individual psychotherapy is useful in examining problems with intimacy and dependency (issues often accompanied by sexual dysfunction).
2. Group therapy, whether behaviorally, educationally, or psychodynamically oriented, may be useful adjuncts to other forms of therapy.
3. Masters and Johnson
   a) Masters and Johnson are mostly responsible for the sex therapy movement.
   b) Their programs attempted to focus on reduction or elimination of the fears of sexual performance and to take the couple "out of their maladaptive spectator role."
   c) The emphasis in the treatment is on the relationship, not on the particular difficulties in either partner. Whatever the problem, the couple is encouraged to see it as a mutual responsibility.
   d) They introduced the concept of *sensate focus* (attention is diverted from erection and orgasm to mutual, nondemanding, pleasurable experiences with the body; genital stimulation is considered at a later stage.
   e) The treatment leads to a gradual, unthreatening exposure to increasing the intimate sexual encounters for the couple.
4. In psychoanalytically oriented sex therapy, sex therapy is integrated with traditional psychoanalytic techniques.
5. The influential treatment methods of Helen Singer Kaplan combine psychodynamic and cognitive-behavioral approaches. She recognizes that some sexual problems may be quite specific, while others may be complicated by underlying intrapsychic conflicts.
6. Many treatment procedures emphasize training in communication between partners about likes and dislikes in sexual treatment and about sources of anxiety and uncertainty.
7. Focus in hypnotherapy is specifically on the anxiety-producing symptom, that is, the particular sexual dysfunction. Patients are also taught relaxation techniques to use prior to sexual intercourse.
8. Many sexual therapy clinics have evolved in the United States, generally in the Masters and Johnson mode.

## G. Outcome

The most difficult treatment cases involve couples with severe marital discord.

## References

Adson, P. R., ed. "Paraphilias and Related Disorders." *Psychiatric Annals* 22, no. 6 (June 1992): 299 ff.

American Psychiatric Association. *Diagnostic and Statistical Manual of Mental Disorders.* 3d ed., rev. Washington, D.C.: APA, 1987.

Campbell, R. J. *Psychiatric Dictionary.* 6th ed. New York: Oxford University Press, 1989.

Davison, G. C., and J. M. Neale. *Abnormal Psychology.* 4th ed. New York: Wiley, 1990.

Gabbard, G. O. *Psychodynamic Psychiatry and Clinical Practice.* Washington, D.C.: American Psychiatric Association Press, 1990.

Goodwin, D. W., and S. B. Guze. *Psychiatric Diagnosis.* 2d ed. New York: Oxford University Press, 1979.

Hastings, D. W. *Impotence and Frigidity.* Boston: Little, Brown, 1963.

Kaplan, H. S. *The New Sex Therapy: Active Treatment of Sexual Dysfunction.* New York: Brunner/Mazel, 1974.

Kaplan, H. I., and B. J. Sadock, eds. *Comprehensive Textbook of Psychiatry/V.* 5th ed. Baltimore: Williams & Wilkins, 1989.

Kolb, L. C., and H. K. H. Brodie. *Modern Clinical Psychiatry.* 10th ed. Philadelphia: Saunders, 1982.

Marmor, J. "Sexual Deviancy: Part 1." *Journal of Continuing Education in Psychiatry* 39, no. 7 (July 1978): 123–34.

_____. "Sexual Deviancy: Part 2." *Journal of Continuing Education in Psychiatry* 39, no. 8 (August 1978).

Masters, W. H., and V. E. Johnson. *Human Sexual Response.* Boston: Little, Brown, 1966.

_____. *Human Sexual Inadequacy.* Boston: Little, Brown, 1970.

# 19 Psychoactive Substance Use Disorders

Some fell by laudanum, and some by steel
and death ambush lay in every pill.

**Sir Samuel Garth, *The Dispensary***

## I. Definition

A. According to *DSM*-III-R, this diagnostic class deals with the symptoms and maladaptive behavioral changes associated with more or less regular use of psychoactive substances that affect the central nervous system. Disorders in this section are to be distinguished from psychoactive substance-induced organic mental disorders because psychoactive substance use disorder refers to the maladaptive behavior associated more or less with the regular use of the substances whereas, psychoactive substance-induced organic mental disorder describes the direct, acute, or chronic effect of substances on the central nervous system.

B. Classes of psychoactive substances
There are nine classes of psychoactive substances that are associated with both abuse and dependence. These include alcohol; amphetamine or similarly acting sympathomimetics; cannabis; cocaine; hallucinogens; inhalants; opioids; phencyclidine (PCP) or similarly acting arylcyclohexylamines; and sedatives, hypnotics, or anxiolytics. A tenth drug, nicotine, shows dependence but not abuse. These ten classes may be grouped into those that share similar features: 1. alcohol and sedatives (anxiolytics and hypnotics); 2. cocaine and amphetamine or similarly acting sympathomimetics; 3. hallucinogens and phencyclidine (PCP) or similarly acting arylcyclohexylamines.

C. The psychoactive substance use disorders are subdivided into substance abuse and substance dependence.

1. Psychoactive substance dependence (*DSM*-III-R)
   a) At least three of the following must be present:

(1) Substance often taken in larger amounts or over a longer period than the person intended

(2) Persistent desire or one or more unsuccessful efforts to cut down or control substance use

(3) A great deal of time spent in activities necessary to get the substance (e.g., theft), taking the substance (e.g., chain smoking), or recovering from its effects

(4) Frequent intoxication or withdrawal symptoms when expected to fulfill major role obligations at work, school, or home (e.g., does not go to work because hung over, goes to school or work "high," intoxicated while taking care of his or her children), or when substance use is physically hazardous (e.g., drives when intoxicated)

(5) Important social, occupational, or recreational activities given up or reduced because of substance use

(6) Continued substance use despite knowledge of having a persistent or recurrent social, psychological, or physical problem that is caused or exacerbated by the use of the substance (e.g., continuing to use heroin despite family arguments about it, cocaine-induced depression, or having an ulcer made worse by drinking)

(7) Marked tolerance: Need for markedly increased amounts of the substance (i.e., at least a 50 percent increase) in order to achieve intoxication or desired effect, or markedly diminished effect with continued use of the same amount. Note: The following items may not apply to cannabis, hallucinogens, or phencyclidine (PCP).

(8) Characteristic withdrawal symptoms

(9) Substance often taken to relieve or avoid withdrawal symptoms

b) Some symptoms of the disturbance have persisted for at least one month or have occurred repeatedly over a longer period of time.

2. Psychoactive substance abuse (*DSM*-III-R)

a) A maladaptive pattern of psychoactive substance use is indicated by at least one of the following:

(1) Continued use despite knowledge of having a persistent or recurrent social, occupational, psychological, or physical problem that is caused or exacerbated by use of the psychoactive substance

(2) Recurrent use in situations in which use is physically hazardous (e.g., driving while intoxicated)

b) Some symptoms of the disturbance have persisted for at least one month or have occurred repeatedly over a longer period of time.

c) Never met the criteria for psychoactive substance dependence for this substance.

## II. Prevalence

A. Substance abuse is a major public health problem in this country. Use of psychoactive substances, including illegal drugs, continues to increase.

B. Prior to the 1960s, the nonmedical use of drugs other than alcohol and tobacco was relatively low. (For example, only 1 percent of Americans aged twelve to seventeen ever used marijuana, and only 4 percent of those aged eighteen to twenty-five had ever used this drug.)

C. In the late 1960s and early 1970s, nonmedical drug use reached epidemic proportions (e.g., marijuana use in the twelve- to seventeen-year-old population rose to 31 percent in 1979, and 68 percent of Americans aged eighteen to twenty-five reported that they had used marijuana at least once. In 1978, nearly 11 percent of American high school seniors reported using marijuana every day of their senior year). In the years since, the rates of illicit drug use have leveled off and, in some cases, declined but none have fallen to the levels characteristic of the years before 1962.

D. Epidemiologic studies during 1981 to 1983 indicate that 5 to 6 percent of the adult population has met *DSM*-III criteria for some type of drug abuse or dependence (other than alcohol) sometime in their life (Kaplan and Sadock 1989).

E. Epidemiologic studies have shown that the onset of the nonmedical drug use is all but limited to the teenage years. The progression is as follows: drug use begins with alcohol (the gateway into recreational, nonmedical use of intoxicants for adolescents). This is followed by the use of marijuana (the gateway into the use of illicit drugs), and moves on to the nonmedical use of dependence-producing pharmaceuticals (many anxiety agents, analgesics, and hypnotics) and cocaine. The final step is to the most stigmatized and least commonly used drugs, such as heroin and phencyclidine.

F. Youths who do not use cigarettes and alcohol during their teenage years are virtually immune to the nonmedical use of other dependence-producing drugs (DuPont 1985).

G. Most drug-dependent people become so by their association with other people who are also drug dependent. Their lives prior to substance use have usually been ones of unsatisfactory or marginal adjustments.

H. Medications that reduce pain, diminish anxiety, or produce euphoria may be taken by those who seek relief from physical or psychological symptoms or feelings of inadequacy.

## III. Etiology

A. Many of the etiological and psychopathological factors found in substance use disorders are also associated with alcoholism (see chapter 20).

B. There are a number of theories as to the cause of drug abuse.

1. Availability

This is considered the sine qua non for drug dependence. In other words, the drug has to be available before one can become addicted. An example of this would be the availability of all kinds of drugs in urban ghettos and the availability of sedatives, narcotics, and psychoactive drugs in the medical community. (Yet, the majority of both of these communities do not take drugs. Thus, availability by itself does not fully explain drug dependency.)

2. Psychological

There is no single personality type who becomes drug dependent. According to *DSM*-III-R, personality disturbance and disturbance of mood are often present, and may be intensified by the psychoactive substance use disorder. For example, antisocial personality traits may be accentuated by the need to obtain money to purchase illegal substances. Anxiety or depression associated with borderline personality disorder may be intensified as the person uses a psychoactive substance in an unsuccessful attempt to treat his or her mood disturbance.

In chronic abuse or dependence, mood lability and suspiciousness, both of which can contribute to violent behavior, are common (*DSM*-III-R).

There are numerous psychological theories (e.g., oral dependence is considered to be etiological in psychoanalytic theory, and some say drugs are used to control anger).

3. Socioeconomic

The incidence is highest in both the lowest and the highest socioeconomic groups, and is lowest in the middle class.

4. Social (e.g., in dictatorships, disapproved drugs are kept out). Russia does not have a drug problem but has a serious problem with alcohol. Sweden and Japan have major problems with amphetamines.

5. Biologic (e.g., opiate addiction is thought to result from an endorphin deficiency).

C. Some people take drugs to overcome feelings of inferiority or inadequacy.

1. The individual who has a reduced tolerance to tension, feelings of inadequacy, and who feels under personal or social stress may take drugs.
2. The availability of drugs and other cultural factors may play a role. Physicians are apt to abuse narcotics and antianxiety agents, housewives are most likely to abuse sedatives and antianxiety agents and adolescents are most apt to abuse marijuana or other street drugs. (The availability of drugs is the most common predisposing factor in substance use.)

D. Some take drugs mostly for the euphoric effect (e.g., cocaine or marijuana).

## IV. Psychopathology

A. Persons who develop drug dependency have subnormal tolerance of tension and above-normal feelings of dependency.
B. Features of various personality disorders are often present in substance abusers. For example, some show traits of antisocial personality, others may show evidences of borderline personality or dysthymic disorder (chronic depression).
C. Some authorities believe that there is absence of a strong father figure in the developmental histories of people who become addicts.

## V. Classes of psychoactive substances

The following are some of the drugs, other than alcohol and nicotine, on which people can become dependent or which they can abuse.

A. Amphetamine or similarly acting sympathomimetic compounds. This group includes all of the substances of the substituted phenylethylamine structure, such as amphetamine, dextroamphetamine, and methamphetamine ("speed"), and those with structures different from the substituted phenylethylamines that have amphetamine-like action, such as methylphenidate and some substances used as appetite suppressants ("diet pills"). These substances are typically taken orally or intravenously, although methamphetamine is frequently taken by nasal inhalation (like cocaine) (*DSM*-III-R).

1. Medical use
   a) They were first used in otolaryngology as a nasal decongestant.
   b) They were also prescribed to relieve fatigue or depression, to control appetite, or to produce wakefulness in those who had to perform tasks of long duration.
   c) There are far fewer legitimate medical indications for their use now, and they have come under much closer

government supervision because of their widespread abuse.

    d) They are used in the treatment of attention-deficit hyperactivity disorder and narcolepsy.

2. Prevalence and course

    a) These drugs are stimulants and produce euphoria.

    b) Sometimes those dependent on sedatives for sleep take them to stay awake during the daytime.

    c) Many people obtain them illicitly.

    d) Acute paranoid psychosis may develop in people who abuse this group of drugs. A urine test for amphetamines is necessary to make the diagnosis of amphetamine intoxication, which may be clinically indistinguishable from acute paranoid schizophrenia.

    e) Abuse occurs in approximately 2 percent of the adult population (*DSM*-III-R).

    f) Many develop abuse or dependence after first using an appetite suppressant.

    g) The amphetamine user often abuses or is dependent on other drugs to counteract unpleasant aftereffects of amphetamine intoxication.

    h) Psychological and behavioral changes include depression, irritability, anhedonia, anergia, and social isolation.

3. Patterns of use

Some people develop amphetamine abuse or dependence after first using amphetamines or amphetamine-like compounds as appetite suppressants.

4. Associated features

Often the user of amphetamine also abuses or is dependent on other drugs, which are taken in an attempt to counteract the unpleasant aftereffects of intoxication.

Psychological and behavioral changes associated with amphetamine abuse and dependence include depression, irritability, anhedonia, anergia, and social isolation.

B. Cannabis

1. This group includes all substances with psychoactive properties derived from the cannabis plant plus chemically similar synthetic substances (marijuana, hashish, and occasionally purified THC; they are almost always smoked).

2. Cannabis, or marijuana, is a leaf that grows wild in most parts of the United States and South America.

3. Medical use

    a) Cannabis was previously used as a treatment for tension headache, dysmenorrhea, and glaucoma.

    b) It was removed from the U.S. Pharmacopoeia in 1935.

c) Generally, it has been prescribed only experimentally (e.g., it has been released for the treatment of glaucoma, and nausea and other side effects of anticancer drugs and anorexia nervosa).

4. Patterns of use

Many people regard this as a substance of low abuse potential, not appreciating its capacity to induce dependence. Dependence is usually characterized by daily or almost daily use. It is used in combination with other substances, particularly alcohol and cocaine. Psychological symptoms associated with cannabis dependency include lethargy, anhedonia, and attentional and memory problems.

5. Course

Chronic use produces the amotivational syndrome.

6. Prevalence

a) About 10 percent of Americans of all ages use marijuana.

b) It remains popular because of its pleasurable effects (usually without the hangover common with alcohol).

C. Cocaine

1. Cocaine has a limited use in medical practice (e.g., as an anesthetic in certain types of nasal surgery).

2. It produces euphoria, loquaciousness, elation, and grandiosity.

3. Sometimes produces somatic hallucinations, including formication, a tactile hallucination or illusion that insects are crawling on the body or under the skin (sometimes referred to as the "cocaine bug").

4. Types

Several different types of coca preparations are used for their psychoactive properties: coca leaves (while a relatively safe practice in South America, with a low concentration of .5–1 percent in the leaves) chewed, coca paste (smoked), cocaine hydrochloride powder (inhaled or injected), and cocaine alkaloid—"freebase" or "crack" (smoked) and which are both deathly destructive. The most commonly used form in the United States is cocaine hydrochloride powder, which is usually inhaled through the nostrils, and then absorbed into the bloodstream through the mucous membranes.

5. Status

a) Prior to the mid-1960s, cocaine was used primarily by heroin addicts and members of the hard-core drug culture, whom Americans regarded as criminals. Thus, cocaine had little appeal or status.

b) During the late 1960s and the early 1970s, it began to be used by a broad segment of American society, when cocaine became viewed as similar to marijuana use. (Possession was illegal, but use was not viewed as criminal behavior.)

c) In the mid-1980s "crack" occurred on the streets. This is available in small, relatively inexpensive doses. Less affluent consumers have experimented and become addicted. Some authorities believe "crack" is the most dangerous and perhaps most addicting of all the illicit drugs.

d) Some feel the mass media played an important role in popularizing cocaine, and it developed an elite status. Perhaps the reduced availability of amphetamines was another factor in popularizing cocaine. Further, cocaine was viewed as "not addicting" because it did not induce physical dependence. (Currently, few still believe this.)

e) It is increasingly reported as the primary drug of abuse among those seeking treatment for addiction in both the private and the public sectors. However, this is misleading because many drug abusers will claim cocaine dependency because it is "fashionable."

f) Bromptom's solution is an oral pain-relieving medication for terminal cancer patients that contains methadone (or morphine), alcohol, and cocaine.

6. Patterns of use

Cocaine abusers often use barbiturates, methaqualone, benzodiazepines, or alcohol to self-medicate for insomnia, agitation, and irritability, which result from the cocaine use.

Cocaine abuse and dependence are associated with two different patterns of use: episodic and chronic daily, or almost daily, use.

"Bingeing" is a common form of episodic use consisting of compressed time periods of continuous high-dose use.

7. Psychological features

Cocaine can produce a broad range of psychological effects, ranging from acute anxiety to full-blown cocaine psychosis with paranoia and auditory or visual hallucinations.

Psychological and behavioral changes include depression, irritability, anhedonia, anergia, and social isolation. Sexual dysfunction, paranoid ideation, attentional disturbances, and memory problems may also occur.

8. Course
   a) Cocaine smoking and intravenous administration of cocaine tend to engender rapid progression from infrequent cocaine use to cocaine abuse or dependence, often within only a few weeks or months.
   b) Progressive tolerance of the desirable effects of the substance leads to use of increasing doses.
   c) With continued use there is a progressive diminution in pleasurable effects and a corresponding increase in dysphoric effects.
   d) Quitting cocaine use causes a severe withdrawal syndrome:
      (1) *Crash,* which can last from nine hours to four days (dysphoria followed by a crash in mood and later sleepiness).
      (2) Withdrawal can last from one to ten weeks (craving returns after periods of "normality").
      (3) Extinction is indefinite (periodic cravings can last a long time).
9. Prevalence
   Cocaine abuse has reached epidemic proportions in this country. Current estimates suggest that 20 to 24 million Americans have experimented with cocaine. Four to five million people are considered to be regular users, and the amount of cocaine used in this country increases by 10 to 20 percent each year (Spitz and Rosecan 1987).
D. Hallucinogens
   1. Definition
      This group includes two types of substances, both of which have hallucinogenic properties:
      a) Substances structurally related to 5-hydroxytryptamine, for example, lysergic acid diethylamine (LSD) and dimethyltryptamide (DMT)
      b) Substances related to catecholamine (e.g., mescaline)
   2. Effect
      a) Most produce a reaction similar to hypomania and schizophrenic withdrawal (preoccupation with own thoughts and perceptions).
      b) Among the perceptual changes are subjective intensification of perceptions, depersonalization, derealization, illusions, hallucinations, or synesthesias (e.g., seeing colors when a loud sound occurs). These occur in a state of full wakefulness and alertness.
      c) These drugs can lead to serious psychological damage.

d) Some of the adverse effects that have been reported from LSD use are
   (1) Long-term psychotic disorders
   (2) Panic from a reaction to the hallucinatory experiences ("bad trip")
   (3) Serious injury and even death from the delusional experiences (e.g., feelings of omnipotence or the feeling that one can fly)
   (4) Long-term intellectual and emotional disorientation
   (5) Flashback phenomenon, a reexperiencing of a trip without further use of the drug

3. Patterns of use
   Most people are introduced to a hallucinogen by "experimenting" with the substance. Some find the hallucinosis extremely dysphoric and stop using the substance, whereas others enjoy the experience and continue its use.

4. Associated features
   Hallucinogens are frequently contaminated with other drugs, such as PCP and amphetamine. In addition, users frequently smoke cannabis and abuse alcohol.

5. Course
   The course is unpredictable and probably related to the nature of the underlying pathology that played a role in onset of its use. Most people rapidly resume their former lifestyle after only a brief period of abuse or dependence.

6. Prevalence
   The use of hallucinogens as the predominant substance is extremely rare (*DSM*-III-R).

E. Inhalants
   1. Included in this classification are disorders induced by inhaling, through the mouth or nose, the aliphatic and aromatic hydrocarbons found in substances such as gasoline, glue, paint, paint thinners, and spray paints. Less commonly used are the halogenated hydrocarbons found in cleaners, typewriter correction fluid, and spray-can propellants and other volatile compounds containing esters, ketones, and glycols.
   2. Most compounds that are inhaled are a mixture of several substances that can produce psychoactive effects. Therefore, under most circumstances, it is difficult to ascertain the exact substance responsible for the disorder.
   3. Several methods are used to inhale intoxicating vapors. Most commonly, a rag soaked with the substance is applied to the mouth and nose, and the vapors are breathed in.

The background of inhalant users is generally marked by considerable family dysfunction (as in school or work adjustment problems).

Generally, inhalants are used by quite young children, nine to thirteen years of age, generally with a group of peers who are likely to use alcohol and cannabis as well.

4. Users of inhalants nearly always use other psychoactive substances as well.

5. Younger children may use inhalants several times a week, often on weekends and after school. Severe dependence in young adults may involve varying periods of intoxication throughout each day.

6. Prevalence is not known.

F. Opioid substances

1. Abuse of or dependence upon opioids generally follows a period of "polydrug use."

2. Course

a) Once the pattern is established, substance procurement and its use generally dominate the individual's life.

b) The course is a function of the context of the addiction; that is, the vast majority of persons who became dependent on heroin in Vietnam did not return to their addiction when back in the United States. In contrast, it is believed that most individuals who become dependent on opioids in the United States become involved in a chronic behavioral disorder, marked by remissions while in treatment or prison or when the substance is scarce, but relapses on returning to a familiar environment where these substances are available and friends or colleagues use these substances (*DSM*-III).

c) In the United States, persons with opioid dependence have a high annual death rate (approximately ten per one thousand).

3. Case examples

a) Thomas De Quincey (1785–1859), essayist and critic, reported his experiences in *Confessions of an English Opium Eater*. While still in college, he took his first opium to relieve the pain of facial neuralgia and several years later became a "regular and confirmed opium eater." Though he wrote "these troubles are passed," he actually remained an opium user for the rest of his life.

b) Samuel Taylor Coleridge (1772–1834), who was the author of *The Rime of the Ancient Mariner, Kubla Khan,* and *Christabel,* in his later years was dejected and became addicted to opium.

G. Phencyclidine or similarly acting arylcyclohexylamine compounds
   1. Phencyclidine is a white powder, commonly called PCP ("peace pill").
   2. Although available as a veterinary anesthetic, most of the illicit supply comes from home laboratories.
   3. On the street it is called "angel dust."
   4. It is sold in powder and tablet form, both in many colors.
   5. It is often sprinkled on marijuana or parsley leaves and smoked in a "joint."
   6. It may well be that the use of PCP is quite common among abusers of other drugs.
   7. PCP is stronger than marijuana, perhaps more comparable to LSD.
   8. The diagnosis of overdosage is frequently missed because the presenting symptoms often closely resemble those of an acute schizophrenic episode.
   9. Some authorities feel that phenothiazines should not be used to manage a patient during the acute stage of overdose because of the anticholinergic potentiation.
H. Sedative, hypnotic, or anxiolytic substances
   1. Types
      Hypnotics, or "sleeping pills," include benzodiazepines such as flurazepam, triazolam, and temazepam, and other substances unrelated to benzodiazepines, such as ethchlorvynol, glutethimide, chloral hydrate, methaqualone, and the barbiturates. Benzodiazepines are also used for the treatment of anxiety and are the most commonly prescribed psychoactive medications (*DSM*-III-R).
   2. Although these psychoactive substances differ widely in their mechanisms of action, rates of absorption, metabolism, and distribution in the body, at some dose and at some duration of use, they are all capable of producing similar syndromes of intoxication and withdrawal. Substances in this category are usually taken orally (*DSM*-III-R).
   3. Patterns of use
      There are two patterns.
      a) The person originally obtained the psychoactive substance by prescription from a physician for treatment of anxiety or insomnia, but gradually increases the dose in frequency of use on his or her own.
      b) A second pattern more frequent than the first that leads to the dependence involves young people in their teens and early twenties who, with a group of peers, use substances obtained from illegal sources. The initial

objective is to obtain a "high" or euphoria on the substances used alone.
4. Course

The most common course is heavy daily use that results in dependence. A significant number of people with dependence eventually stop using the substance and recover completely, even from the physical complications of the disorder (*DSM*-III-R).
5. Prevalence

Approximately 1.1 percent of the adult population have had sedative, hypnotic, or anxiolytic abuse or dependence at some time in their lives.

Epidemiologic data gathered over the last fifteen years show that the U.S. benzodiazepine use is not higher than that of other developed nations and that most patients who use these drugs do so with symptomatic relief and restraint in terms of amount, dose, and duration of treatment. On the other hand, the same data show that almost 2 percent of the adult population use these agents more or less chronically.

For many patients suffering from anxiety disorders, continued use of a benzodiazepine is preferable to enduring the underlying anxiety symptoms (DuPont 1986).

## VI. Treatment

A. Treatment of the underlying personality disorder
   1. This is often extremely difficult, because the substance abuser and the substance-dependent person, like the alcoholic, have reduced tolerance for tension.
   2. Psychotherapy
      a) Psychotherapy is of help in many cases.
      b) Support and reassurance are important.
      c) Group psychotherapy has been helpful in some cases.
B. Treatment of the drug dependence
   1. Self-help groups

   Groups such as AA or other groups composed of drug-dependent people are often the most helpful.
   2. Withdrawal
      a) At present, most withdrawal treatment is fairly abrupt and uses the principles of supportive treatment. Sometimes people who are intoxicated or stuporous are taken to detoxification centers or to hospitals.
      b) Supportive treatment involves
         (1) A detoxification period during which certain drugs are judiciously prescribed. The drugs include methadone (see the following), chlordiazepoxide (Librium), diazepam (Valium), or phenobarbital. They

are continued for several days after the patient has discontinued using the abused drug.

(2) Adequate diet and fluid intake.

(3) Often, placement in chemical dependency units where patients are treated much like alcoholics (units like the Minnesota Model). Such persons often need more "attention" than other patients.

(4) A therapeutic, supportive, and reassuring attitude. The therapist avoids being judgmental or moralistic.

c) Methadone

Methadone (Dolophine) is the drug used to treat addicts of opiate and opiate-like agents. It is administered in two ways.

(1) Methadone substitution

In this approach, the addict takes a regular dose of methadone, given orally, after which the methadone is progressively withdrawn over a period of a few days.

(2) Methadone maintenance

In this method, the methadone is prescribed indefinitely.

(3) Methadone withdrawal

Clonidine (Catapres) has been used with reported success in withdrawing people from methadone.

3. Therapeutic communities demanding total commitment from the patient are residential treatment programs that attempt to deal with the psychological causes of addiction by changing the addict's personality and character (not suitable for very many).

4. Those who abuse substances are at risk as a result of their behavior—for example, automobile accidents, drug-related violence, the sharing of needles for drug injection. This latter carries a risk of hepatitis and AIDS. Also drug abusers increase other kinds of risk-taking behavior including unsafe sexual practices.

5. Rehabilitation of the drug-dependent person must be regarded as a long-term management problem. Refer to chapter 21 for information about follow-up treatment and rehabilitation after the patient leaves the hospital.

## VII. Prognosis

A. The prognosis is often poor.

B. Relapses are common.

C. However, given someone who is well motivated and willing to regard his or her problem as a long-term one that must be dealt with consistently over a protracted period of time, the frequency of relapses can be reduced and the periods of abstinence can be lengthened.

D. Follow-up programs such as AA, halfway houses, and other various group settings have improved the remission rate.

**VIII.** **Case examples**

A. Medical addiction

Mrs. J., a forty-year-old housewife, had suffered from migraine headaches since puberty. They had gradually increased in frequency and severity. At thirty, she began taking codeine. For a few years, this gave some relief, but for five years she had been taking Demerol (a synthetic narcotic drug) in increasingly larger doses. At the time of admission to the hospital, she was using five hundred to six hundred milligrams of Demerol per day (the usual dose is fifty milligrams). She was always very dependent on her mother. Even after her marriage, she never lived farther away from her mother than one block. She had always had a reduced tolerance for any kind of discomfort; for example, she required medication for painful menses, sinusitis, and other pain.

Although Demerol was successfully withdrawn rapidly during her hospitalization, she was never fully able to face her underlying problems of dependency and unexpressed hostility. One month after discharge, she was again beginning to take Demerol for her headaches.

In the foregoing case, note that the patient began taking drugs for a psychosomatic illness (migraine), that she had a reduced tolerance of discomfort, was very dependent, and was unable to express hostile feelings.

B. Self-administration

Mr. D. S., a twenty-three-year-old single male, was referred to the court's psychiatric consultant for evaluation after he had been placed in the county correctional facility for driving after suspension of his license and driving under the influence of drugs. These offenses occurred while he was awaiting trial on a charge of aggravated robbery.

He had received an undesirable discharge from the Marine Corps centering on his possession and use of marijuana, "at my own request." In addition, he reported, he had been court-martialed for disrespect to a noncommissioned officer and had received minor discipline for two other offenses. Concerning his use of drugs, he said that he was first "turned on" by marijuana about three years earlier, while serving with the marines. From then until the time of the arrest that brought him to the attention of the court's consultant, he had used drugs extensively. He had used LSD and other hallucinogenic drugs, but gave these up after he began to have bad trips and flashbacks. He said that he had been hospitalized in Okinawa for four days for withdrawal of hallucinogenic drugs. He suffered minor withdrawal symptoms when he was jailed for the current offenses. Chiefly, he had been "mainlining" heroin, although he also used cocaine. Throughout this whole period, he had never tried to stop smoking marijuana, although he said that for periods of up to one or two months during the preceding four years he had been able to remain off other drugs.

He also admitted that he had used "speed" intravenously. He said that his "habit" was costing him $100 to $120 a day.

Mental-status examination revealed him to be somewhat anxious and superficial, and he seemed to be trying to impress the examiner by his need to be released. He admitted feeling depressed in the past when his freedom was restricted, and also sometimes from the bad effects of drugs. Although he was lucid, appropriate, and free of psychotic mentation, he said that he was aware of paranoid ideation at times in the past when he was on drugs. He also admitted having hallucinatory experiences from LSD, mescaline and, on one occasion, from "Panama marijuana." In all of these instances, he had pleasant and vivid visual and auditory sensations. His later trips had a paranoid content and would last up to five hours. Needle scars were evident over the antecubital areas of both arms. Treatment in a hospital was recommended.

## References

American Psychiatric Association. *Diagnostic and Statistical Manual of Mental Disorders.* 3d ed., rev. Washington, D.C.: APA, 1987.

DuPont, R. L. "Substance Abuse." *Journal of the American Medical Association* 254 (1985): 2335–37.

———. "Substance Abuse." *Journal of the American Medical Association* 256 (1986): 2114–16.

Eaton, M. T., Jr., M. H. Peterson, and J. A. Davis. *Psychiatry.* 4th ed. Garden City, N.Y.: Medical Examination Publishing, 1981.

Farnsworth, D. L., and F. J. Braceland, eds. *Psychiatry: The Clergy and Pastoral Counseling.* Collegeville, Minn.: Saint John's University Press, 1969.

Gawin, F. H., and H. D. Kleber. "Abstinences Symptomatology and Psychiatric Diagnosis in Cocaine Abusers." *Archives of General Psychiatry* 43 (1986): 107–13.

Goodwin, D. W., and S. B. Guze. *Psychiatric Diagnosis.* 2d ed. New York: Oxford University Press, 1979.

Kaplan, H. I., and B. J. Sadock, eds. *Comprehensive Textbook of Psychiatry/V.* 5th ed. Baltimore: Williams & Wilkins, 1989.

Kolb, L. C., and H. K. H. Brodie. *Modern Clinical Psychiatry.* 10th ed. Philadelphia: Saunders, 1982.

Spitz, H. I., and J. S. Rosecan, eds. *Cocaine Abuse.* New York: Brunner/Mazel, 1987.

# 20 Nicotine Dependence

A custom loathsome to the eye, harmful to the brain, dangerous to the lungs, and in the black stinking fume thereof, nearest resembling the horrible Stygian smoke of the pit that is bottomless.

James I of England; *Counterblaste to Tobacco,* (1604)

## I. Introduction

Alcoholism and nicotine dependence are being discussed separately because both of these substances are legal, and yet a recent report showed that about 30 percent of all deaths in the United States are premature because of the use of these two dependence-producing drugs. Additionally, "youths who do not use cigarettes and alcohol during their teenage years are virtually immune to the nonmedical use of other dependence-producing drugs" (Dupont 1985).

## II. Tobacco

According to the *Encyclopedia Britannica,* the native Indians were using tobacco in much the same manner as it is used in modern times when Christopher Columbus discovered the Americas. The American Indians believed it possessed medicinal properties, which was the chief reason it was introduced into European countries. The Indians also used tobacco in ceremonies (for example, smoking a peace pipe).

Nicotine and related alkaloids furnish the narcotic effect of the substance.

Studies suggest that smoking begins from curiosity, desire to conform, and need to achieve status and self-assurance, as well as parents' example and advertising that encourages smoking. The habit seems to persist because it reduces tension and because it is thought to be pleasurable.

## III. Definition

A. Nicotine withdrawal

The essential feature of this disorder is a characteristic withdrawal syndrome due to the abrupt cessation of or reduction in the use of nicotine-containing substances (e.g., cigarettes, cigars, and pipes, chewing tobacco, or nicotine gum) that has been at least moderate in duration and amount. The syndrome includes craving for nicotine; irritability, frustration, or anger; anxiety; difficulty concentrating; restlessness; decreased heart rate; and increased appetite or weight gain (*DSM*-III-R).

B. Nicotine dependence

The most common form of nicotine dependence is associated with the inhalation of cigarette smoke. Pipe and cigar smoking, the use of snuff, and the chewing of tobacco are less likely to lead to nicotine dependence. People with this disorder are often distressed because of their inability to stop nicotine use (*DSM*-III-R).

1. Course

The course of nicotine dependence is variable. Most people repeatedly attempt to give up nicotine use without success.

2. Complications

The most common complications are bronchitis, emphysema, coronary artery disease, peripheral vascular disease, and a variety of cancers.

## IV. Prevalence

A. In 1987, approximately 33 percent of U.S. adults regularly used some form of tobacco (38.9 percent were men, 27.2 percent women).

B. Cigarette smoking: 28.8 percent of adults smoked cigarettes (31.2 percent were men, 26.5 percent women).

C. Smoking was most prevalent among the twenty-five to forty-four years age group.

D. Cigarette/alcohol consumption

1. People who smoke cigarettes were much more likely to drink beer frequently (10.7 percent versus 3 percent of people who never smoked and 8.5 percent of former smokers).

2. Of all beverage types, smokers were more likely than nonsmokers to consume large quantities of alcohol.

## V. Treatment

A. The most effective treatment programs are those that combine the use of nicotine chewing gum, or the nicotine patch (Transdermal Therapeutic System), in conjunction with a behavioral program.

B. Nicotine blockade therapy (Mecamlamine): Attenuates the effect of nicotine and is safe at doses that affect cigarette smoking. This blockade strategy may prove helpful in a subpopulation of cigarette smokers.

C. Recent reports have suggested the use of buspirone, in conjunction with cessation of smoking.

D. When Surgeon General Koop retired as surgeon general of the U.S. Public Health Service, he expressed before the U.S.

Congress—and later wrote about this in the *Journal of the American Medical Association*—his concern for the effect of tobacco advertising and children's access to tobacco products on the incidence of nicotine abuse. Koop was concerned about the fact that cigarette advertising does increase cigarette consumption. He also expressed concern for the audiences he felt that advertising targeted (while acknowledging that the issue is complex).

# References

American Psychiatric Association. *Diagnostic and Statistical Manual of Mental Disorders.* 3d ed., rev. Washington, D.C.: APA, 1987.

"Commentary." *Journal of the American Medical Association* 2622, no. 17 (November 3, 1989): 2364–65.

"Commentary." *Journal of the American Medical Association* 2622, no. 20 (November 24, 1989): 2894–95.

DuPont, R. L. "Substance Abuse." *Journal of the American Medical Association* 254 (1985): 2335–37.

Gawin, F., A. Comptom, and R. Byck. "Selective Therapeutic Index: Potential Use Abuse Forum as Treatment for Smoking Cessation, a Preliminary Trial." *Family Practice Recertification* Vol. 11, no. 9, supplement (September 1989).

Henningfield, J. E. "Pharmacologic Basis and Treatment of Cigarette Smoking." *Journal of Clinical Psychiatry* 45, no. 12 (December 1984): 24–33.

Hughs, J. R., and D. Hatsukami. "Signs and Symptoms of Tobacco Withdrawal." *Archives of General Psychiatry* 63 (March 1986): 289–94.

# 21 Alcoholism

There is no doubt that not to drink wine is a great deduction from life; but it may be necessary.

Samuel Johnson

## I. Introduction

Although alcohol is listed as one of the psychoactive substances in chapter 19 and technically could be included in that chapter, it, along with nicotine, is being discussed separately because they both are *legal* drugs, and recent reports show that about 30 percent of all deaths in the United States are premature because of the use of these two dependence-producing drugs.

## II. Definition

A. Alcoholism is a disorder characterized by excessive use of alcohol to the point of habituation, overdependence, or addiction.

B. Many definitions of alcoholism have been formulated by various authorities, partly because of the complexity of the disorder and partly because of the divergent orientations of the investigators. Some have stressed operational aspects, whereas others have attempted to describe causal factors.

1. The World Health Organization regards excessive drinking to be any form of drinking that goes beyond traditional and customary use or ordinary compliance with the customs of the community. By the definition, alcoholics are those excessive drinkers whose dependence upon alcohol has attained such a degree that it causes a noticeable mental disturbance or interferes with their bodily and mental health, their interpersonal relationships, or their smooth and economic functioning.

2. The *Manual of Alcoholism* of the American Medical Association defines alcoholism as "an illness characterized by a significant impairment that is directly associated with persistent and excessive use of alcohol. Impairment may involve physiological, psychological, or social dysfunction."

3. E. M. Jellinek (1960) defines alcoholism as any use of alcoholic beverage that causes damage to the individual or society or both. He delineates five subgroups.
   a) *Alpha alcoholism*—a purely psychological, continual dependence upon the effects of alcohol, which is used to relieve bodily or emotional pain (sometimes called *problem drinking* or *thymogenic drinking*).
   b) *Beta alcoholism*—similar to Alpha with the added complication of physiological derangements, such as gastritis, neuritis, liver and vascular disease (sometimes called *somatopathic*).
   c) *Gamma alcoholism*—characterized by the traditional pharmacological criterion of addiction, including both tolerance (a diminished effect with repeated use) and dependency. This is the usual type of alcoholism seen in the United States, Canada, and other Anglo-Saxon and hard-liquor-drinking countries. It is the form most commonly seen in courts, large municipal hospitals, and correctional institutions (also known as *essential alcoholism*).
   d) *Delta alcoholism*—characterized by the inability to abstain from drinking for even short periods of time; continuous speed drinking. This is the usual type of alcoholism seen in wine-drinking countries such as France (also known as *inveterate drinking*).
   e) *Epsilon alcoholism*—characterized by paroxysmal drinking bouts, during which the alcoholic drinks for varying periods of time, ranging from days to weeks (also known as *periodic drinking* and formerly called *dipsomania*).
4. In *DSM-III-R*, three main patterns of chronic alcohol abuse or dependence are listed: regular daily intake of large amounts; regular heavy drinking limited to weekends; and long periods of sobriety interspersed with binges of daily heavy drinking lasting for weeks or months.
C. Alcoholics have lost the power of choice in the matter of their drinking, and their drinking interferes with their health, work, or personal relationships. Generally, one can say that persons are alcoholics if their drinking interferes in any way with their lives.
D. Technically, abuse of and dependence on alcohol belong in chapter 19, but for previously stated reasons are treated separately here.

## III. Prevalence of alcoholism

A. Alcohol is widely used socially. As of 1985, 86 percent of the population consumed alcohol and about 12 percent reported using it twenty or more times each month (NIDA 1988).

B. It is difficult to accurately estimate the prevalence of alcoholism. Not everyone who occasionally becomes drunk (or even fairly often) can be considered an alcoholic. Drinking is considered pathological only when it is prolonged and excessive.

C. No adequate prevalence rates of alcoholism are available, partly because of the lack of agreement about the definition of the disorder.

D. Most people with drinking problems do not seek professional help (however, alcoholics do constitute a significant portion of admissions to general and mental hospitals).

E. One basis of current estimates uses the Jellinek (1960) definition and relates the prevalence to death from cirrhosis of the liver. Of the estimated 120 million people in the United States who drink alcohol, perhaps as many as 9 or 10 million of these could be considered alcohol dependent.

F. Other estimates are that one of every thirteen alcohol users becomes a problem drinker.

G. There are about five to six times as many male alcoholics as female alcoholics (probably because of the different role expectations of the two sexes). This ratio has remained fairly constant in the United States for many years, even though recent estimates suggest that the proportion of female alcoholics is increasing.

H. Much of the absenteeism in industry is related to alcoholism.

I. Alcoholism is an important factor in traffic accidents, and studies have indicated that about 50 percent of fatal accidents involve alcohol abuse. In general, state legislatures and courts are becoming much firmer in dealing with drivers who are under the influence of alcohol.

J. Many alcoholics are unrecognized because their drinking is done secretly and their problem does not become manifest for a long time.

K. Many very responsible people are alcoholics. This is often one of the reasons why spouses are reluctant to identify them as such.

L. People with other kinds of emotional disorders are more predisposed to alcoholism; for example, some persons with bipolar disorder may use alcohol excessively.

## IV. Sociocultural factors

A. Functions of alcohol

The many purposes for which various groups employ alcohol can be divided into four general categories. These purposes influence drinking patterns greatly.

1. Religious (e.g., wine in Roman Catholic and Jewish services)
2. Ceremonial (e.g., toasting the bride with champagne, drinking wine at the bar mitzvah or bas mitzvah ceremony)
3. Utilitarian (e.g., in cooking, in medicines, as a psychic balm, and at business and social functions)
4. Hedonistic (e.g., as a social lubricant and especially for the euphoria produced)

B. McCord, McCord, and Gudeman (1960) demonstrated the difference in ethnic and cultural backgrounds of American males who developed alcoholism. For example, American Indians and Eastern and Western European and Irish men were alcoholic more often than those of Latin and Italian background. Also, more alcoholics were from the middle class than the lower class.

C. Asians, such as Chinese, have low rates of alcoholism. As ethnic groups become more acculturated in their behavior patterns in drinking, they are much more like their larger peer groups (an exception to this seems to be some Chinese and Japanese, who apparently get a "flush" with the ingestion of small amounts of alcohol). Irish Americans tend to use alcohol for personal goals (promotion of fun and pleasure, physical states of well-being, and the release of inner tension) rather than for social functions, and they have few, if any, strong sanctions against heavy drinking.

D. Other studies have shown a low incidence of alcoholism among first-generation Italians, but this is not true of those in the third generation.

E. Studies have indicated that if persons who come from a Protestant background of strict abstinence from drinking, there is a relatively high likelihood that they will become problem drinkers.

F. More men than women drink, and men drink larger amounts and more frequently. This sex difference in the rate of alcoholism is sometimes explained in terms of the different role expectations of the two sexes. There is less social pressure on women to drink, and they are expected to drink in fewer kinds of situations. Women do not have to prove their femininity by drinking. In addition, the negative social sanctions against female drunkenness are much greater than for male drunkenness.

Recent estimates are that of women over eighteen years of age, 60 percent drink and 40 percent do not drink; and that 6–10 million women are alcoholics.

G. Studies of industrial populations reveal that American industry numbers about 2 million alcoholics on its collective payroll, of whom 90 percent are in the thirty-five to forty-five age group. The alcoholic's accident rate is twice that of others, and he or she loses twenty-five to thirty working days each year because of drinking. The direct costs of alcoholism include high rates of absenteeism and accidents, higher medical expenses, higher disability payments, and pension payments to alcoholics who retire prematurely. The indirect costs include low efficiency of employees with hangovers, slowdown in production, and adverse effects on safety standards and the morale of other workers. Some have referred to the alcoholic in the industrial setting as the "hidden half-man."

## V. Etiology

A. Many theories about the etiology and psychopathology of alcoholism have been offered, but the causes are not really known.

B. Generally, alcoholics show more depression, paranoid thinking, and aggressivity; they also have lowered self-esteem, a lowered sense of responsibility, and less self-control when compared with nonalcoholic populations. In the not-so-distant past, the public—including many physicians and other professionals—thought that alcoholics were simply weak individuals who lacked willpower and could really control their drinking if they wished to. Some naively assumed that alcohol itself was responsible and that if no alcoholic beverages were available, there would be no alcohol problem. (The eighteenth amendment to the U.S. Constitution was an attempt to solve the drinking problem on this basis.)

C. Most adults in the Western world drink alcohol, but only one in twelve or less develop serious problems from drinking. There is no good explanation for this.

D. Although the cause of alcoholism is unknown, a number of risk factors have been identified. Included are:

1. Family history
   There is little dispute that there is a strong family aspect to alcoholism. There is six times the incidence of alcoholism in children of families of which one parent is an alcoholic—but this may be an environmental factor rather than a genetic factor. However, children of alcoholics become alcoholic about four times more often than children of nonalcoholics, and there is some evidence that this is true even if they are not raised by the alcoholic parents.

2. Genetics
   The importance of genetics in vulnerability to alcoholism is supported by evidence from family, twin, and adoption

studies in humans. Studies suggest that genetic influences are important in alcoholism and reflect multiple genes interacting with environment to produce a final level of risk. In this theory, no one is predestined to become an alcoholic, but genetic factors increase or decrease this level of vulnerability toward this disorder (Schuckit 1985).

   3. Sex

     Men are more frequently alcoholic than women, in a ratio of 3:1.

   4. Age

     Alcoholism develops later in women than in men.

   5. Developmental factors

     Childhood history of conduct disorder, attention deficit disorder, or both, apparently increases a child's risk of becoming an alcoholic, especially if there is alcoholism in the family.

   6. Some Asians develop a "flush," the basis for which is undoubtedly genetic. The alcoholism rate in Asian countries is lower than that in the Western world.

   7. Theories of etiology

     a) Psychoanalytic perspectives: Most psychoanalytic theories view alcoholism as a fixation at the oral stage of psychosexual development in a child. Drinking is sometimes seen as a means of releasing aggressive and angry feelings and the guilt associated with these impulses.

     b) Learning theories: Based on the idea that consuming alcohol reduces stress (supported by animal research that interprets drinking as a learned response that is acquired and maintained because it reduces stress and discomfort).

     c) Genetics: See Genetics above.

 E. In summary, alcoholism should probably be regarded as resulting from a complex interaction of psychological, sociocultural, biological, and possibly genetic factors. An eclectic and empirical approach to this problem is indicated.

## VI. Symptoms

 A. Efforts to establish diagnostic criteria for alcoholism have included definitions based on: 1. the quantity imbibed, 2. the degree of loss of control, 3. social consequences, 4. psychophysiological and biochemical criteria, and 5. psychological factors.

 B. There is a high incidence of various types of psychopathology among alcoholics. Included in these are depression, impulsivity, poor reality testing, struggle with dominance-submission issues, and activity-passivity conflict. None of these factors is specific for alcoholics.

C. There is no constellation of psychological factors that is uniquely specific for alcoholism per se. One can only say that a well-adjusted person is unlikely to drink regularly to excess and is even less likely to become an alcoholic.

D. Some alcoholics have symptoms of other emotional disorders (e.g., anxiety or depression). One must distinguish between emotional conditions that are symptoms of premorbid psychopathology and those that are the psychiatric consequences of the alcoholism.

E. Some alcoholics have symptoms of character defects (e.g., borderline antisocial or passive-aggressive personality). The strongest relationship is with the antisocial personality. Some studies indicate that 15 percent of male alcoholics are antisocial.

F. Others seem to have no obvious symptoms apart from the excessive drinking.

G. Toxic effects may accompany alcoholism (see case example A at the end of chapter—section XI).

H. Generally, alcoholics, in attempting to cope with their environment and their drinking, overuse the defenses of:
   1. Rationalization (that is, they give "reasons" to explain their drinking)
   2. Denial (an inability or unwillingness to be able to admit to themselves that they have a drinking problem)
   3. Projection (blaming factors outside of themselves for their drinking)
   4. Dissociation

I. Patterns: The patterns of drinking are usually of two types:
   1. Spree or periodic drinkers drink excessively for a period of time, alternating with periods of sobriety. Included in this group are those who plan drinking episodes carefully.
   2. Others are continual drinkers. Such alcoholics sip every day and although never obviously intoxicated, are nearly always under the influence of alcohol. Some alcoholics restrict their drinking to weekends (these are considered as a subtype of continual drinkers).

J. Some authorities divide alcoholism into three types:
   1. Essential alcoholism
      Included here are those people who have drifted across the line from social drinking without any other obvious emotional problems. Also known as addictive drinking, compulsive drinking, and alcoholism simplex.

2. Symptomatic alcoholism

The drinking is a symptom of a serious emotional disorder, such as anxiety disorder, affective disorder, or schizophrenic disorder.

3. Reactive drinking

The drinking is in response to some particular emotional stress such as the death of a loved one; the alcohol helps the individual "work through" his or her feelings of grief.

K. Sheldon Bacon (1959) has given three criteria for determining the presence of alcoholism in individuals.

1. They ingest more alcohol (and in different ways) than their appropriate associates.

2. So-called problems, especially of an intrapersonal and emotional nature, that are clearly related to the deviant use of alcohol emerge chronically.

3. There is a growing loss of rational, socially mature self-control over the ingestion of alcohol.

## VII. Course

The progression into alcoholism often proceeds as follows:

A. The drinking is at first social and masquerades as a companionable or relaxing activity.

B. Then the drinkers turn to alcohol for escape from stress and anxiety and feelings of inadequacy.

C. Later, their self-control diminishes and their need for alcohol increases.

D. As control lessens, their work begins to suffer, and so also does their health, family, and social relationships, and all other aspects of their lives.

E. Detection of alcoholism

Four clinical questions, CAGE, have proved useful in diagnosing alcoholism. These are:

1. Have you ever felt you ought to *C*ut down on your drinking?

2. Have people ever *A*nnoyed you by criticizing your drinking?

3. Have you ever felt bad or *G*uilty about your drinking?

4. Have you ever had a drink first thing in the morning to steady your nerves or get rid of a hangover (*E*ye-opener)?

## VIII. Alcohol-induced organic mental disorders (*DSM*-III-R)

A. Alcohol intoxication

The essential feature of this disorder is maladaptive behavioral changes due to recent ingestion of alcohol. These changes may include aggressiveness, impaired judgment, impaired attention, irritability, euphoria, depression, emotional lability, and other manifestations of impaired social or occupational functioning.

Characteristic physiologic signs include slurred speech, incoordination, unsteady gait, nystagmus, and flushed face (*DSM*-III-R).

B. Alcohol idiosyncratic intoxication

This has also been called pathological intoxication. The essential feature of this disorder is a marked behavioral change—usually to aggressiveness—that is due to the recent ingestion of an amount of alcohol insufficient to induce intoxication in most people. There is usually subsequent amnesia for the period of intoxication. The behavior is atypical of the person when not drinking; for example, a shy, retiring, mild-mannered person, after one weak alcoholic drink, may become belligerent and assaultive.

C. Uncomplicated alcohol withdrawal

The essential features of this disorder are certain characteristic symptoms such as a coarse tremor of hands, tongue, or eyelids; nausea or vomiting; malaise or weakness; autonomic hyperactivity (such as tachycardia, sweating, and elevated blood pressure); anxiety, depressed mood, or irritability; transient hallucinations (generally poorly formed) or illusions; headache; and insomnia. These symptoms follow within several hours after cessation of or reduction in alcohol ingestion by a person who has been drinking alcohol for several days or longer.

D. Alcohol withdrawal delirium

The essential feature of this disorder is a delirium-reduced ability to maintain attention to external stimuli; disorganized thinking, as indicated by rambling, irrelevant, or incoherent speech; and at least two of the following: reduced level of consciousness; perceptual disturbances; misinterpretations, illusions, or hallucinations; disturbance of sleep-wake cycles with insomnia or daytime sleepiness; increased or decreased psychomotor activity; disorientation to time, place, or person; memory impairment. It usually develops within one week after a recent cessation of a reduction in alcohol consumption.

E. Alcohol hallucinosis

The essential feature of this disorder is an organic hallucinosis in which vivid and persistent hallucinations develop shortly (usually within forty-eight hours) after cessation of or reduction in alcohol ingestion by a person who apparently has alcohol dependence. The hallucinations may be auditory or visual. The auditory hallucinations are usually voices and, less commonly, unformed sounds such as hissing or buzzing.

In the majority of cases, the content of the hallucinations is unpleasant or disturbing. However, the hallucinatory content may be benign and leave the person undisturbed. The voices may address the person directly, but more often they discuss him or her in the third person.

F. Alcohol amnestic syndrome

The essential feature of this disorder is an amnestic syndrome (demonstrable evidence of impairment in both short- and long-term memory) apparently due to the vitamin deficiency associated with prolonged, heavy ingestion of alcohol. Alcohol amnestic disorder due to thiamine deficiency is also known as Korsakoff's syndrome.

1. Course

Alcohol amnestic disorder often follows an acute episode of Wernicke's encephalopathy, a neurologic disease manifested by confusion, ataxia, eye-movement abnormalities (gaze palsies, nystagmus), and other neurologic signs.

2. Wernicke's disease

Wernicke's syndrome is a rare disorder of central nervous system metabolism, associated with a thiamine deficiency and seen chiefly in chronic alcoholics. It is characterized by irregular eye movements, incoordination, impaired thinking and, often, sensory-motor deficit. Korsakoff's psychosis, with accompanying confabulation, commonly accompanies Wernicke's syndrome.

G. Dementia associated with alcoholism

The essential feature of this disorder is the development of a dementia, following prolonged and heavy ingestion of alcohol, for which all other causes of dementia have been excluded. In order to exclude transient effects of intoxication and withdrawal, this diagnosis should not be made until at least three weeks have elapsed since cessation of alcohol ingestion.

Features

1. Demonstrable evidence of impairment in short- and long-term memory.

2. At least one of the following:

a) Impairment in abstract thinking

b) Impaired judgment

c) Other disturbances of higher cortical function, such as aphasia (disorder of language), apraxia (inability to carry out motor activities despite intact comprehension and motor function), agnosia (failure to recognize or identify objects despite intact sensory function), and "constructional difficulty" (e.g., inability to copy three-dimensional figures, assemble blocks, or arrange sticks in specific designs)

d) Personality change

3. The disturbance in 1 and 2 significantly interferes with work or usual social activities or relationships with others.

## IX. Treatment

A. Treatment of the alcoholic can be considered under two headings:
   1. Treatment of withdrawal and the underlying alcohol organic mental disorders
   2. Treatment of the underlying personality disorder

B. Treatment of withdrawal and the underlying alcohol organic mental disorder
   1. Treatment of acute alcohol organic mental disorder
      a) Those people who are unable to stop their drinking and have to be withdrawn from alcohol often have to spend time in the hospital or a detoxification center.
      b) Attention must be directed to the alcoholic's nutrition and electrolyte intake, but the use of intravenous fluids is usually not indicated.
      c) Adequate vitamin intake, especially thiamine and niacin, must be provided. These can be administered parenterally or orally, as indicated.
      d) Psychotropic drugs
         Medications are often useful in the management of withdrawal. A number of medications have been used, but perhaps the most commonly employed at the present time is chlordiazepoxide (Librium) in fairly substantial doses for several days; diazepam (Valium) may be used instead. If a withdrawal seizure (convulsion) is anticipated, an anticonvulsant such as Dilantin may be added.
      e) Corticotropin
         Used intramuscularly or intravenously, this drug has been helpful in some cases of acute hallucinosis or delirium tremens.
   2. Treatment of the chronic mental disorders secondary to alcoholism
      a) Hospitalization is sometimes necessary.
      b) Maintenance of intake of fluids, vitamins, and nutrition is important.
      c) Various psychotropic drugs may help to relieve certain symptoms.
         Antidepressants are used to relieve depression; antipsychotic agents are used if there is psychotic behavior.
      d) Since the brain damage is irreversible, treatment is only palliative.

C. Treatment of the underlying personality disorder
  1. Treatment of the personality disorder underlying the compulsion to drink is usually much more difficult than is hospital management of the acute organic mental disorders, especially since many alcoholics deny that their drinking problem exists and tend to resist intervention. Many alcoholics can be treated as outpatients if they present themselves during a period of sobriety. The physician can use certain medications to assist the patient in coping without alcohol. Most commonly employed drugs used to help the patient through the withdrawal period are chlordiazepoxide (Librium) and diazepam (Valium). These must be used with caution and for only a short period of time because of the possibility of creating dependence on them. Various other psychotropic drugs might be indicated when the physician finds there is another underlying psychiatric disorder (e.g., Lithium for major mood disorders).
  2. Chemical dependency treatment centers
      a) Estimates are that almost 95 percent of the treatment centers in the United States are based, at least loosely, on the "Minnesota Model" approach: thirty-day impatient stay, abstinence, and Alcoholics Anonymous–based inpatient treatment. This program assumes that alcoholism is a primary illness, not a symptom of something else.
      b) Patients in this program are in an extremely structured environment with a program that is short termed and focused. It deals directly with the problem of alcoholism. Patients attend lectures and groups and individual counseling sessions all day, and in the evenings there is another lecture or AA meeting.
      c) Additionally, the Minnesota Model program is multidisciplinary and in addition to the focus on the "disease" model of alcoholism acknowledges mental, emotional, physical, spiritual, and social aspects and makes attempts to treat them. Following discharge from the program, aftercare programs and follow-up are usually provided.
      d) Generally, outpatient programs are similar except the patients go home at night.
      e) The overall approach, techniques, and methods have remained essentially the same for many years. Patients are provided with information about the disease of alcoholism and are also provided personal and emotional counseling.

f) The harsh confrontational approach once part of the treatment in the early days is no longer popular. In addition, there is a trend toward outpatient care, apparently as a result of younger persons and persons with families and jobs who are seeking treatment.

3. Pharmacological treatment

a) Disulfiram therapy

This is the Antabuse treatment. Following its introduction in 1948, this therapy gained wide acceptance, but it, too, seems to have had only limited use in the treatment of alcoholism. The drug tetraethylthiuram disulfide when combined with alcohol, produces distressing vasomotor symptoms. No conditioned response is established. This is not an aversion therapy; the unpleasant effects are produced by mixing Antabuse and alcohol. Patients must take the Antabuse each day; if they stop for several days, they can drink alcohol without the distressing symptoms. Patients who receive this treatment must be in good physical health.

b) Tranquilizing drugs

Various types of psychotropic drugs are sometimes helpful in the management of alcoholism, either for facilitating psychotherapy or for mitigating anxiety or the symptoms of overindulgence. Neuroleptics are also used in the management of acute psychotic conditions related to alcoholic excesses. Among the tranquilizing medications that have been used in alcoholism are chlordiazepoxide (Librium), diazepam (Valium), chlorpromazine (Thorazine), and promazine (Sparine).

c) Aversive therapy

This was once widely used. The aim of treatment is to produce a conditioned response such that the odor or taste of alcohol will immediately lead to nausea and vomiting. The drugs used to set up such a response are emetine and apomorphine, both of which are emetics (agents that induce vomiting). This form of treatment is seldom used now.

4. Dual focus (or dual treatment) programs

In some communities there are special programs for the treatment of people with alcoholism or other substance use disorders, in association with another psychiatric disorder (i.e., schizophrenia, bipolar disorder, or other affective disorders, including depression). Many times these are not AA oriented but more likely to be based on the behavior modification model. The dual program needs to be integrated treatment and to simultaneously address each of the disorders.

5. Psychotherapy
   a) Any psychotherapeutic approach must operate from the premise that alcoholism is a personality problem and not a moral one.
   b) The ideal treatment goal should be the elimination of the desire to drink, rather than restraint.
   c) It is also important to keep in mind that the alcoholic is usually a dependent person who often has hostile, anxious, and guilty feelings.
   d) Psychotherapy has had only limited success, one reason being that the uncovering of conflicts produces anxiety, whereas the alcoholic has a reduced tolerance for tension.
   e) Certain authorities emphasize the importance of "surrender" versus "submission" in any psychotherapeutic approach; that is, alcoholics must *accept* the fact that they are alcoholics, and not just admit it.

6. Group therapy
   Group therapy is often useful in the treatment of alcoholics. Sometimes, but not always, such therapy is moderated by a professional person, such as a psychiatrist, clinical psychologist, or social worker.

7. Community resources
   a) Continued care following discharge from the hospital or a chemical dependency unit is crucial. It is true that a "supportive network" is needed by all alcoholics, but it is especially necessary for those who lack close personal relationships. It is also important to keep in mind that the family, or other people affected by the alcoholic's disorder, may also need assistance.
   b) There are many agencies and organizations concerned with this problem.
      (1) Most states have a department for alcoholism or substance use disorder.
      (2) In the past, many communities had an alcoholism information center that acted as the coordinator of available resources for the understanding and treatment of alcohol problems. Currently, most helping agencies know of treatment resources in the community, so there is less need for this particular kind of facility now.
   c) Alcoholics Anonymous (AA) is an informal, worldwide fellowship of groups of alcoholics who help each other

to stay sober and to remain abstinent. The basic philosophy is based on twelve steps and twelve traditions. The basic source of AA's strength is the relationship with God as the individual understands Him. For those who fit well into formal group activity, this approach has proven effective in maintaining sobriety. Of all the available resources, it has easily been the most helpful. However, there are some who cannot accept this approach, particularly those who have difficulty accepting a personal God.

Various attempts have been made to explain why the program has been so useful. Some think the evangelistic theme and religious overtones are important; others view the program as a resocialization process. Most local AA groups have telephone listings and place referral information in the personal columns in the newspapers.

d) Alanon and Alateen are groups that help the significant others in the alcoholic's life. They often need help to understand the problem and to help the recovering alcoholic maintain his or her health and sobriety. These people are sometimes referred to as "near" or "coalcoholics," or "codependents."

e) Since the decriminalization of drunkenness and the enactment of the Uniform Alcoholism and Intoxication and Treatment Act of 1970, detoxification centers for the treatment of alcoholics have been established in many communities. One significant advantage of such a place is that it is usually tied into the therapeutic network for alcoholics.

f) Many communities have established various types of halfway houses where alcoholics who have no place to live may go to avoid a life-style that is conducive to drinking. Such halfway houses usually have various support groups, including local AA groups.

g) Many churches and religious groups sponsor other active programs. Among them are Calix, a group for Catholic alcoholics, and social agencies such as the Salvation Army. The local mental health association is also a possible source of information.

## X. Prevention

A. Very little is known about the prevention of alcoholism, mainly because we know very little of its natural history or distribution of its psychosocial determinants.

B. Alcoholism, like mental illness, has been negatively viewed by the general public. However, in recent years there has been a greater acceptance of alcoholism as a disorder.

C. Alcoholism is one of the four major public health concerns in the United States (the others are mental disorders, cardiovascular disease, and cancer).

D. There is a need to identify and discover cases of alcoholism *early* if we are to make any progress in controlling this disorder. Case findings should be active rather than passive. Many of the community programs, including those in industry, have this orientation.

E. Research in social, psychological, and biological areas is a continuing need.

## XI. Case examples

A. Alcoholism with hallucinations

> J. P. C., a thirty-eight-year-old single man, was referred to the court's psychiatric consultant for evaluation after he had pleaded guilty to a charge of drunkenness, growing out of an incident in which he was arrested for behaving in a strange manner near a neighbor's apartment building. When questioned by the police who were called, he said he was looking for his sister who was in a tree. He said that he had dropped her child in a culvert and that he had retrieved the baby. He explained that his sister, while changing the baby's diaper, was snatched up into the tree. The man appeared to be intoxicated and admitted to the officers that he had been drinking.
>
> When interviewed by the psychiatric consultant, he admitted that he had been drinking excessively for years. For about a week before his arrest, he was aware that he was "acting screwy," that is, imagining things, but whenever he ceased drinking temporarily, he hallucinated. For example, he recalled that he believed that two men had crawled through the transom of his room at a cheap downtown hotel. This was so real that he phoned the police to complain.
>
> Following his arrest, he experienced other vivid hallucinations. For example, he thought there were cockroaches in his cell and that the jailer was throwing ants into his cell to eat the cockroaches. In addition, he was certain that he had seen his drinking companion in jail with him, and he insisted, when he was bailed out by his brother, that the companion was still there (which was not true).
>
> His background history revealed that he had been arrested about twenty times, mostly for drinking, including one arrest for drunken driving and another for petty theft committed while he was drinking. He had been hospitalized on three occasions for his drinking problem. He believed that his drinking had been a serious problem for a least thirteen or fourteen years and said, "It continually gets worse." He had been in Alcoholics Anonymous programs at various times but regarded AA as a married man's organization and considered it populated by many people who were not really alcoholics.
>
> In addition, he complained of nervousness, uneasiness, and anxiety, which he said antedated his first drinking. His Minnesota

Multiphasic Personality Inventory profile revealed a high level of anxiety and indicated that he was worried, apprehensive, and tense.

He admitted to a very poor employment record over the years because of his drinking problem and had been unemployed for six months prior to his arrest. For approximately a year before that, he had worked as an unskilled laborer.

This case is one of severe, chronic alcoholism in which the person also has symptoms of an anxiety disorder. In addition, he experienced a bout of acute alcoholic hallucinosis, which brought him to the attention of the police. The prognosis is poor.

B. Alcoholism with depression

C. T., a fifty-two-year-old woman, was admitted to the hospital, at the request of her personal physician, for depression and a drinking problem. Her husband, who brought her to the hospital, reported that when he returned home from a business trip, he found his wife drunk, and she said she was unable to control her compulsive drinking. Her physician was summoned and arrangements were made for her admission to the hospital.

Her background history revealed that she had always been a passive person and had difficulty with recurrent depressive feelings. She had made two suicide attempts, once with barbiturates, and, on another occasion, with carbon monoxide in her automobile. She had been hospitalized for psychiatric treatment on at least four other occasions.

Prominent among her symptoms while she was in the hospital were social uneasiness and the ease with which she could feel rejected. Feelings of dependency, inferiority, and inadequacy were also evident. She said that for a number of years while she was struggling with her depressed feelings and her compulsion to drink, she blamed her difficulty on her husband. About three or four years earlier, she had finally come to realize that the problem was within her and not the fault of her husband. She had gone to AA meetings a number of times but, because of her passivity, she did not follow through very faithfully.

In this case, alcoholism complicates a recurrent depressive reaction. She was placed on antidepressants and psychotherapy and was referred to a local AA group for supportive help. A follow-up evaluation, six months following her discharge from the hospital, revealed that she had done reasonably well and had had only three minor slips, when she drank a few beers over a one- or two-day period.

# References

American Medical Association. *Manual on Alcoholism*. 3d ed. Chicago: AMA, 1977.

American Psychiatric Association. *Diagnostic and Statistical Manual of Mental Disorders*. 3d ed., rev. Washington, D.C.: APA, 1987.

Bacon, S. D. "The Interrelatedness of Alcoholism and Marital Conflicts." *American Journal of Psychiatry* 24 (1959): 153.

Campbell, R. J. *Psychiatric Dictionary*. 5th ed. New York: Oxford University Press, 1981.

Dupont, R. L. "Substance Abuse." *Journal of the American Medical Association* (1985): 2335–37.

———. "Substance Abuse." *Journal of the American Medical Association* (1986): 2114–16.

Goodwin, D. W., and S. B. Guze. *Psychiatric Diagnosis*. 2d ed. New York: Oxford University Press, 1979.

Jellinek, E. M. *The Disease Concept of Alcoholism*. Highland Park, N.J.: Hillhouse Press, 1960.

Keller, M. "The Definition of Alcoholism and the Estimation of Its Prevalence." In *Society, Culture, and Drinking Patterns*, edited by D. D. J. Pittman and C. R. Snyder. New York: Wiley, 1962.

Kirn, T. F. "Advances in Understanding of Alcoholism Initiate Evolution and Treatment Programs." *Journal of the American Medical Association* 256 (September 19, 1986): 1405–12.

McCord, W., J. McCord, and J. Gudeman. *Origins of Alcoholism*. Stanford: Stanford University Press, 1960.

Mirian, S. M., ed. "Alcohol Abuse." *Psychiatric Annals* 19, no. 5 (May 1989): 235 ff.

Schuckit, M. A. "Genetics and the Risk for Alcoholism." *Journal of the American Medical Association* (1985): 2614–17.

World Health Organization, Expert Committee on Alcohol. *First Report*. W.H.O. Technical Report Series, no. 84. Geneva, 1955.

Yandow, V. "Alcoholism in Women." *Psychiatric Annals* 19, no. 5 (May 1989): 253.

# 22 Adjustment Disorders

Mankind is made up of inconsistencies, and no man acts invariably
up to his predominant character.
The wisest man sometimes acts weakly and the weakest sometimes wisely.

**Philip Dormer Stanhope, fourth Earl of Chesterfield,**
*Letters to His Son* (1748)

## I. Definition

The essential feature of this disorder is a maladaptive reaction to an
identifiable psychosocial stressor, or stressors, that occurs within
three months after onset of the stressor and has persisted for no
longer than six months. The maladaptive nature of the reaction is
indicated either by impairment in occupational (including school)
functioning or in usual social activities or relationships with others
or by symptoms that are in excess of a normal and expectable reaction to the stressor. The disturbance is not merely one instance of a
pattern of overreaction to stress or an exacerbation of one of the
mental disorders. It is assumed that the disturbance will remit soon
after the stressor ceases or, if the stressor persists, when a new level
of adaptation is achieved. This category should not be used if the
disturbance meets the criteria for a specific mental disorder, such as
a specific anxiety or mood disorder, or represents uncomplicated bereavement (*DSM*-III-R).

## II. Stressors

A. The stressors may be single (e.g., an uncomplicated divorce) or
   multiple (e.g., marked business difficulties or marital problems).
   They may be recurrent, as with seasonal business crises, or continuous, as with chronic illness or residence in a deteriorating
   neighborhood.
B. The severity of the reaction is not completely predictable from
   the severity of the stressor. People who are particularly vulnerable may have a more severe form of the disorder following
   only a mild or moderate stressor, whereas others may have only
   a mild form of the disorder in response to a marked and continuing stressor.

## III. Prevalence

   A. This disorder is apparently very common, but confirmatory data are limited (Kaplan and Sadock 1989).
   B. It may occur at any age.
   C. Studies in consultation/liaison psychiatry indicate that adjustment disorder is a commonly used diagnosis (for example, adjustment disorder with depressed mood in AIDS).
   D. This disorder is presumedly caused by psychic overload (Goldman 1988).

## IV. Course

By definition, this disorder begins within three months of onset of a stressor and lasts no longer than six months.

## V. Types

This disorder may manifest itself in a number of ways; hence there are several different types, according to the predominant symptoms, and include:

   A. Adjustment disorder with anxious mood
   This is manifested as symptoms of anxiousness, such as nervousness, worry, and jitteriness.
   B. Adjustment disorder with depressed mood
   Predominant manifestation involves depressive symptoms such as depressed mood, tearfulness, and feelings of hopelessness.
   C. Adjustment disorder with disturbance of conduct
   This is manifested chiefly in violation of the rights of others or of major age-appropriate societal norms and rules (e.g., truancy, vandalism, reckless driving, fighting, defaulting on legal responsibilities).
   D. Adjustment disorder with mixed disturbances of emotions and conduct
   The predominant manifestations of both emotional symptoms, such as depression or anxiety, and a disturbance of conduct, such as those listed under C.
   E. Adjustment disorder with mixed emotional features
   This disorder shows various combinations of depression and anxiety or other emotions.
   F. Adjustment disorder with physical complaints
   The predominant manifestation is physical symptoms—for example, fatigue, headache, backache, or other aches and pains that are not diagnosable as specific Axis III physical disorder or condition.
   G. Adjustment disorder with withdrawal
   The predominant manifestation is social withdrawal without significant depressed or anxious mood.

H. Adjustment disorder with work (or academic) inhibition

Predominant manifestation here is an inhibition in work or academic functioning, occurring in a person whose previous work or academic performance has been adequate.

I. Adjustment disorder not otherwise specified

This category is for disorders involving maladaptive reaction to psychosocial stressors that are not classifiable as specific types of adjustment disorder.

## VI. Treatment

A. Some believe that because the stressor is clearly identifiable and the condition will have a spontaneous remission, psychotherapy or other kinds of treatment are not indicated.

B. Generally, treatment for disorders in this group is time limited. The goals are to remove the stressor if possible, to relieve symptoms, and to assist the person in achieving a level of adaptation that existed prior to the stressful event.

C. Psychosocial treatment methods most commonly recommended are:

1. Individual psychotherapy, specifically, brief psychodynamic therapy focusing on the meaning of the stressful event to the individuals and its possible activation of underlying conflict. Supportive or expressive psychotherapy (or both) may be appropriate.

2. Behavior therapy may be helpful.

3. Group therapy, including self-help groups with others who have undergone similar stresses, may be useful.

D. Psychopharmacological treatment

Generally, psychotropic medications are not used in adjustment disorders because the condition is often self-limited and there is always the possible risk that the person may develop psychological or physical dependency on the agents.

However, in some cases antianxiety agents or perhaps antidepressant agents may be useful for short periods of time to help bring the stress under control, permitting the person to reerect his or her defenses or develop other means of coping.

## VII. Case examples

A. A forty-four-year-old single female bank clerk was referred for psychiatric evaluation by her gynecologist because she complained of "depression alternating with nervousness." She described the depression as "heavy feelings associated with sadness" and described the nervousness as "tenseness in her arms, legs, and shoulders." She related that these symptoms had been present for about three months and were related to (1) a stressful work environment and (2) a stressful living situation. Concerning her job, she reported that she was the oldest of twelve women in a "dead-end job," in an office where she felt "snubbed and ignored" by the younger women. In addition, she felt she had a moody supervisor.

When describing her living situation, she reported that she resided in one-half of a double house, where the family in the adjoining portion of the house had noisy children who disturbed her in the evening when she went home. Thus, she felt under stress both in her workplace and in her home.

She described herself as being shy and extremely sensitive and admitted it was difficult for her to forget hurts.

She always enjoyed good health, although about six months before the onset of her symptoms, she had undergone a hysterectomy for uterine fibroids and endometriosis. She had never experienced any nervous symptoms in the past.

This seemed to be an adjustment disorder with mixed emotional features (with depressed and anxious mood). She elected to explore feelings and the issues in a few psychotherapeutic sessions.

B. A thirty-eight-year-old male management engineer sought evaluation with a psychiatrist because of anxiety and dissatisfaction, which were secondary to divorce proceedings in progress at the time of his initial consultation.

He reported that he had been married fourteen years to a woman of the same age. He described her as a loving, unselfish person, but one who wanted to control. He said, "We were in competition, and without communication and without intimacy." He had decided on the divorce when his wife refused to join him in seeking counseling in an effort to work out their marital relationship.

There was no history of previous mental illness or emotional disturbance of any kind.

This seems to be an example of adjustment disorder with mixed emotional features (with anxious and depressed mood).

He was seeking counseling to aid him in adjusting to his divorce and to assist him in working out a continuing relationship with his two children.

# References

American Psychiatric Association. *Diagnostic and Statistical Manual of Mental Disorders.* 3d ed., rev. Washington, D.C.: APA, 1987.

Goldman, H. H. *Review of General Psychiatry.* Los Altos, Calif.: Lange Medical Publications, 1988.

Kaplan, H. I., and B. J. Sadock, eds. *Comprehensive Textbook of Psychiatry/ V.* 5th ed. Baltimore: Williams & Wilkins, 1989.

# 23 Mood Disorders (Affective Disorders)

Hence, loathed melancholy,
Of Cerberus and blackist midnight born,
In Stygian cave forelorn,
'Mongst horrid shapes, and shrieks and sights unholy!

John Milton, *L'Allegro* (1632)

## I. Introduction

A. The main characteristic is a primary pervasive disturbance in mood.

B. The affective disorders are characterized by pathologically elevated or depressed mood and should be regarded as existing on a continuum with normal mood. The mood changes, to depression or elation, differ from other mood swings chiefly in degree and duration. The change may occur without apparent cause, seem disproportionate, or persist too long.

C. Many times the abnormality of activity, affect, and thought appears to have a plausible relationship to the immediate social environment. Any concomitant disturbances in thought or behavior are appropriate to the mood.

D. Mood disorders, chiefly depression, are the most common disorders seen in outpatient practice. They are the principal disorders associated with suicide.

E. Generally, when people speak of depression, they are referring to the *emotion* of feeling sad, blue, or unhappy (i.e., dysthymia). When clinicians speak of depression they are usually referring to a *syndrome* or mental disorder of depression consisting of many symptoms and signs, including anorexia, anhedonia, hopelessness, insomnia, and dysthymia.

F. Much recent research has been concerned with mood disorders. The awesome rate at which knowledge has been accruing about these disorders makes it virtually impossible for one person to keep abreast of all the new developments in the field.

G. Many improvements have been developed in various drug treatments, including the tricyclic antidepressants, the monoamine oxidase inhibitors (MAOI), lithium, and the newer second- and third-generation antidepressant medications (see XI—the treatment section of this chapter).

## II. Terminology

In *DSM*-III-R, the following terms are used in the classification of mood disorders.

A. *Mood syndrome* (depressive or manic) is a group of mood and associated symptoms that occur together for a minimal period of time. (For example, major depressive syndrome is defined as a depressed mood or loss of interest of at least two weeks' duration, accompanied by several associated symptoms, such as weight loss and difficulty concentrating.) Mood syndromes can occur as part of a mood disorder, as part of a nonmood psychotic disorder (for example, schizoaffective disorder), or as part of an organic mental disorder (for example, organic mood disorder).

B. *Mood episode* (major depressive, manic, or hypomanic) is a mood syndrome that is not due to a known organic factor and is not part of a nonmood psychotic disorder (e.g., schizophrenia, schizoaffective disorder, or delusional disorder). For example, a major depressive episode is a major depressive syndrome (as defined earlier) in which it cannot be established that an organic factor initiated and maintained the disturbance, and the presence of a nonmood psychotic disorder has been ruled out.

C. *Mood disorder* is determined by the pattern of mood episodes. For example, the diagnosis of major depression is made when there have been one or more major depressive episodes without a history of a manic or unequivocal hypomanic episode.

## III. Degrees of depression

Depressions can range from "normal" to "mood variance" (for example, sadness, gloominess, or dejection) through uncomplicated bereavement on to severe delusional depression. One way to classify depressions according to degree would be to divide them into the following:

A. A depression is a normal human emotion. Such "normal" depression is characterized by feelings of sadness, disappointment, despair, frustration, or unhappiness. It is a universally experienced emotion and is not considered abnormal.

B. Grief (uncomplicated bereavement)

Bereavement is a normal, appropriate, affective sadness in response to a recognizable external loss. It is realistic and appropriate to what has been lost; it is self-limiting and gradually subsides. It seldom leads to serious disorder in one's personal life.

It usually occurs in three stages: numbness (or impact), depression, and recovery (Clayton 1990).

The reaction to the loss may not be immediate but rarely occurs after the first two or three months. The duration of "normal" bereavement varies considerably among different cultural groups (*DSM*-III-R).

C. Major depressive disorder

The etiological factor is less obvious than normal grief or the depression is more severe or persists unduly long. The situation that occasions the reaction is often more of a precipitating event than a causal factor. The individual usually realizes that the response is excessive but does not recognize the underlying cause.

The degree of depression can range from mild (only slightly more severe than "normal" depression) to profound depression in which the patient may lose contact with reality, develop delusions, and may be of serious suicidal risk. Such a person is often said to be psychotic.

## IV. Descriptive types of depression

A. It should be kept in mind that depression is really a syndrome and that modern researchers suggest multiple etiologies (a spectrum disorder) with a variety of symptoms.

B. Aside from the official diagnostic classification of the various depressive disorders, certain clinical types of depression are often described.

C. Symptom complex (subtypes)

Among the descriptive subtypes that have been described are the following:

1. Primary-secondary affective disorders
   a) *Primary affective disorders* are those that occur in persons who have never had an episode before or whose only previous psychiatric illnesses were episodes of depression or mania.
   b) *Secondary affective disorders* occur in persons who have had other psychiatric illnesses (e.g., schizophrenia or alcoholism) or who have suffered an affective disorder related to a medical condition.

2. Bipolar-unipolar dichotomy
   a) The *bipolar* group consists of patients who have had both depressive and manic episodes.
   b) The *unipolar* group consists of those who have only had depressive episodes.
   c) Genetic studies indicate that persons with a bipolar affective disorder have families with a greater frequency of a similar illness and are more likely to develop

hypomanic responses to administration of the tricyclic antidepressants.

3. The psychotic-neurotic dichotomy
   a) This distinction has lost its importance in recent years.
   b) The frequency of depressions of psychotic proportions has greatly decreased in recent years. Perhaps this is in part accounted for by the fact that people with signs of depression receive early treatment; hence, the fully developed psychotic syndromes described in the past do not occur. More recent use of the term *psychotic* has become synonymous with severe impairment of social and personal functioning. But even using these criteria, psychotic depressions are relatively infrequent in current clinical practice.

4. Endogenous-reactive dichotomy
   a) This subdivision of depression is based on whether or not the depression seemed to develop "from within" (endogenous) or was related to life events (reactive).
   b) Those who have endogenous depressions usually show a central group of symptoms including psychomotor retardation, early morning awakening (terminal insomnia), weight loss, guilt, and unreactivity. It is more likely to occur in older patients, and people with endogenous depressions show more stable non-neurotic premorbid personality.
   c) Those with reactive depression show a correlation with light stress.
   d) Recent studies suggest that a valid definition of endogenous depression is one in which the endogenous group is characterized by the following:
      (1) A greater family history of depression
      (2) A lower family history of alcoholism
      (3) A lower family history of antisocial personality
      (4) Older age
      (5) Higher scores on symptom severity indexes
      (6) Less frequent, nonserious suicide attempts
      (7) A lower prevalence of divorce or marital separations
      (8) Fewer life events
      (9) Fewer premorbid personality disorders
      (10) Better social support
      (11) Less cognitive distortion
      (12) A higher frequency of neuroendocrine or other biologic abnormalities
      (13) A better response to somatic therapy
      (14) A poorer response to psychotherapy

5. Agitated-retarded dichotomy
   This subdivision is based on whether or not the symptoms include
   a) Uneasiness, mental perturbation, and motor restlessness (agitation)
   b) Slowing down of mental and physical activity (retardation)
6. Early versus late onset
   This includes "pure" versus "spectrum" depression, involutional depression, chronic characterological depression, and hysteroid dysphoria.
D. Life events and stress as precipitating factors
   1. Not all persons who experience loss and separation subsequently develop depression.
   2. Loss and separation are demonstrable in only about a quarter of people with depressions.
   3. Loss and separation may precipitate a wide variety of psychiatric conditions.
   4. Predisposing factors, as well as precipitating factors, must be taken into account. Genetic factors (e.g., in the bipolar affective disorder) or early life experiences may render the individual sensitive to losses or separations.
E. Melancholia
   1. This is a term used since ancient times to refer to a severe form of depression.
   2. In *DSM*-III-R, the term *major depressive episode, melancholic type,* refers to a severe depression that includes anhedonia (loss of pleasure), lack of reactivity to usually pleasurable stimuli, depression regularly worse in the morning, early morning awakening (terminal insomnia), psychomotor retardation or agitation, significant anorexia, weight loss, no significant personality disturbance before the first major depressive episode, one or more previous major depression episodes followed by complete or nearly complete recovery, and previous good response to specific and adequate somatic antidepressive therapy.
   3. Involutional melancholia
      a) The term *involutional melancholia* was used to describe a depression of initial onset occurring during the involutional years (forty to fifty-five in women and fifty to sixty-five in men), with symptoms of marked anxiety, agitation, restlessness, somatic concerns, hypochondriasis, occasional somatic or nihilistic delusions, insomnia, anorexia, and weight loss (Brown et al. 1984).

b) This disorder characteristically occurred in an obsessive-compulsive personality (narrow range of interests, difficulty adjusting to change, limited capacity for sociability and friendship, rigid adherence to a strict ethical code, etc.).

c) Such patients who experience the first depressive episode in the involutional period have more somatic symptoms and hypochondriasis.

d) This diagnosis was excluded in *DSM*-III and *DSM*-III-R, and a recent study (Brown et al. 1984) does not support the clinical picture of the previously outlined involutional melancholia. However, even if involutional melancholia does not stand as a separate entity, it may be useful to recognize that elderly patients may present a clinical picture that differs somewhat from that of their younger counterparts (Brown et al. 1984).

F. Seasonal affective disorder (SAD)

This term is new in *DSM*-III-R. The diagnostic criteria for seasonal pattern are: a regular temporal relationship between the onset of an episode of bipolar disorder or recurrent major depression and a particular sixty-day period of the year; full remission or change from depression to mania or hypomania also occurred within a particular sixty-day period of the year; there have been at least three episodes of mood disturbance three separate years that demonstrated the temporal seasonal relationship; seasonal episodes of mood disturbance outnumbered any nonseasonal episodes of such disturbance that may have occurred by more than three to one (*DSM*-III-R).

An example of this type of disorder would be the person who becomes depressed every winter.

G. Atypical depression

This term originally referred to a depressive syndrome responsive to a monoamine oxidase inhibitor (MAOI). It does not really describe a discrete or homogeneous group of patients. Rather, it describes a variety of nonendogenously depressed patients. Some reports have emphasized the importance of atypical neurovegetative signs (e.g., increased sleep and increased appetite); however, others have stressed the coexistence of anxiety symptoms, generalized or phobic anxiety, or panic disorder; and others described atypical depression as being nonendogenous or neurotic depression. Atypical depression has a chronic course if there's no treatment intervention. Although MAOI antidepressants are considered to be specific for this condition, tricyclic antidepressants are now considered useful. (The MAOIs seem to have a special efficacy for atypical depression with prominent anxiety or panic attacks.) Atypical depression is not an official *DSM*-III-R diagnosis.

H. Other types have also been described. For example:
1. Anxious depression, a condition in which both symptoms of anxiety and depression are prominent. It could also be considered a milder form of agitated depression.
   a) The *DSM*-IV task force is considering the utility of a category for anxiety/depression, reported to be encountered frequently in primary care and outpatient settings (Frances et al. 1990)

## V. Classification of mood disorder

A. Cases of mood disorder really fall along a continuum varying from mild, short-lived, subclinical depressions and elations on one end, to severe delusional depressions and delirious manias on the other.

B. In *DSM*-III-R the mood disorders are classified as follows:
1. Depressive disorders
   a) Major depression, in which there is one or more major depressive episodes (major depressive disorder, single episode; or major depressive disorder, recurrent)
      (1) It is estimated that 50 percent of people who have a single episode of depression will subsequently have another episode.
      (2) People who have recurrent depression are more apt to develop the bipolar disorder.
      (3) The course of recurrent depression is variable as some have episodes separated by many years of normalcy, others have clusters of episodes, and still others have increasingly frequent episodes with aging. In 20 to 35 percent of the cases there is a chronic course (*DSM*-III-R).
   b) Dysthymia is a chronic disturbance of mood in which there is a history of depressive mood (or irritable mood in children or adolescents) for more days than not for at least two years and which during the first two years of the disturbance the condition does not meet the criteria for major depressive disorder. In some cases there are superimposed major depressions ("double depressions") (*DSM*-III-R).
2. Bipolar disorders
   The essential feature is the presence of one or more manic or hypomanic episodes (usually with a history of major depressive episodes). There are two bipolar disorders.
   a) Bipolar disorder, in which there is one or more manic episodes (usually with one or more major depressive

episodes). With subclasses: Bipolar disorder, manic; bipolar disorder, mixed; bipolar disorder, depressed.

b) Cyclothymia, in which there are numerous hypomanic episodes and numerous periods with depressive symptoms (do not meet the criteria for major depressive or manic episodes).

c) "Bipolar II" disorders with hypomanic and full major depressive episodes are included in the residual category of bipolar disorder NOS (not otherwise specified).

## VI. Symptoms of affective disorders

A. Depression

1. The chief clinical complaints of patients with depression are psychological.

   a) The mood is either depressed or, possibly, in children or adolescents, irritable; or loss of interest or pleasure in almost all activities. The person will usually describe feeling sad, hopeless, discouraged, "down in the dumps," or some other colloquial equivalent.

      (1) The vast majority of depressed patients complain of this.

      (2) Behavior is consistent with the verbally expressed depression. But sometimes the presence of the depressed mood can be inferred from the person's sad or depressed appearance.

      (3) A small number of patients do not spontaneously complain of depression, but the disorder is manifested as two other symptom complexes. Such covert depression may appear as

         (a) Chiefly hypochondriacal symptoms

         (b) Neurasthenic symptoms of exhaustion, fatigue, or weakness

      (4) A few cases are "smiling depression."

      (5) Pleasurelessness (anhedonia) or loss of interest is often present. Previous interests no longer gratify the patient. A depressed person may not complain of this, but it will be manifested to family members and friends as his or her withdrawal from socializations and neglect of avocations.

      (6) Adolescents often show negativistic or "acting-out" behavior. These are sometimes referred to as "behavioral correlates" and include running away from home, school problems, vandalism, verbal assaultiveness, physical assaultiveness, petty theft, major theft, forgery, dealing in illicit drugs, property break-ins, sexual promiscuity, extortion, lying, gambling,

court involvement; teasing, taunting, or abusing domestic animals; sadistic actions; masochistic actions; fire setting; assault with weapon; substance abuse; and so forth.

(7) Elderly patients often show symptoms of impaired memory and disorientation (not due to organic factors and termed "pseudodementia"—an exaggerated indifference to one's surroundings without actual mental impairment).

b) Anorexia

Most depressed patients suffer loss of appetite and often lose weight. A small number, usually adolescents, have increased appetite (bulimia).

"Atypical" depressed patients exhibit hyperphagia.

c) Insomnia

Most patients experience some type of sleep disturbance. This may involve difficulty falling asleep (initial insomnia), difficulty remaining asleep (middle insomnia), or early morning awakening (terminal insomnia). A few, usually adolescents, sleep excessively (hypersomnia). It may be manifest as sleeping for longer periods of time than usual, daytime sleepiness, or taking excessive naps. Patients with "atypical" depression also have hypersomnia. Sometimes a sleep disturbance, rather than a depressed mood or anhedonia, is the main symptom. Some endogenously depressed patients show a pattern of entering rapid eye movement (REM) sleep earlier in their sleep than is usual for normal sleepers and concentrate more REM sleep in the first half of the night.

d) Psychomotor retardation or psychomotor agitation

Depressive patients may appear retarded or agitated.

(1) Retarded depressions are manifested by decreased activity.

(a) Slowed speech, increased pauses before answering, soft or monotonous speech, and verbal frugality.

(b) Inactivity: slowed body movements. In stuporous depression, the patient may be mute, immobile, and severely regressed.

(2) Agitated depressions are manifested by increased psychomotor activity.

(a) Restlessness, inability to sit still, jitteriness, pacing, handwringing, pulling or rubbing hair, skin, or clothing

(b) Difficulty in concentration—the patients report that thinking is slowed down or that their minds are blank, and they often complain of loss of memory.

(c) Sense of worthlessness

This may vary from lowered self-esteem with accompanying feelings of inadequacy and incompetence and poor self-concept, or the patient may reproach him- or herself for underlying feelings that are exaggerated, or this guilt may be expressed as an excessive reaction to either current or past feelings, or a sense of worthlessness or guilt may be of delusional proportions (*DSM*-III-R).

(d) Difficulty in concentrating, slowed thinking, and indecisiveness are frequent. The patient may complain of memory difficulties; this is more a function of inability to concentrate because of the depressed affect.

(e) Thoughts of death (not just the fear of dying) are common. Many times the person feels that he or she may be better off dead. There may be suicidal thoughts with or without a specific plan or suicidal attempts.

2. Associated features

   a) Anxiety, irritability, or obsessive rumination may occur.

   b) When hallucinations are present their content is usually consistent with a predominant mood (mood congruent). Less commonly the hallucinations or delusions are unrelated to the mood disturbance (mood incongruent).

3. Somatic symptoms

   a) These may be manifested as a mild physiological response of any body system, hypochondriacal preoccupation, definite physical symptoms, or somatic delusions.

   b) Often it is the somatic symptom that first concerns the patients and leads them to seek medical examination. This is especially true of elderly depressed patients.

   c) Thus, depressed persons may complain of any one of a variety of physical complaints, such as headache, cramps, nausea, constipation, or indigestion.

   d) In clinical practice many patients emphasize the somatic symptoms and minimize the psychological ones to the point where they can be considered to have "masked" depression.

4. Depression as a syndrome

a) A depressed patient usually has a constellation of the previously mentioned symptoms but does not manifest all of them.

b) Thus, we may speak of three depressive syndromes:
   (1) Ideational depressions (depressed mental content and few, if any, physical or motor symptoms)
   (2) Retarded depressions
   (3) Agitated depressions

B. Mania

1. Generally, the essential feature of a manic episode is an elevated euphoric, expansive, or irritable mood. Associated symptoms include inflated self-esteem or grandiosity (which may be delusional), decreased need for sleep, pressure of speech, flight of ideas, distractibility, increased involvement in goal-directed activity, psychomotor agitation, and excessive involvement in pleasurable activities that have a high potential for painful consequences that the person often does not recognize (*DSM*-III-R). This diagnosis is made only if it cannot be established that an organic factor initiated and maintained the disturbance (*DSM*-III-R).

2. In addition, other symptoms may be prominent.
   a) Inflated self-esteem or grandiosity
   b) Decreased need for sleep
   c) Loquaciousness or pressure of speech
   d) Flight of ideas or racing thoughts
   e) Distractibility
   f) Increase in goal-directed activity (in one of several areas, socially, work or school, or sexually) or psychomotor agitation
   g) Excessive involvement in pleasurable activities that have a high potential for painful consequences (e.g., unrestrained buying sprees, foolish business investments, or sexual indiscretions)

3. Absence of organic factor that might initiate a manic episode (toxic or metabolic factors).

## VII. Suicide

A. Introduction

1. Since the possibility of suicide is frequently raised by depressive disorders of all types, it is considered here.

2. However, it should be kept in mind that suicide is not exclusively limited to people with such diagnoses. Nearly everyone has had death wishes and suicidal thoughts, but only the suicidal ruminate about them.

3. The number of suicidal attempts is much smaller than the number of people who have contemplated suicide, and the

percentage of successful suicides is even smaller. It is variously estimated that attempts are five to fifty times more common than successes (the most common estimate seems to be ten attempts for every successful suicide).

4. The care and management of the suicidal patient presents a therapeutic challenge.

B. Prevalence
   1. Suicide is a major public health problem (constituting .4 percent to .9 percent of all deaths).
   2. Suicide is the tenth major cause of death in the United States (officially, 50,000 people kill themselves each year; however, an estimate of 100,000 would probably be a more realistic figure). These figures do not include unconsciously motivated ''fatal accidents'' or numerous other self-destructive behaviors, such as alcoholism. Among white males aged fifteen to nineteen, it is the second major cause of death.
   3. Throughout the world, the annual number of suicides is equivalent to the population of Edinburgh, Scotland, and the number of people who try to kill themselves each year is equal to the population of London or Los Angeles.
   4. Some studies indicate that it is rare for people to make more than one suicide attempt.
   5. Although more attempts are made by women in the United States, more men are successful. (Completed suicides are twice as high for men, although attempted suicides are twice as high for women.)
   6. Suicide prevention centers have apparently not affected the suicide rate.

C. Risk factors
   1. The presence of psychiatric disorders (especially those who have depressions or alcoholism, but there is also an increased incidence in personality disorders and drug dependence).
   2. Social factors.
      a) Suicidal rates are low in the less prosperous Catholic countries and higher in the more affluent countries and in the Eastern European countries.
      b) Suicide rates are higher in the spring and early summer.
      c) Suicide rates are lowest in married people and higher in divorced, separated, and widowed people.
      d) Suicide is higher among Protestants and lower among Catholics and Jews.
   3. Physical disorders.

Physical disorders with attendant mood disturbances have higher rates of suicide (for example, Huntington's chorea and epilepsy).

4. Genetic factors.

   Suicide is more common in families where there is a history of suicide; it is also more common in the second of two identical twins where the first one has committed suicide (this is supported by adoption studies, too). Generally, one can say that "suicide runs in families."

5. Biological factors: The central serotonin system has been implicated in suicide.

6. Previous suicidal behavior: A past suicidal attempt is perhaps the best indicator of the increased risk in a patient.

D. Psychodynamic factors

1. Most authorities believe that suicide rarely results from a single cause. Several factors may be operant in a cumulative way.

2. Any serious loss may be a possible etiological factor (e.g., loss of a loved one, a job, money, health, beauty, independence).

3. The anniversary of an important event (e.g., the death of a loved one) may initiate a suicide attempt.

4. Karl Menninger regarded suicide as self-murder. In *Man against Himself,* he also described other self-destructive behaviors that stop short of suicide (invalidism, alcoholism, self-mutilation, and accident proneness).

5. Beck was not able to substantiate the earlier dynamic formulation of internalized aggression.

6. Schneidman and Faberow (1961) have classified people who commit suicide into four general groups:

   a) Those who view suicide as a means to a better life or as a means of saving reputation

   b) Those who are psychotic and commit suicide in response to delusions or hallucinations

   c) Those who commit suicide as revenge against a loved person

   d) Elderly and infirm people who use suicide as a release from pain

7. What prods a person from contemplation to action is not really known.

8. Some authorities feel that suicide attempts may be understood in terms of suicidal patients' fantasies. Included in these are:

   a) A wish for revenge

   b) A wish for power control

   c) A wish for atonement, sacrifice, or restitution

9. Others feel that suicide attempts are motivated by:
   a) Feelings of hopelessness
   b) Fantasies of reunion (anniversary suicide)

E. Danger signs
   1. History of previous suicide attempts or threats
   2. Suicide note
   3. Psychotic reactions with suspiciousness, paranoid delusions, or panic
   4. Chronic illness (especially the attitude toward the illness)
   5. Alcoholism or drug dependency
   6. Advancing age, especially in men
   7. Recent surgery or childbirth
   8. Hypochondriasis
   9. Unaccepted homosexuality

F. Evaluation of suicidal risks
   Most suicidal patients will admit their intentions to a physician. When estimating the possibility that a person will attempt suicide, the following questions are helpful.
   1. Have you thought of suicide?
   2. Have you thought of what way you would take your life? Do you have a plan?
   3. Have you already made preparations?
   4. Do you trust yourself?

G. Self-injury
   Self-injury is really a different issue than suicide or attempted suicide, but it is discussed here since it often has to be evaluated in the context of the psychiatric setting.
   1. Four percent of patients in psychiatric hospitals have *cut* themselves (female-to-male ratio of 3:1).
   2. They have usually done this in private with a razor blade, knife, or some other sharp object such as broken glass.
   3. The great majority of the patients who do this are personality disordered (with alcohol and drug abuse commonly associated). It is also true that they may, in the past, have attempted suicide.

## VIII. Course

A. Depression
   1. Depressive episodes
      a) The onset is variable, with symptoms developing over a period of a few days to weeks.
      b) Many depressive episodes are self-limiting and remit without specific treatment.
      c) With treatment, the duration of episodes has been reduced from several months to a few weeks.

d) It is estimated that at least half of the individuals with a major depressive episode will eventually have another one.
　　　e) It should be kept in mind in dealing with depressive people that one can usually be optimistic that the depression will remit.
　　2. Chronic depression
　　　a) About 15 percent of depressive disorders run a chronic course.
　　　b) The patients continue to experience depressed mood, sleep disturbances, and various bodily symptoms.
　B. Manic episodes (or elations)
　　1. Most patients with manic episodes also have depressions.
　　2. Before the advent of the psychotropic drugs (neuroleptic agents, antianxiety agents, lithium) and electroconvulsive therapy, the episodes were usually longer.
　　3. Manic episodes are frequently recurrent.
　　4. Before the introduction of lithium, only about 25 percent of manic patients had a single episode.
　　5. The prophylactic administration of lithium therapy often prevents further attacks.
　C. Diagnostic categories
　　1. Depressive disorders
　　　a) Major depression, recurrent, or major depression, single episode. The essential feature is one or more major depressive episodes without a history of either a manic episode or unequivocal hypomanic episode (unipolar depression).
　　　　(1) Although some people have a single episode, estimates are that over 50 percent will eventually have another major depressive episode (major depression, recurrent).
　　　　(2) People with the recurrent type of the illness are more likely to develop bipolar disorder (discussed later).
　　　　(3) The course of recurrent depression varies from episodes separated by many years of normal functioning, those having "clusters of episodes," and others who have increasingly frequent episodes as they grow older.
　　　b) Dysthymia (or depressive neurosis)
　　　　(1) The central feature is the chronic disturbance of mood involving depressed mood (or possibly an irritable mood in children or adolescents), for most

of the day more days than not, for at least two years (one year for children and adolescents).

(2) The following associated symptoms may be present (*DSM*-III-R):
   (a) Poor appetite or overeating
   (b) Insomnia or hypersomnia
   (c) Low energy or fatigue
   (d) Low self-esteem
   (e) Poor concentration or difficulty making decisions
   (f) Feelings of hopelessness

(3) Other predisposing factors
   Chronic, nonmood Axis I or Axis III disorder (e.g., anorexia nervosa, somatization disorder, psychoactive substance dependence, rheumatoid arthritis). Such cases are referred to as secondary types. Cases unrelated to any preexisting condition are called primary types.

(4) There are no clear boundaries between dysthymia and major depression.

(5) This disorder often begins in early life and hence is referred to as a depressive personality.

2. Bipolar disorder (mixed; manic; depressed)
The essential feature is one or more manic episodes usually accompanied by one or more major depressive episodes.

a) Course
   (1) Manic episode is usually the initial episode that leads to hospitalization.
   (2) Often a manic or depressive episode is followed immediately by a short episode of the opposite kind (''rapid cycling'').
   (3) Cases of bipolar with mixed or rapid-cycling episodes are much more often chronic.
   (4) Familial pattern: occurs at a much higher rate in first-degree biological relatives of people with bipolar than in the general population.

b) Prevalence
   .4 percent to 1.2 percent of the adult population

c) Sex ratio
   Equally common in males and females (unlike major depression, which is more common in females).

d) Both manic and depressive episodes may be intermixed or rapidly alternate every few days (mixed bipolar disorder).

3. Cyclothymia

This is a chronic mood disturbance of at least two years' duration (one year for children and adolescents), involving hypomanic episodes and numerous periods of depressed mood or loss of interest or pleasure of insufficient severity or duration to meet the criteria for major depressive or a manic episode. The boundaries between this disorder and bipolar disorder are not well defined. Some consider cyclothymia a mild form of bipolar disorder.

    a) Course

       Usually a chronic course without clear onset. Oftentimes the person develops bipolar disorder.

    b) Prevalence

       .4 percent to 3.5 percent

    c) Sex ratio

       Equally common in males and females

    d) Onset

       Usually begins in adolescence or early adult life

## IX. Epidemiology

A. Depression is a very common symptom. It is at least ten times as prevalent as schizophrenia. Severe depression affects fully 2 percent to 3 percent of the world's population—some 100 million individuals—and recent figures indicate that this figure is probably an understatement.

B. In the United States alone, some 10 to 14 million people are estimated to be afflicted by moderate or severe depression. Other estimates are that 15 percent of Americans experience depressive episodes.

C. Depending on the studies, indications are that perhaps 15 to 30 percent of adults in a general population experience depressive episodes.

D. The incidence (the number of new cases per year) varies from 1.8 per thousand to 4.5 per thousand per year.

E. Its "ripple effect" extends in varying degrees to family members, friends, and work associates.

F. For every severely or moderately depressed person who has been diagnosed as such, there are many more ill who have not been diagnosed or treated.

G. Depression occurs two to four times more frequently in women than in men. As noted earlier, bipolar disorder afflicts both sexes equally.

H. In the past, it was thought that manic-depressive disease was a disorder of the upper-middle and the upper classes, but subsequent investigators have found no relationship between social class and bipolar affective disorders (when occupational level and educational achievement are used as indexes of social status).

## X. Etiology

Most researchers consider mood disorders to be a heterogeneous group of disorders. Thus, any consideration of etiology of mood disorders, as with the etiology of most mental disorders, must take into consideration all the factors that could possibly play a role in the development of the mood disorder, including genetic and biological factors, environmental stress and life events, and psychodynamic factors.

A. Genetic factors

Genetic studies have included family pedigree studies, twin studies, adoption studies, population surveys, and linkage studies using known genetic markers. Generally, they have shown the following:

1. There is an increased frequency of affective illness, particularly bipolar affective illness or disorder, in the relatives of affectively disordered patients. Generally, these studies indicate that families with histories of unipolar illness are at risk for unipolar disease, and families with histories of bipolar disorder are more at risk for bipolar disorders.

2. Studies show a concordance of 72 percent for monozygotic (identical) twins and 14 percent for dizygotic (fraternal) twins in the incidence of manic-depressive disorder.

3. Depression also occurs in families, and studies indicate that relatives are also at greater risk for other types of disorders: alcoholism, panic disorders, and phobias (suggesting that these disorders belong to the same "genetic cluster" or "depressive spectrum").

4. Studies also support the use of a bipolar-unipolar classification.

B. Biological factors

Introduction of antidepressants in the 1950s led to investigation of the study of the neurotransmitter biochemistry of these disorders. And certain biological factors, other than genetic, seem to be important:

1. Catecholamine hypothesis
   Biogenic amines are the neurotransmitters that have been implicated with having roles in schizophrenia and affective disorders.

2. The term *biogenic amine* generally refers to four compounds: norepinephrine, epinephrine, and dopamine, which are catecholamines; and serotonin, which is an indolemine. According to the catecholamine hypothesis, a deficiency of norepinephrine leads to depression and over activity of

norepinephrine leads to mania (this theory is incomplete for mania).

3. The biogenic amine permissive hypothesis holds that a functional underactivity of serotonin is necessary for every affective disorder. But the level of norepinephrine determines whether elation or depression exists. (Some investigators report low levels of serotonin metabolites in the spinal fluid of some depressed patients. Others have noted increased incidence of completed suicide, suicidal attempts, or acts of aggression and a lower level of cerebral spinal fluid serotonin metabolites.)

4. The adrenergic-cholinergic imbalance hypothesis maintains that the ratio of acetylcholine to catecholamines in the brain is low in mania and high in depression.

5. The electrolyte-membrane potential disturbance theory asserts that depression is accounted for in part by an accumulation of intracellular sodium.

C. Environmental stress and life events

1. Most clinical psychiatrists believe there is a relationship between the onset of depression and environmental stress. Some believe that such events play the major role.

2. Some recent research confirms a relationship between stressful environmental factors (e.g., death or losses) and the onset of depression.

D. Psychodynamic factors

1. In the past, it was believed that the dependent person with low self-esteem and a strong superego was more prone to depression. Subsequent clinical findings have not supported the existence of a single personality type or constellation of personality traits (under appropriate conditions, anyone can become depressed).

2. In the past, it was assumed that hostility turned inward was important in the development of the depression. Although this dynamic formulation enjoys wide clinical acceptance, research supporting it is still being developed (Nicholi 1988).

3. Some regard mania as a "running away from" depression.

4. At present, the psychodynamic hypotheses that are based on reactions to loss or hostility turned inward and with the presence of guilt in ongoing dynamic conflicts are chiefly of empirical value, assisting the therapist to formulate a therapeutic program.

5. Once started, the episode *usually* does not respond to interpretation and thus the person usually requires somatic therapy, such as antidepressant medication and even

electroconvulsive therapy. However, once the episode is controlled with appropriate somatic therapy (usually antidepressants), psychotherapy may be helpful in dealing with the secondary consequences of the illness and will foster avoidance of precipitants or help the individual cope with contributing underlying psychological problems.

6. Cognitive model of depression: The cognitive triad consists of the patient's negative views of: a) self, b) experience, and c) the future.

7. Most psychosocial theories of depression involve loss of self-esteem. This loss can also trigger mania. It should be remembered that successful events may also trigger depression (e.g., "promotion depression").

## XI. Treatment

A. Depression

There are many effective treatments for the depressive disorders, including various psychotherapy modalities, antidepressant medications, and electroconvulsive therapy. A pluralistic approach seems indicated.

1. Psychotherapy

a) A number of treatment modalities may be used with acutely depressed patients. Most respond to some type of supportive treatment (for details, see chapter 9).

b) Two approaches seem to be especially useful in a psychotherapeutic approach to the depressive disorders.

(1) Psychodynamic psychotherapy that is based on assumptions that are derived from psychoanalytic theory. For general purposes, the aim is to produce insight by uncovering emotional conflicts, chiefly unconscious, so that they can be dealt with in a way that does not hamper current relationships and activities.

(2) Cognitive therapy is an approach aimed at directing the cognitive distortions (negative view of self, experience, and future) and the specific habitual errors in thinking (cognition).

c) Most important in the psychotherapeutic management of the acute depressive episode is that the therapist be available and active.

d) A word of caution: Advice should be used very sparingly. One usually does not know all the nuances of the situation under consideration, and further, the depressed individual does not want advice but rather someone to listen with respect, understanding, and without criticism.

e) Frequently, depressed patients present themselves as markedly dependent. This is a feeling that must be handled delicately because they frequently are ambivalent about such strivings. (As Maxmen [1986] has said: "Dispense hope, not saccharin.") Also, it should be remembered that most depressions remit (the advantage of treatment is that it shortens the periods of depression).

f) Appropriate and prompt attention should be paid to suicidal issues. Sometimes hospitalization may be necessary, not so much because of the actual suicidal potential but more because the depressed person has no networks of supportiveness.

2. Pharmacological therapy

a) Although direct stimulants, primarily the amphetamines, were used by physicians for the treatment of depression for many years, the modern pharmacological treatment of depression dates back to the early 1950s, when the tricyclic antidepressants and the monoamine oxidase inhibitors (MAOI) were introduced.

b) Of all of the antidepressant agents available, the tricyclic antidepressants are the ones that have been the most employed. With the introduction of second- and third-generation antidepressants following continuing research, the newer ones are somewhat replacing the tricyclics and the MAOI drugs. Generally, the tricyclics are effective and act by blocking the neuronal uptake of amines into the presynaptic nerve endings. MAOI antidepressants are drugs of choice for treating atypical depression (especially with panic attacks).

c) Recently introduced antidepressants are gaining popularity. Among these are amoxapine (Asendin), maprotiline HCL (Ludiomil), trimipramine maleate (Surmontil), trazodone HCl (Desyrel), and recently, fluoxetine hydrochloride (Prozac)—a blocker of serotonin uptake. More recently, a second selective serotonin reuptake blocker, sertraline (Zoloft), was introduced. Its chemical structure differs from that of fluoxetine. Bupropion (Wellbutrin) is an antidepressant that does not involve brain norepinephrine or serotonin. Generally, the effectiveness of these is similar to the effectiveness of tricyclics, and it is the side effect profiles that often determine which drug is prescribed.

d) Sedatives and antianxiety agents (generally, benzodiazepines) are prescribed for coexisting symptoms of anxiety and tension.

e) Neuroleptics (e.g., the phenothiazines, thioxanthenes, butyrophenones) are also used if psychotic symptoms are present. They are sometimes helpful in treating depressed people with agitation.

3. Electroconvulsive therapy
   a) Since the introduction of the antidepressants in the early 1960s, the use of electroconvulsive therapy (ECT) has declined.
   b) However, it remains an effective treatment and is still prescribed for severe depressions, especially patients with whom suicide is a major concern.
   c) Remission rates with this treatment are 85 percent and higher (in contrast to 70 percent and higher with tricyclic antidepressants).

4. Hospitalization
   a) Most depressed patients can be treated outside of the hospital.
   b) Patients with severe depressions, suicidal urges—especially if these are accompanied by plans—medical conditions that require extensive evaluations, or patients who have failed at outpatient attempts should probably be hospitalized.
   c) With modern treatment approaches, the average stay is less than a month.

5. Clinical treatment
   Generally, the treatment of depressions is successful—given the availability of effective treatments, including various types of psychotherapy, pharmacological therapy, and so on. An eclectic approach seems appropriate (the use of compatible aspects from diverse systems into an integrated whole).

6. Maintenance therapy
   For those with recurrent episodes or chronic symptoms, maintenance therapy consisting of antidepressants or psychotropics as appropriate, plus supportive psychotherapy, seems to be effective. Lithium is often used (see treatment of mania, which follows).

7. Dexamethasone Suppression Test (DST)
   Recent studies have suggested some clinical value to the use of this test. It is theorized that in normal individuals, the administration of dexamethasone suppresses cortisol secretion (from the hypothalamus). In some depressed patients, dexamethasone often does not suppress cortisol secretion. It is usually considered that patients with *endogenous* types of depression fail to suppress their cortisol after

their DST. A positive DST is also found in nondepressed patients and a negative DST in depressed ones. Thus, conflicting published reports suggest that this test lacks sufficient specificity for a place in the *routine* assessment of depression.

B. Mania
   1. Persons with hypomania, or mild elations, can often be treated as outpatients.
   2. Hospitalization is indicated for patients who are acutely manic. Aside from specific treatment for the episodes, patients need to be protected from the social consequences of their expansive behavior and poor judgment.
   3. Pharmacological therapy
      a) Lithium carbonate shortens periods of elation and helps prevent attacks of either depression or elation when administered as part of a maintenance program. (Lithium citrate as a liquid may be prescribed for people who have difficulty swallowing tablets or for whom there is some suspicion they may be "cheeking" their lithium.)
      b) In clinical practice, since it usually takes several days for lithium to become effective, neuroleptics, especially phenothiazines, thioxanthenes, and the butyrophenones are prescribed to provide early control of maniacal systems. These are gradually withdrawn when the elation comes under control.
      c) Recently, evidence is growing for the antimanic efficacy of anticonvulsants such as carbamazepine (Tegretol). Other anticonvulsants such as clonazepam (Klonopin) or valproate (Depakene) have also been suggested as supplementary medications.
      d) Clinical studies would suggest a trial of carbamazepine, rather than traditional antipsychotics, is indicated.
   4. Occasionally, when the episode does not respond to drugs, electroconvulsive therapy is prescribed.

C. Bipolar disorders
   1. The goal is to prevent recurrences of acute episodes, relieve chronic low-grade disturbing symptoms, and improve the patient's adjustment.
   2. The most effective clinical approach seems to be combined drug therapy and psychotherapy.
   3. Pharmacological therapy
      a) Lithium carbonate for acute elations plus prophylactic use to prevent further episodes; and other neuroleptics

and anticonvulsants as noted earlier under the treatment of mania.

b) Antidepressants must be administered judiciously to people who have manic episodes, since it is possible to precipitate an elation in the course of long-term maintenance therapy.

c) Some recent studies indicate that the combining of lithium with either carbamazepine (Tegretol) or isoptin (Verapamil) is useful in the management of "rapid-cycling" bipolar disorder.

4. Occasionally, electroconvulsive therapy is used on a maintenance basis to prevent relapses. Such treatment is given at intervals of four, six, or eight weeks for several months or years. It has proved effective in some cases that have not responded to direct maintenance alone.

## XII. Organic mood syndrome

A. In *DSM*-III-R, a separate category is listed for mood disturbances due to specific organic factors.

B. The essential feature is a prominent and persistent depressed, elevated, or expansive mood, resembling either a manic episode or a major depressive episode, which is due to a specific organic factor.

C. The clinical phenomenology of this syndrome is similar to that of manic or major depressive episode described earlier in this chapter.

D. Etiology

This is usually caused by toxic or metabolic factors (e.g., reserpine, methyldopa, and some of the hallucinogens are apt to cause a depressive syndrome). Certain endocrine disorders, such as hyper- and hypothyroidism and hyper- and hypoadrenocorticalism, may produce either depressive or manic episodes. Carcinoma of the pancreas is sometimes associated with depression (possibly due to neuropeptides in the gastrointestinal tract that are identical to those found in the brain). Viral illness may also cause a depressive illness. Structural disease of the brain, such as may result from hemispheric strokes, is a common cause of organic mood syndrome.

E. Treatment

1. Treatment of the underlying specific cause.

2. Sometimes treatment will also have to be directed at depression if that is not resolved by treatment of the specific underlying condition.

## XIII. Case examples

A. Major depressive disorder, single episode

Mrs. S., a thirty-five-year-old housewife, was admitted to the hospital complaining of nausea, vomiting, crying, and depression. Her symptoms had begun four months earlier, following an incident that should have made her feel hostile toward her husband. However, because of guilt related to an extramarital affair a few years earlier, she was unable to express her hostile feelings, and these became redirected against herself and produced the depressive symptoms.

On admission, she appeared depressed and cried rather easily when discussing her illness and her husband. There was no obvious psychomotor retardation, but she did complain of some difficulty in concentration. In the hospital, she ate poorly and had difficulty sleeping. She responded promptly to treatment and has remained free of symptoms for several years.

This patient had a single depressive episode, with symptoms common to most depression, namely, depressed mood, difficulty in concentration, disturbance of appetite and sleep, and somatic symptoms.

## B. Major depressive disorder, recurrent

Mr. N., a fifty-five-year-old accountant, was admitted to the hospital with a severe depression, which had begun following the accidental injury of his son nine months earlier. He showed marked psychomotor retardation, refused to eat, and was mute most of the time. When he did speak, he expressed delusions of worthlessness, hopelessness, and nihilism. His history revealed three previous episodes of depression, beginning at age twenty. Only the first attack had been severe enough to require hospital treatment. During the other episodes, he was able to work, but with reduced efficiency. He was described as a quiet, shy, conscientious, sensitive person who worried unduly about his work and family.

This is a case of major depressive disorder characterized by several episodes of depression and an absence of personality deterioration between attacks. The marked psychomotor retardation, the muteness, the refusal to eat, and the delusions characterize the last attack as a stuporous depression.

## C. Manic disorder, single episode

A forty-three-year-old married man was admitted to a closed psychiatric unit at the request of his family, after "uncontrolled" behavior. On admission, he was agitated, hyperactive, uncooperative, and out of touch with reality, and had flight of ideas and rambling, incoherent speech. He angrily ordered the nurses around. These symptoms had developed over a period of a few weeks, during which he was on strike. He first became insomniac and drank excessively.

Physical and laboratory examinations were normal. A brain scan was reported as within normal limits. He responded to treatment, including lithium and Haldol.

He had never had any previous affective symptoms. His family history revealed one sister who had a schizophrenic disorder.

It was not clear whether his excessive alcoholic intake was causal or symptomatic of the manic episode. At any rate, this seems to be an example of a single manic episode.

D. Bipolar disorder

Mr. S., a forty-one-year-old attorney, was admitted to the hospital in an acute manic episode. He was extremely hyperactive, distractible, irritable, and demanding. He had a marked flight of ideas and expressed hostility toward his wife for what he described as infidelity. Eight years earlier, he had developed a depressive episode following his wife's severe infectious disease, and since that time he had developed manic symptoms every spring and depressive symptoms every fall. Prior to the onset of his illness, he was described as perfectionistic, egotistical, and outgoing. Between episodes, he practiced law with above-average skill and showed no evidence of personality deterioration.

This is a classical case of manic-depressive illness. The patient's behavior on admission—elated mood, flight of ideas, and increased activity—was typical of acute mania. Note, also, the absence of personality deterioration between attacks.

E. Other examples of bipolar disorder
   1. John Ruskin (1819–1900), writer, critic, artist, and author of *Modern Painters,* was an example of a bipolar disorder, swinging from elation to misery, always sensitive and always expressive.
   2. Vincent Van Gogh (1853–1890), Dutch painter, suffered from mood swings, alternating between profound depression and extreme exuberance. On Christmas Eve, 1888, he cut off part of his left ear, and in July 1890, he committed suicide.

# References

Aarons, S. F., et al. "Atypical Depression: A Review of Diagnosis and Treatment." *Hospital and Community Psychiatry* 36 (March 1985): 275–82.

American Psychiatric Association. *Diagnostic and Statistical Manual of Mental Disorders.* 3d ed., rev. Washington, D.C.: APA, 1987.

Brown, R. P., et al. "Involutional Melancholia Revisited." *American Journal of Psychiatry* 141 (January 1984): 24–28.

Clayton, P. J. "Bereavement Depression." *Journal of Clinical Psychiatry* 51 (July 1990 Supplement): 34–38.

Frances, A., H. A. Pincus, T. A. Widiger, W. W. Davis, and N. B. First. "DSM-IV: Work in Progress." *American Journal of Psychiatry* (November 1990): 1439–48.

Kaplan, H. I., and B. J. Sadock, eds. *Comprehensive Textbook of Psychiatry/V.* 5th ed. Baltimore: Williams & Wilkins, 1989.

Kolb, L. C., and H. K. H. Brodie. *Modern Clinical Psychiatry.* 10th ed. Philadelphia: Saunders, 1982.

Maxmen, J. S. *Essential Psychopathology.* New York: Norton, 1986.

Nicholi, A. M., Jr., ed. *The New Harvard Guide to Modern Psychiatry.* Cambridge, Mass.: Belknap Press, 1988.

Schneidman, E. S. "Suicide." In *Comprehensive Textbook of Psychiatry, vol. 2,* 2d ed., edited by A. M. Freedman, H. I. Kaplan, and B. J. Sadock. Baltimore: Williams & Wilkins, 1976.

Schneidman, E. S., and N. L. Faberow. *A Cry for Help.* New York: McGraw-Hill, 1961.

Zimmerman, M., W. Coryell, B. Pfohl, and D. Stangl. "The Validity of Four Definitions of Endogenous Depression." *Archives of General Psychiatry* (March 1986): 234.

# 24 Schizophrenic Disorders

We are prone to the malady of the introvert, who, with the manifold spectacle of the world spread out before him, turns away and gazes only upon the emptiness within. But, let us not imagine that there is anything grand about the introvert's unhappiness.

Bertrand Russell, *The Conquest of Happiness* (1930)

I. **Historical notes**
   A. The syndromes that are now classified as schizophrenia have been recognized for at least 3,400 years, although in the past they have carried varying labels.
   B. Greek physicians in the fifth century B.C. termed it *dementia* and distinguished it from mania and melancholia.
   C. In 1683, Thomas Willis reported a patient whose personality had changed in early life.
   D. Benedict Augustin Morel (1860) introduced the term *demence precoce* to describe psychosis in a fourteen-year-old boy.
   E. Ewald Hecker (1871) described *hebephrenia* as a progressive psychotic illness of rapid onset in adolescence.
   F. Karl Kahlbaum (1874) described *catatonia*, or *tension insanity*, and assumed it to be a symptom of some organic brain disease. His description was of a condition characterized by muteness, immobility, waxy flexibility, and so forth.
   G. Emil Kraepelin (1896), believing that all of the previously mentioned syndromes were related, classified them into one group called *dementia praecox*. He reserved the diagnosis for a relatively small group of psychotic patients whose prognosis was poor.
   H. Subsequently, American investigators broadened the concept of schizophrenia. Among these investigators were the following:
   I. Adolf Meyer (1906) theorized that dementia praecox was a type of reaction to environmental experiences (*parergastic reaction*).
   J. Eugen Bleuler (1911) coined the term *schizophrenia* to emphasize the "splitting" of the personality (from the Greek *schizo*, "to split," and *phren*, "mind"). He recognized that dementia

praecox does not always lead to deterioration, but he regarded it as a syndrome, a group of disorders.

K. Jacob Kasan (1933) described *schizoaffective psychosis.*

L. Gabriel Langfeldt (1949) described *reactive schizophrenia,* or *schizophreniform psychosis* and emphasized a relatively good prognosis and good response to treatment.

M. Paul Hoch and P. Polatin (1949) described *pseudoneurotic schizophrenia* to apply to those patients whose defense mechanisms seemed neurotic but on close investigation showed basic schizophrenic mechanisms. Symptomatically they showed pan anxiety and pan neurosis.

N. Paul Hoch and S. L. Dunaif (1955) coined the term *pseudo psychopathic schizophrenia* to describe the anxious withdrawn person with serious interpersonal problems and psychopathic or neurotic symptomatology.

## II. Definition

A. The American Psychiatric Association's *Psychiatric Glossary* defines schizophrenia as a large group of disorders, usually of psychotic proportion, manifested by characteristic disturbances of language and communication, thought, perception, affect, and behavior, which last longer than six months. Thought disturbances are marked by alterations of concept formation that may lead to misinterpretation of reality, misperceptions, and sometimes to delusions and hallucinations. Mood changes include ambivalence, blunting, inappropriateness, and loss of empathy with others. Behavior may be withdrawn, regressive, and bizarre. The clinical picture is not explainable by any of the organic mental disorders.[1]

B. *DSM*-III-R describes the essential features as "the presence of characteristic psychotic symptoms during the active phase of the illness and functioning below the highest level previously achieved (in children or adolescents, failure to achieve the expected level of social development), and a duration of at least six months that may include characteristic prodromal or residual symptoms. At some phase of the illness schizophrenia always involves delusions, hallucinations, or certain characteristic disturbances in affect and the form of thought. The diagnosis is made only when it cannot be established that an organic factor initiated and maintained the disturbance. The diagnosis is not made if the symptoms are due to a mood disorder or schizoaffective disorder" (*DSM*-III-R).

    1. Clinical criteria include:

1. American Psychiatric Association, *A Psychiatric Glossary,* 5th ed. (Washington, D.C.: APA 1980).

        a) Functioning below a highest level previously achieved in such areas as work, social relations, and self-care.

        b) Characteristic symptoms involving multiple psychological processes including: content and form of thought, perception, affect, sense of self, volition, impaired interpersonal functioning and relationship to the external world and psychomotor behavior.

        c) For elaboration on these descriptions, see IV. Symptoms.

## III. Conceptions of schizophrenia

A. Over the past century, many widely divergent concepts of schizophrenia have been held by different psychiatrists in different countries. Under I. Historical notes, many of these have been listed.

B. Emil Kraepelin believed that dementia praecox resulted from injury to the germ plasm or from some metabolic disorder, which caused autointoxication. Thus, he thought of it as an organically caused disease. He was the first to include hebephrenic, catatonic, and paranoid reactions under one category.

C. Eugen Bleuler's concept was broader than Kraepelin's. Although he believed this illness to be primarily of physical origin, he did consider certain secondary symptoms (such as delusions, hallucinations, and mannerisms) to be psychogenic (an indicative attempt at adaptation to the primary disturbance). He emphasized the "splitting of the various mental functions" (i.e., the coexistence of disharmonious complexes). He regarded the formal mechanism underlying schizophrenic symptoms as the loosening of association.

D. Adolf Meyer regarded this as a maladaptive reaction ("the accumulation of lifelong faulty habits of adaptation in the setting of an inferior psychobiological endowment"). That is, he saw it as a habit disorganization. He emphasized longitudinal (versus cross-sectional) psychological factors.

E. Sigmund Freud regarded schizophrenia as withdrawal and regression associated with a weak ego, a return to early narcissism (e.g., the libido is withdrawn from external objects and directed toward the ego).

F. Carl Jung believed that schizophrenia arises when the psyche is unable to rid itself of a complex and can no longer adapt to the surroundings. Thus, separation from reality results. He thought that delusions, hallucinations, and other schizophrenic symptoms were due to an autochthonous complex (i.e., a group of ideas that, because they were disturbing, were removed from consciousness and maintained in an independent existence).

G. Harry Stack Sullivan regarded schizophrenia as the indirect outcome of unhealthy interpersonal relationships between the child (who later becomes schizophrenic) and the parents.

H. Emil Kraepelin and Eugen Bleuler are the two progenitors of the modern concept of schizophrenia.

I. *DSM*-III and *DSM*-III-R have moved from the broadened definitions to new definitions that narrow the range of patients who are currently diagnosed with schizophrenia.

## IV. Symptoms

A. Since our present-day concept of this disorder includes varying clinical types, it is difficult to present a "typical" cluster of symptoms.

B. Bleuler

1. Bleuler (1950) described four main symptoms: disturbance of association, disturbance of affect, autism, and heightened ambivalence. These are often called the "four A's."

   a) Disturbance of association is looseness of association (cognitive slippage or derailment). In schizophrenic speech, successive ideas appear to be unrelated or only slightly related to each other.

   b) Disturbances of affect usually take the form of flatness, bluntness, or inappropriateness.

   c) Autism is fantasy and daydreaming that substitutes for reality.

   d) Heightened ambivalence is exaggeration of coexisting opposite feelings or emotions for the same person, thing, situation, or goal.

2. In addition, Bleuler believed that the main accessory or secondary symptoms need to be present. In severe or advanced cases they are usually found. They are delusions, hallucinations, and ideas of reference. Ideas of reference include feelings of thought control and feelings of influence.

C. According to *DSM*-III-R, the essential features of this group of disorders are

1. Presence of characteristic psychotic symptoms during the active phase of the illness

2. Functioning below the highest level previously achieved in such areas as work, social relationships, and self-care and a duration of at least six months

3. Characteristic symptoms involving multiple psychological processes

   a) Content of thought

   The major disturbance involves delusions that are multiple, fragmented, or bizarre.

   (1) Persecutory and referential delusions

(2) Delusions of thought broadcasting (belief that one's thoughts are broadcast to the external world)

(3) Thought insertion (belief that one's thoughts are not one's own but inserted into the mind)

(4) Thought withdrawal (belief that thoughts have been removed from one's head)

(5) Delusions of being controlled (belief that one's feelings, impulses, thoughts, or actions are imposed by external force)

(6) Somatic, grandiose, religious, and nihilistic delusions—less common

b) Form of thought

A disturbance in the form of thought is frequently present ("formal thought disorder").

(1) Most commonly this is manifest as loosening of associations (cognitive slippage), in which ideas shift from one subject to another on completely unrelated or only on obliquely related subject.

(2) When loosening of association is severe, speech may become incoherent and incomprehensible.

(3) There also may be poverty of content of speech (that is, speech conveys little information because it is vague, overly abstract, or stereotyped).

(4) Less common disturbances include neologisms, perseveration, clanging, and blocking.

c) Perception

The major perceptual disturbances are varieties of hallucinations.

(1) Although these occur in all modalities, the most common are auditory hallucinations, frequently involving voices the individual perceives as coming from outside the head. These voices often make insulting remarks and speak directly to the person or comment on his or her ongoing behavior (including command hallucinations).

(2) Tactile and somatic hallucinations are much less common.

(3) Visual, gustatory, and olfactory hallucinations may occur (but always raise the possibility of the presence of an organic mental disorder).

d) Affect

(1) Blunting, flattening, or inappropriateness are common.

(2) Antipsychotic drugs have effects that may appear similar to affective blunting and affective flattening.

e) Sense of self
   (1) The sense of self that gives the normal person a feeling of individuality, uniqueness, and self-direction is frequently disturbed.
   (2) This is sometimes referred to as a loss of ego boundaries and is frequently manifested by extreme perplexity.
f) Volition
   (1) Disturbance in self-initiated, goal-directed activity, which may grossly impair work or other role functioning.
   (2) This may take the form of inadequate interest or drive or inability to follow a course of action to its logical conclusions.
   (3) Ambivalence regarding alternative courses of action can lead to near cessation of goal-directed activity.
g) Relationship to the external world
   (1) Frequently there is a tendency to withdraw from involvement with the external world and become preoccupied with egocentric illogical ideas and fantasies in which objective facts are obscured, distorted, or excluded.
   (2) Severe forms of this condition are referred to as "autism."
h) Psychomotor behavior
   Various disturbances in psychomotor behavior are observed.
   (1) A marked decrease in reactivity to the environment.
   (2) The individual may appear unaware of the nature of his or her environment (as in catatonic stupor).
   (3) The individual may maintain a rigid posture, resisting efforts to be moved (as in catatonic rigidity).
   (4) The individual may make apparently purposeless and stereotyped, excited motor movements (as in catatonic excitement).
   (5) The individual may voluntarily assume inappropriate or bizarre postures (as in catatonic posturing).
   (6) The individual may resist and actively counteract instructions or attempts to be moved (as in catatonic negativism).
   (7) In addition, there may be mannerisms, grimacing, or waxy flexibility.
4. Associated features
   Almost any symptom can occur as an associated feature.

a) Perplexed, disheveled, or eccentric grooming and appearance may occur.
b) Symptoms can include abnormalities of psychomotor activity—for example, pacing, rocking, or apathetic immobility.
c) Frequently, there is poverty of speech.
d) Ritualistic or stereotyped behavior associated with magical thinking may occur.
e) Dysphoric mood is common and may take the form of depression, anxiety, anger, or a mixture of these.
f) Depersonalization, derealization, ideas of reference, and illusions are often present, as are hypochondriacal concerns.
g) Usually there is no disturbance in sensorium.

5. Positive and negative symptoms
The diagnosis of schizophrenic disorders under the present classification (Kraepelinian) is extremely difficult, which often means reduction in diagnostic reliability. Because of this symptomatic variability, there is continuing interest in establishing subtypes. The present system tries to distinguish between **positive** and **negative** symptoms.
a) Positive symptoms consist of excesses, such as delusions, hallucinations and bizarre behavior.
b) Negative symptoms consist of behavioral deficits (affective flattening; alogia—language deficit including poverty of speech, poverty of content of speech, lacking in long delays before responding; avolition-apathy—a lack of interest, drive, and energy manifested as inattention to grooming and hygiene, difficulty in seeking and keeping a job, and a low level of general activity; anhedonia-asociality—inability to experience pleasure and feel intimacy, together with little interest in recreational activities, sex, and social relationships (Andreasen and Olsen 1982).
c) The importance of the distinction between negative and positive symptoms is related to the role of dopamine and brain pathology and the etiology of schizophrenia and is of clinical importance in the prescription of neuroleptic medication (for example, the recent introduction of clozaril as a medication that has effects on the negative symptomatology).

## V. Types

Because of the varied clinical picture, cases are classified into different clinical types depending upon the predominant symptomatology. In *DSM*-III-R, the following phenomenological subtypes are described:

A. Catatonic type

The essential feature is marked psychomotor disturbance, which may involve stupor, negativism, rigidity, excitement, or posturing. Sometimes there is rapid alternation between the extremes of excitement and stupor (*DSM*-III-R).

1. The five different types of catatonic symptomatology described in *DSM*-III-R are
    a) Catatonic stupor or mutism
       Characterized by marked decrease in reactivity to environment, reduction of spontaneous movements and activity, or mutism
    b) Catatonic negativism
       Characterized by an apparently motiveless resistance to all instructions or attempts to be moved
    c) Catatonic rigidity
       Characterized by maintenance of a rigid posture against efforts to be moved
    d) Catatonic excitement
       Characterized by excited motor activity, apparently purposeless and not influenced by external stimuli
    e) Catatonic posturing
       Characterized by voluntary assumptions of inappropriate or bizarre posture

2. Onset and course
    The onset of catatonic schizophrenia is usually sudden, and the course is usually short.

3. Prognosis
    Good for recovery from the episode, but guarded about future recurrences.

4. Case example, catatonic stupor

> Miss J., a thirty-nine-year-old secretary, was brought to the hospital by her two sisters because her behavior had been bizarre for a week. She was described as a quiet, reserved person who had few friends and preferred to remain by herself. Although she danced occasionally, she was generally shy in the company of men. She had no symptoms of emotional illness until seven days earlier, when she suddenly began to abstain from food. Five days later she expressed religious delusions, became self-condemnatory, refused to go to bed at night, and demanded to see a priest at 3:00 A.M. A few hours later, she was admitted to a general hospital and given intravenous feedings because of her

refusal to eat. She would not remain in bed and left the hospital against advice. At home she continued to refuse food. Finally, her sisters sought her admission to the hospital.

On admission she was negativistic, refusing food, medication, and nursing care. She was mute most of the time, and when she did speak she expressed religious delusions and hallucinations. She postured, that is, assumed uncomfortable postures for long periods, and exhibited waxy flexibility, that is, her extremities would remain in positions in which they were placed.

She recovered from this episode after a course of electroconvulsive therapy and was discharged to her home at the end of one month. A few weeks later, the symptoms recurred. This second episode also responded rather promptly to treatment, and she was discharged after six weeks. She has remained well for several years.

The characteristic features in the foregoing case of catatonic stupor are the sudden onset of negativism, mutism, posturing, and waxy flexibility; the good response to treatment in both instances; and the prepsychotic schizoid personality.

5. Case example, catatonic excitement

P. H., a twenty-year-old college student, was brought to the hospital in restraints by the police. His illness had become manifest the previous day, when he began expressing delusions of grandeur and persecution. He left his fraternity house without telling anyone where he was going and remained away all night. About two hours before admission, the police were summoned to pick him up in a nearby suburb because of bizarre behavior characterized by agitation, assaultiveness, and disrobing. Before the onset of his illness he was described as conscientious, compulsive, and meek. He resisted accepting responsibility and had an "inferiority complex."

On admission he was uncooperative, mute, belligerent, agitated, and assaultive. He refused food, medications, and nursing care, and was careless of his excreta. After a series of electroconvulsive treatments, he became cooperative and calm. Treatment was continued in another hospital to which he was transferred in order to be nearer his parents.

Mutism, negativism, agitation, assaultiveness, and violent behavior characterized this case as catatonic excitement.

6. Periodic catatonic type
This is a rare form of episodic catatonia that is related to shifts in the individual's metabolic nitrogen balance. Maintenance on neuroleptic drugs prevents recurrence.

B. Disorganized type
Also called *hebephrenic,* after Hebe, the Greek goddess of youth.
1. The essential features are marked incoherence, marked loosening of associations or grossly disorganized behavior,

flat or grossly inappropriate affect, and fragmentary, unsystematized delusions or hallucinations with an incoherent theme.

2. Associated features include grimacing, mannerisms, hypochondriacal complaints, extreme social withdrawal, and other oddities of behavior.
3. It is usually associated with extreme social impairment and poor premorbid personality, insidious onset, and chronic course without significant remissions.
4. Case example

Mary, a twenty-one-year-old stenographer, was brought to the hospital by the police, who had been called after she had entered a strange residence at 1:00 A.M. in response to an uncontrollable urge to urinate. She had always been a shy, introverted, and intensely religious girl. Three years earlier, after high school graduation, she had had a "nervous breakdown" that required six months' hospitalization. She showed improvement following that treatment, but still seemed shy and self-contained, and behaved inappropriately at times.

Three days before her second admission to the hospital, she became restless and sleepless, and spent the night on her knees in continuous prayer. The following morning she seemed elated and became upset by several commonplace incidents. She started out for work, but in response to a "voice" went instead to religious services at a nearby church. The second night was likewise spent in continuous prayer. The following morning, she again started out for work but became confused and returned home. The evening preceding admission, she boarded a bus to attend church but became confused "because my friend Anne prayed that I would get mixed up," and she left the bus far from church. She wandered about aimlessly, finally entering a strange residence at 1:00 A.M.

On admission she was obviously disturbed. She was preoccupied with religious and moral ideas and said that God was talking to her through the newspapers, radio, and television. She repeatedly misidentified the ward personnel as apostles, disciples, and other biblical characters. Her affect was euphoric and inappropriate. She was physically active, making frequent changes in posture and moving about the room aimlessly. She was unkempt and continuously disrobed.

Despite a three-month stay in the hospital, during which time she received thirty electroconvulsive treatments, there was no sustained improvement in her behavior and she was committed to a state hospital for prolonged care.

In this case, note the schizoid premorbid personality, the rather definite onset of psychotic symptoms in adolescence, the obvious emotional disturbance at the time of admission, the bizarre nature of her symptoms, and her bizarre delusions and hallucinations.

C. Paranoid type
  1. The essential feature is preoccupation with one or more systematized delusions or with frequent auditory hallucinations related to a single theme.
  2. Symptoms characteristic of catatonic and disorganized types are absent.
  3. Associated features include unfocused anxiety, anger, argumentativeness, and violence. Interpersonal interactions are often stilted or extremely intense.
  4. The onset is abrupt and usually occurs in adult life, later than the other subtypes.
  5. Case example

> Mrs. L., a thirty-year-old housewife, was brought to the hospital by her family because she had behaved strangely for the preceding seven months. The behavior was characterized by withdrawal, inappropriate mood, preoccupation with religious ideas, and delusions that her husband and the family physician were "trying to poison the food." In preschool years she had been overly attached to her mother, but she subsequently became so interested in outdoor activities that she was considered a tomboy.
>
> In the hospital, she was markedly suspicious of the entire staff, accusing them of poisoning her food, talking about her, gambling, and so forth. She said she received messages from Christ, whose voice came to her over the radio. Much of the time she was withdrawn, but at times she talked readily, though inappropriately. Her affect was flattened.
>
> Following a course of electroconvulsive therapy, she improved, and returned home. Eighteen months later, the same symptoms recurred and she was readmitted to the hospital. Though the second episode was more refractory to treatment, she did improve sufficiently to return home after eight months.

D. Undifferentiated type
  The essential features are
  1. Permanent psychotic symptoms (delusions, hallucinations, incoherence, or grossly disorganized behavior) that cannot be classified as catatonic, disorganized, or paranoid, or
  2. Meets the criteria for more than one category
E. Residual type
  1. This category is for those who have at least one episode of schizophrenia. The clinical picture that occasioned the evaluation or admission to clinical care is without permanent psychotic symptoms, though signs of the illness persist.
  2. This is equivalent of the category *in partial remission*.
  3. Examples of persistent symptoms are emotional blunting, social withdrawal, eccentric behavior, and persistent but

inconspicuous delusions or hallucinations—but not accompanied by strong affect.

    4. The course is either chronic or subchronic.

## VI. Epidemiology

A. Since schizophrenia is very likely an etiologically heterogenous group of disorders, there are variations in the epidemiologic studies published.

B. Estimates of prevalence and incidence depend not only on the population studied but also on the criteria used for the diagnosis.

C. Over the past one-hundred years, many widely divergent concepts of schizophrenia have been held by different psychiatrists in different countries.

D. British figures report the annual incidence is probably seen between .1 and .5 per thousand population; lifetime risk of developing schizophrenia is reported as between 7 and 9 per thousand population; the point prevalence in European countries is probably between 2.5 and 5.3 per thousand (*Oxford Textbook of Psychiatry,* 2d ed., 1989).

E. The National Institute of Mental Health, ECA program, which reported on a survey of 18,572 persons residing in New Haven, Connecticut; Baltimore, Maryland; St. Louis, Missouri; the North Carolina Piedmont area; and greater Los Angeles, California, during the period 1980–1985, gave figure prevalence data of lifetime prevalence rates varying from .6 per thousand in Los Angeles to 1.9 per thousand in New Haven.

F. The prevalence rate is about 1 percent for most population studies.

G. The NIMH-ECA studies found that when potential confounding factors such as education are controlled, the difference in racial prevalence disappears.

H. Although schizophrenic disorders affect a small percentage of the population, patients with these disorders occupy a significant proportion of mental hospital beds.

## VII. Etiology

A. The etiology of schizophrenia is not clearly understood.

    1. Conflicting findings by different investigators lead to the belief that schizophrenia is really several different disorders.

    2. Others describe two major types: a) "process," which does not respond to treatment, has a poor prognosis, and is probably biologically determined, and b) "reactive," a remitting type that has a more favorable prognosis and is probably related to experiential factors.

B. Theories of etiology can be divided into

    1. Organic

2. Sociocultural
3. Experiential, or psychological

C. Organic considerations

There seems little doubt that biological factors play a role in the cause of schizophrenia. What factors are significant and the importance of the role remain controversial.

1. Brain structure and function

   a) The possibility that schizophrenia is an organic disorder with accompanying cerebral pathology has been a point of focus for many researchers for virtually as long as the disorder has been studied.

   b) Postmortem studies for many years did not implicate any single underlying neuropathological or neurological factor.

   c) During the years immediately following World War II, emphasis was on psychological and social factors in conceptualizations about schizophrenic disorders.

   d) In recent years a renewed interest in the possible neuropathological basis of schizophrenia has developed. There seem to be two forces fostering this:

      (1) Success of the psychopharmacological treatments that have evolved since the fifties (see 3. Biochemical predisposition and XI. Treatment of schizophrenia)

      2) Development of nuclear magnetic resonance imaging (also called MRI—magnetic resonance imaging)

   e) Brain imaging is a computer-assisted graphic representation of brain structure and function. A computer graphic uses color to represent a range of numbers in measuring the phenomenon under study. Tomographic methods of brain imaging include X-ray computed tomography (CT scan), magnetic resonance imaging (MRI), and positron emission tomography (PET). These technologies made possible the improved study of the structure and function of the brain.

   f) Concomitant with the introduction of these technologies, direct examinations of the brain have provided the development of reliable and precise diagnostic criteria, which helped overcome methodological problems in many of the earlier research studies.

   g) Thus, there seems to be increasing consensus that schizophrenia is probably a group of organic disorders. No single neuropathological or neurophysiological factor has so far been delineated (but this would be consistent with etiological heterogeneity).

2. Genetic predisposition
   a) The current psychiatric literature points to a genetically transmitted *predisposition* for schizophrenia.
   b) The major methods have included family, twin, and adoptive studies.
   c) The risk of schizophrenia in the general population is somewhat on the order of 1 percent.
   d) Family studies: Relatives of schizophrenics are at increased risk for the disorder, and the risk increases as the genetic relationship between the proband (an original case in genetic studies) and the relative becomes closer (but environmental influences cannot be completely discounted) (Gottesman, McGriffin, and Fornier 1987).
   e) Twin studies: The concordance for MZ (monozygotic, identical) twins was 44.3 percent, which is clearly greater than DZ (dizygotic, fraternal), which was 12.08 percent—but this is obviously less than 100 percent (Gottesman, McGriffin, and Fornier 1987).
   f) Adoptee studies: Heston (1966) reported a study of forty-seven people born to schizophrenic mothers in state mental hospitals, separated at birth and reared by adoptive or foster parents and compared them with fifty controls (from the foundling homes that placed the children of the schizophrenic mothers); 16.6 percent of the offspring of the schizophrenic mothers developed schizophrenia; and thirty-one of the forty-seven (66 percent) were given psychiatric diagnoses (compared to nine of the controls, equaling 18 percent), and none of the controls developed schizophrenia.
   g) Evaluation of genetic studies: All the data indicates that genetic factors play an important but not complete role in development of schizophrenia.
   h) A diathesis-stress model seems appropriate (see chapter 5). Thus, a *predisposition* is genetically determined, but a subsequent stress is required.
3. Biochemical predisposition
   a) There has been a remarkable increase in our knowledge of brain biochemistry and psychopharmacology in recent years.
   b) Biochemical abnormalities are present in many, if not all, the cases.
   c) Many findings of early biochemical investigations turned out to be related to diet or medication rather than the disorder.

d) Several hypotheses have been suggested. Most attention has been paid to those concerned with transmethylation, serotonergic transmission, and dopaminergic transmission.

   (1) Transmethylation hypothesis

Harley-Mason theorized that since many hallucinogens are methylated substances, an accumulation of methylated substances might occur in schizophrenia. Methylated indoleamine has been found in the blood and urine of schizophrenics. Recent studies indicate that methylated substances have been found in people with other mental disorders, so the specific relationship to schizophrenia seems doubtful.

   (2) Serotonergic transmission

Earlier studies suggested that serotonergic transmission might be reduced in schizophrenia. Subsequent brain studies have not revealed any consistent abnormality of serotonin.

   (3) Dopamine hypothesis

     (a) Schizophrenia is assumed to reflect a defect in dopamine-mediated brain systems, particularly mesolimbic and mesocontical systems.

     (b) Amphetamines, which stimulate release of catecholamines, can also produce psychotic symptoms that resemble schizophrenia and exacerbate psychotic symptoms of acute schizophrenia.

     (c) The class of antipsychotics (phenothiazines) most effective in treating schizophrenic symptoms acts to inhibit or block dopamine-mediated transmissions. (Although altered levels of dopamine are not considered a "cause" of schizophrenia, they do seem to be implicated in the manifestation of symptoms. Also, such drugs are equally effective in reducing psychotic symptoms and other types of psychosis.)

     (d) The advent of clozapine and other "atypical" antipsychotic drugs has limited the generality of the original dopamine hypothesis by raising questions about the types and specificity of dopamine receptors involved in symptom reduction and by implicating neurotransmission systems (e.g., serotonin, glutamate) in their effects.

4. Neurodevelopmental factors
   a) Many investigators have noted the frequency with which prenatal and perinatal developmental adverse events occur in the histories of schizophrenic patients.
   b) Some of these events can cause hypoxic ischemic damage to the ventricles and surrounding tissue, which is associated with later ventricular enlargement.
   c) Some researchers currently suggest that prenatal and perinatal events that affect neural development may interact with predisposing genetic factors or by themselves may contribute to the latent expression of schizophrenia.
D. Sociocultural theories
   1. There is a high density of schizophrenics in urban ghettos and other underprivileged areas of the city. This finding has led to two contradictory theories.
      a) The "downward-drift" theory states that schizophrenics drift to such areas because they are socially and economically incompetent.
      b) These areas "breed" schizophrenics because they are populated by people laden with severe socioeconomic problems. In other words, the schizophrenic has never experienced achievement.
      c) It seems more likely that people who are developing schizophrenia tend to move into areas that provide solitary and unsatisfactory accommodations.
   2. Many studies confirm the association of schizophrenia and lower socioeconomic class. Social and economic limitations prevent the achievement of fundamental gratification, thus poverty and crowding may be factors that produce greater stress and reduce flexibility in the choice of personal response to stress.
   3. There is a higher incidence of broken homes in the lower socioeconomic areas.
E. Psychodynamic theories
   These theories assume that psychopathology is functional—that is, that symptom formation can be explained in part, or entirely, by psychology rather than by physiology or organic factors. These theories originated from psychoanalytic or psychodynamically oriented psychotherapy. Among those who have proffered psychodynamic theories are the following:
   1. Sigmund Freud emphasized the role of sexual regression in the development of this disorder.
   2. Melanie Klein emphasized the importance of early mother-child relationships (British object relations school).

3. Harry Stack Sullivan emphasized the patient's deeply disturbed interpersonal relationships, rather than the intrapsychic mechanisms emphasized by Freud and Klein (the interpersonal school).
4. Margaret Mahler related schizophrenia to her autistical phase of development (development school).
5. Gregory Bateson suggested that repeated exposure to double-bind experiences makes the potential schizophrenic perceive the entire environment as a double bind.
6. Please refer to chapter 2, Psychodynamic Foundations, for additional elaboration of these views.

## VIII. Psychopathology

A. Most psychiatrists regard schizophrenic disorder as regression (see the Freudian concept discussed earlier and the section on regression in chapter 6).
1. There is withdrawal of interest from the environment and loss of interest in objects and other persons.
2. According to psychoanalytic theory, this is regression to a level at which schizophrenics, like infants, are incapable of distinguishing themselves from the environment (i.e., regression to primary narcissism).
B. Those having paranoid delusions are also overusing the mechanism of projection (see chapter 6).
C. The prepsychotic personality is often schizoid (introverted), schizotypal, or borderline.
D. Precipitating factors may or may not be evident, and their effect varies with the individual's vulnerability. They are evident in the so-called reactive types of schizophrenia.
E. The onset may be gradual, occurring in the absence of obvious precipitating factors, as in so-called process schizophrenia.

## IX. Cultural influences

A. Records suggest that the incidence of schizophrenia in this country has probably remained essentially unchanged during the past century, perhaps even longer.
B. Cultural factors, however, have had an influence on the relative frequency and character of schizophrenic *symptoms*.
C. Prior to the publication of *DSM*-III-R, there had been a classification of simple schizophrenia. Such cases are probably now classified as schizoid personality or schizotypal personality.
D. Catatonic forms of schizophrenia seem less frequent.
E. Schizophrenics are less aggressive than they were a quarter of a century ago, perhaps in part because of the early prescription of antipsychotic medications that reduce assaultive and antisocial behavior.

F. Although paranoid reactions have increased, delusions of grandeur, witchcraft, and other magic have become less frequent, whereas ideas of being hypnotized or influenced by electronics or radiation have increased.

G. The content of delusions has become more realistic and plausible.

## X. Course and prognosis

A. Schizophrenia was once regarded as a progressive disorder with a poor or hopeless prognosis.

B. As can be noted from the *DSM*-III-R classification, episodic types of the disorder are now recognized. These are many times followed by symptom-free periods, long periods of remission. Occasionally, individuals have been observed to have a single, mild schizophrenic (or schizophrenic-like) attack, without any recurrence.

C. As noted earlier, schizophrenic disorders can occur either in attacks or as a progressive disease; thus, we speak of "reactive" and "process" schizophrenic disorder.

D. Schizophrenic patients do much less well than patients with mood disorder; thus, schizophrenia must be regarded as a tenacious disorder.

E. Currently, there is more optimism about arrest and recovery in this illness, chiefly because of the favorable effect of psychotropic drugs.

F. In general, however, the prognosis is guarded.

G. Certain criteria have become more or less accepted for prognosticating the outcome of any case of schizophrenic disorder.

1. The following are considered favorable prognostic signs:
   a) Sudden or acute onset
   b) Conspicuous precipitating factors
   c) Catatonic symptoms
   d) The presence of affective symptoms, that is, depression or elation; perhaps these cases are more properly classified as schizoaffective disorders in the present nomenclature
   e) The presence of confusion
   f) History of a good previous social adjustment
   g) Married schizophrenics have a better outlook than single, divorced, or widowed ones
   h) Stable employment (the schizophrenic has a job to which to return)
   i) Cooperativeness (the patient cooperates with the treatment regime)
   j) An empathic therapist
   k) Positive symptoms
   l) Good support system

2. The following are considered unfavorable prognostic signs:
   a) History of previous episodes
   b) Schizoid or schizotypal personality
   c) Absence of conspicuous precipitating factors
   d) Family history of mental illness
   e) Persistence of the symptoms for more than one year
   f) The presence of sustained emotional withdrawal, aloofness, and shallow or inappropriate affect, which makes the patient less cooperative about taking maintenance medication
   g) Onset in childhood or early puberty (recovery is unlikely)
   h) Negative symptoms
   i) Numerous relapses

## XI. Treatment of schizophrenia

A. Since schizophrenia is probably a heterogenous group of disorders and etiology is incompletely understood, the treatment has been largely empirical. Presently, there is no known cure for the disorder.

B. The type of treatment depends upon the type and severity of the disorder. It can be divided into
   1. Milieu therapy
   2. Various psychotherapies (psychoanalytic, supportive, and behavioral)
   3. Somatic (electroconvulsive therapy)
   4. Psychopharmacology (chemotherapy with antipsychotic drugs)

C. Milieu therapy
   The exact plan varies according to the individual needs of the patient. Included are:
   1. Various inpatient hospital programs
      In a token economy utilizing the principles of operant conditioning, developed by B. F. Skinner, a system of rewards and punishment can increase or decrease the frequency of specific human behaviors and specified contexts. These programs are usually most effective in inpatient or halfway house settings where therapeutic staff can control the rewards and punishment. It is helpful to pair the earning of tokens with social reinforcement (for example, praise and affection).
   2. Various outpatient arrangements, individually arranged. These include:
      a) Various living arrangements, such as halfway houses, apartments, board-and-care facilities, foster homes, and family care.

      b) Vocational arrangements, such as sheltered workshops, day activity centers, and vocational rehabilitation placements.

      c) Social skills training: This training is usually performed with groups of patients and tends to teach social behaviors such as listening skills, assertiveness, conversation, and so on.

   3. Behavioral family therapy

      Unlike other family therapy, this context does not assume that the schizophrenia is caused by family deviance. Rather the orientation is to assume that the family members do have impact on the course of the illness and to help the family reduce stresses in the patient's life. There are three components to this: education, communication, and problem solving.

D. Psychotherapeutic treatment

   1. Psychoanalytic psychotherapy (see chapter 9).

   2. In general, therapists should be active and positive in their approach.

   3. Establishing a relationship may be difficult because of the schizophrenic's distrust and inability to become close.

   4. The patient's ability and willingness to collaborate in treatment often is largely determined by the bond that forms in the doctor-patient relationship.

   5. Behavioral therapy is mostly based on the operant conditioning principles of B. F. Skinner. This type of treatment has almost always been used in conjunction with the use of antipsychotic medications.

   6. Supportive therapy

E. Somatic therapy (electroconvulsive therapy)

   Its status is uncertain, although it has been successfully used in two types of cases: those that have not responded to drugs, and acute attacks.

F. Psychosurgery is a rare form of treatment (see chapter 10).

G. Megavitamin therapy

   This treatment involves the administration of large doses of niacin. Major controlled studies indicate that niacin is no better than a placebo.

H. Psychopharmacology (chemotherapy, antipsychotic agents)

   1. Antipsychotic agents: There are a large number of these including:

      a) Phenothiazines

         (1) Chlorpromazine (Thorazine)

         (2) Mesoridazine besylate (Serentil)

         (3) Thioridazine HCL (Mellaril)

        (4) Fluphenazine hydrochloride (Prolixin and Permitil)

        (5) Perphenazine (Trilafon)

        (6) Trifluoperazine hydrochloride (Stelazine)

    b) Thioxanthenes

        (1) Thiothixene (Navane)

        (2) Chlorprothixene (Taractan)

    c) Butyrophenones

        (1) Haloperidol (Haldol)

    d) Dibenzazepines

        (1) Loxapine succinate (Loxitane, Daxolin)

        (2) Clozapine (Clozaril) was recently released in the United States and is marketed as a drug that has proved helpful in schizophrenics who have responded poorly to other antipsychotic medications. It favorably influences negative symptoms. It can cause agranulocytosis, and hence white blood cell counts must be checked frequently.

    e) Indolones

        (1) Molindone HCl (Moban, Lidone)

        This antipsychotic has the unique property of being effective without associated weight gain but with weight reduction.

2. Intramuscular injections of long-acting phenothiazines (such as Prolixin Decanoate) or butyrophenones (Haldol Decanoate) may be necessary until the patient becomes cooperative. Or it may be necessary in those patients who find it easier to receive an injection once every two to four weeks rather than to take oral or injected medications daily.

3. Lithium carbonate. Although lithium has been primarily indicated in elations and sometimes depressions, it has sometimes been used in schizophrenia and occasionally patients have responded to it, perhaps because they had affective symptoms combined with the thought disorders.

4. It should be kept in mind, however, that a large percentage (two-thirds or more) of schizophrenics do not comply with the drug regime after discharge.

5. Maintenance therapy may be necessary.

    a) In many cases, drugs can eventually be discontinued.

    b) However, a significant number of patients relapse when antipsychotic agents are withdrawn.

I. Combined psychotherapy and drug therapy

Antipsychotic drugs plus ''the therapeutic alliance'' seem helpful to most schizophrenics.

J. The most effective treatment program is usually one combining psychotropic, psychotherapeutic, and milieu therapy.

K. Results of treatment
1. About one-third of the patients will do relatively well.
2. One-third will become severe and persistent.
3. The remainder will occupy an intermediate status.

## References

American Psychiatric Association. *Diagnostic and Statistical Manual of Mental Disorders*. 3d ed., rev. Washington, D.C.: APA, 1987.

Andreasen, N. C., and S. A. Olsen. "Negative Versus Positive Schizophrenia Definition and Validation." *Archives of General Psychiatry* 39 (1982): 789–94.

Arieti, S. *Interpretation of Schizophrenia*. New York: Basic Books, 1975.

Bleuler, E. *Dementia Praecox or the Group of Schizophrenias*. New York: International Universities Press, 1950.

Davison, G. C., and J. M. Neale. "Schizophrenia." Chap. 14 in *Abnormal Psychology*. 5th ed. New York: Wiley, 1990.

Gelder, N., D. Gath, and R. R. Mayou. *Oxford Textbook of Psychiatry*. 2d ed. Oxford: Oxford Medical Publications, 1989.

Goldman, H. H. *Review of General Psychiatry*. Los Altos, Calif.: Lange Medical Publications, 1988.

Goodwin, D. W., and S. V. Guze. *Psychiatric Diagnosis*. 2d ed. New York: Oxford University Press, 1979.

Gottesman, I. I., P. McGriffin, and A. E. Fornier. "Clinical Genetics as Clues to 'Real' Genetics of Schizophrenia." *Schizophrenia Bulletin* 13 (1987): 23–47.

Heston, L. L. "Psychiatric Disorders in Foster Home Reared Children of Schizophrenic Mothers." *British Journal of Psychiatry* 112 (1966): 819–825.

Kaplan, H. I., and B. J. Sadock, eds. *Comprehensive Textbook of Psychiatry/V*. 5th ed. Baltimore: Williams & Wilkins, 1989.

Nicholi, A. M., Jr., ed. *The New Harvard Guide to Modern Psychiatry*. Cambridge, Mass.: Belknap Press, 1988.

Richelson, E. "Psychopharmacology of Schizophrenia: Past, Present, and Future." *Psychiatric Annals* 20, no. 11 (November 1990): 640.

# 25 Delusional (Paranoid) Disorders

What is madness: To have erroneous perceptions and to reason correctly from them.

Voltaire, "Madness," in *Philosophical Dictionary* (1764)

## I. Introduction
A. Virtually throughout psychiatric history, the term *paranoia* or *paranoid disorder* was used to describe a psychotic disorder with prominent delusions as the only manifestation of the illness. Otherwise, the personality of the individual was intact, and he or she clung tenaciously to the fixed false set of beliefs.
B. Karl Kahlbaum used the term *paranoia* to describe a chronic delusional deterioration of the belief system but spared the intellect. The delusions were persecutory and grandiose.
C. Emil Kraepelin emphasized an insidious onset and chronic course in agreement with Kahlbaum. He distinguished paranoia from dementia praecox (schizophrenia). He emphasized the chronic, unremitting nature of paranoia and its lack of other features such as hallucinations common in schizophrenia.
D. This category was labeled paranoid disorder in *DSM*-III, but since in this disorder delusions are the primary symptoms and the term *paranoid* has multiple other meanings, the term *delusional disorder* was used in *DSM*-III-R.

## II. Definition
A. The essential feature of this disorder is the presence of a persistent, nonbizarre delusion that is not due to any other mental disorder, such as schizophrenia, schizophreniform disorder, or a mood disorder.
B. Organic factor as an etiological determinant must also be excluded (drug intoxication, delirium) (*DSM*-III-R).
C. Apart from the delusion or its ramifications, there is no obvious or odd behavior.

## III. Types
A. Common delusional themes are
   1. Erotomanic

The central theme is an erotic delusion that one is loved by another, usually of a higher status, such as a famous person or a superior at work. It usually concerns idealized romantic love and spiritual union rather than sexual attraction. Efforts to contact the object of the delusion, through telephone calls, letters, gifts, visits, and so forth, are common.

2. Grandiose

These delusions center on the person's conviction that he or she possesses great unrecognized talent or insight or has made some important discovery. They seem to represent a regression to an earlier phase of development in which children regard themselves as omnipotent. An example is Cervantes's *Don Quixote,* who roamed the world righting wrongs and tilting windmills—his combat against the villainous foe. Grandiose delusions may have a religious content, and sometimes people with this delusion can become leaders of religious cults.

3. Jealous

The jealousy is usually more persistent and profound than normal jealousy. There is usually some grain of truth in the pathological jealousy, but the constructs on which it rests are based on inadequate evidence. The delusionally jealous person may find bits of "evidence" to substantiate his or her delusion. Shakespeare's Othello becomes furiously jealous of his innocent wife, Desdemona, and his loyal lieutenant, Michael Cassio, and executes Desdemona with his own hands. When he learns of her innocence, he judges and executes himself.

4. Persecutory

This is the most common type. The paranoid person feels conspired against, cheated, spied upon, followed, poisoned or drugged, maliciously maligned, harassed, or obstructed in the pursuit of long-term goals (*DSM*-III-R). Sometimes the focus of the delusion is some injustice that must be corrected (querulous paranoia).

5. Somatic

Such delusions can take one of several forms: most common ones involve beliefs that the person emits a foul odor from his or her skin, mouth, rectum, or vagina; there's an infestation of insects on his or her skin; he or she has an internal parasite; certain parts of the body are misshapen or ugly; or certain parts of the body are not functioning.

6. Litigious

This is not listed in *DSM*-III-R as a type of delusional disorder. Such people's delusions produce disputatiousness,

contentiousness, fondness for litigation, or proneness to engage in lawsuits.
   7. Unspecified types
      This is a delusional order that does not fit into any of the previous categories—for example, persecutory and grandiose themes without a predominance of either.
   B. Delusions in such disorders usually involve a single theme or a series of connected themes. Aside from the delusional system, there are no signs of mental disorder in the paranoid person. There is no withdrawal or regression (as in the schizophrenic disorders), or any affective changes (as in affective disorders or schizoaffective disorders).
IV. **Prevalence**
   A. Delusional disorders are relatively uncommon (.03 percent of the population).
   B. Immigration, emigration, deafness, and other severe stresses may predispose to this disorder.
V. **Psychopathological factors**
   A. The cause is unknown, but there have been a number of theories, most of which emphasize a psychological (experiential) and possible psychoanalytical theory.
   B. There is overuse of denial and projection as defenses against underlying conflicts, feelings of insecurity, repudiated impulses, and other conflictual factors.
   C. In the grandiose type, there is also overuse of rationalization. The behavior may be a response to a need to improve self-esteem or to enhance prestige.
   D. Paranoid, schizoid, or avoidant personality may be more likely to develop this disorder.
   E. The individual may form a projective defense structure (the paranoid system) in response to conscious and unconscious perceptions of him- or herself as weak and inadequate ("power anxiety," according to Ovesey and others).
   F. In the shame-humiliation theory, the individual develops a series of defenses eschewing underlying shame and assigning blame to others for any underlying failure (Colby).
   G. According to psychobiological theory, delusions are the consequence of anomalous perceptual experience—that is, within the central nervous system, the sensory apparatus, or the environment.
   H. Sex ratio
      Delusional disorders are apparently somewhat more common in females, with the exception that in forensic cases, most are males.

## VI. Course and prognosis

The published studies suggest about half the cases experience a remission, while the other half show chronic relapsing patterns (Nicholi 1988).

## VII. Treatment

A. Treatment of patients in this category would be similar to management of people with paranoid delusions in other diagnostic groups.

B. Denial, projection, and distortion are commonly employed defenses.

C. Most of these people make at least marginal adjustments outside of the hospital and, hence, treatment attempts would focus on treatment within the community (it may be of assistance in helping the patient improve the relationship with his or her family and relatives).

D. The therapist who can accept the delusional person and, at the same time, clearly indicate nonagreement with the delusional system may be of value in a supportive way to the patient. The therapist who is not skilled in dealing with such an individual may run the risk of becoming a part of the patient's delusional system.

E. Various neuroleptic drugs, especially the phenothiazines, butyrophenones, thioxanthenes, and pimozide, may be of some help in modifying patients' delusional preoccupations or assisting them to adapt more comfortably.

F. Sometimes management of such disorders is determined more by the needs of society than by the needs of individual patients.

G. Few patients eventually require institutionalization.

## References

American Psychiatric Association. *Diagnostic and Statistical Manual of Mental Disorders.* 3d ed., rev. Washington, D.C.: APA, 1987.

Goldman, H. H., ed. *Review of General Psychiatry.* 2d ed. Norwalk, Conn.: Appleton & Lange, 1988.

Kaplan, H. I., and B. J. Sadock, eds. *Comprehensive Textbook of Psychiatry V.* 5th ed. Baltimore: Williams & Wilkins, 1989.

Nicholi, A. M., Jr., ed. *The New Harvard Guide to Modern Psychiatry.* Cambridge: Mass.: Belknap Press, 1988.

# 26  Psychotic Disorders Not Elsewhere Classified

There is no great genius without some touch of madness.

Seneca, *Moral Essays* (8 B.C.–A.D. 65)

I. **Introduction**

This class is for disorders that cannot be classified as organic mental disorder, schizophrenia, delusional disorder, or mood disorder with psychotic features. Generally, this chapter reflects the current status of knowledge about these disorders.

II. **Brief reactive psychosis (*DSM*-III-R)**

A. The essential feature is sudden onset of psychotic symptoms of at least a few hours, but no more than one month's duration, with eventual return to premorbid level of functioning.

B. The psychotic symptoms (which may be of various types, such as delusions, hallucinations, loose or disconnected verbalization, common disorganized behavior) appear shortly after one or more events that singly or together would be markedly stressful to almost anyone in similar circumstances. Precipitating events may be any major stress, such as the loss of a loved one or the psychological trauma of combat (e.g., three–day schizophrenia of World War II).

C. Invariably there is emotional turmoil.

D. Behavior may be bizarre; there is often suicidal or aggressive behavior; affect is often inappropriate.

E. Age at onset
Usually begins in adolescence or early adulthood.

F. Incidence and sex distribution are unknown.

G. Predisposing factors
Preexisting psychopathology may predispose to the development of this disorder; individuals with paranoid, histrionic, narcissistic, schizotypal, or borderline personality disorder are thought to be vulnerable to the development of this disorder.

H. Etiology

Considered to be mainly psychological in origin (symptoms may emerge when psychological defenses collapse). For some, only chaotic events such as natural disaster or combat would cause this, whereas others might be overwhelmed by lesser stresses such as physical illness or divorce. Others with certain kinds of character defects might be unable to cope with disappointments that other people would be able to handle.

I. Prognosis

Usually remits

J. Treatment

1. Medication

The general principles of treatment are conservative and individualized. Antipsychotic medicines such as phenothiazines, butyrophenones, and thioxanthenes—or even benzodiazepines for agitation and anxiety.

2. Psychological treatment: including removal from the crisis area; oftentimes the care and attention of the professional staff is enough to be reassuring to the patient.

III. Schizophreniform disorder (*DSM*-III-R)

A. This term was coined by Gabrial Langfeldt in 1939 to describe a disorder that was typical of schizophrenia but did not have the chronic course.

B. In *DSM*-III-R the essential features are identical with those of schizophrenia, with the exception that the duration, including prodromal, active, and residual phases, is less than six months.

C. It is classified outside the category of schizophrenia because the evidence linking schizophreniform disorder to typical schizophrenia remains unclear. There is consistent evidence that people with symptoms of less than six months' duration have a better outcome than those with a more prolonged disturbance.

D. The diagnosis is made under two conditions: 1. an episode of illness of less than six months' duration from which the person has already recovered, and 2. a person who is symptomatic but has been this way for less than six months (qualified as "provisional").

E. Prognosis

In the long term, half will improve or recover (a higher rate than for schizophrenic disorder).

F. Prevalence

Not known (probably less common than schizophrenic disorder).

G. Etiology

The cause is unknown. Some have considered them as atypical affective disorders; some others, however, see them as related more to schizophrenic disorders. Up to 20 percent of patients with this disorder also have unusually large cerebral ventricles—a finding commonly found in schizophrenic disorders.

H. Treatment
1. Somatic treatments rather than psychological treatments are usually employed (this includes neuroleptic medications such as phenothiazines, butyrophenones, thioxanthenes, etc., during the acute phase and also lithium, often in combination with these neuroleptics). Electroconvulsive therapy might possibly be used in the event that there was no response to the psychotropic medications. Prolonged depressive symptoms often follow the clearing of the psychotic elements, and the possibility of suicide must be considered.
2. General measures
Individual psychiatric management of the patient varies from case to case. The patient can be reassured throughout the symptomatic period that his or her disorder will be of limited duration (without residual deficit).

IV. **Schizoaffective disorder (*DSM*-III-R)**
A. This diagnosis has been used in many different ways since it was first introduced.
B. The term was first introduced in 1933 by Jacob S. Kasanin.
C. The approach taken in *DSM*-III-R emphasizes the temporal relationship of schizophrenic and mood symptoms.
D. In the past this has been called atypical schizophrenia, good prognosis schizophrenia.
E. The description of schizoaffective disorder appears to have tentative validity from prognostic treatment and family studies as delimiting an entity that appears to be distinct from mood disorder.
F. Prevalence
Unknown
G. Etiology
Probably not all cases are from a single cause.
H. Course
Some suggest that there is a tendency toward a chronic course but with a prognosis somewhat better than for schizophrenic disorder, but not as good as the prognosis for mood disorder.
I. Treatment
As in schizophrenic disorder, affective disorder, or schizophreniform disorder, treatment is basically empirical and uses neuroleptics alone or with antidepressant medications as well as benzodiazepines (for dramatic or agitated symptoms), or carbamazepine which is sometimes effective, or calcium channel blockers for episodes that do not respond to lithium and/or neuroleptics.

## V. Induced psychotic disorder

A. Definition

The essential feature of this disorder is a delusional system that develops in a second person as a result of a close relationship with another person who already has a psychotic disorder with prominent delusions. The delusions are at least partly shared. Usually, if the relationship with the primary person is interrupted, the delusional beliefs in the second person diminish or disappear (delusions may spread to others as well, but usually only to people in close, intimate relationship).

B. Previously known as shared paranoid disorder, *folie à deux,* or communicated psychosis. It was also sometimes called double insanity or psychosis of association.

C. The delusions are usually persecutory or hypochondriacal, and in some the *perceived* hostility of the world as viewed by those with the delusions.

D. Gralnick, who reviewed the English literature and reported on 103 cases in 1942, defined it as a "psychiatric entity characterized by the transference of delusional ideas or abnormal behavior from one person to one or more others who have been in close association with the primarily affected patient."

E. This is a rare condition, first described in 1877 by Ernest Lasègue and Jean-Pierre Falret.

F. Psychopathology

1. A. A. Brill described the essential psychological process as unconscious identification.

a) There is a communication of delusional ideas from one person to another (both of whom have been closely associated for a long period of time).

b) It frequently involves a parent and child, husband and wife, or two sisters.

c) The identification is a mutual phenomenon.

d) Nothing is ever accepted by the secondary partner that is ego-alien. That is, the delusional material from the primary partner must resemble the unconscious fantasies and fit the defense mechanisms of the secondary partner.

e) The identification in *folie à deux* may be more akin to identification with the aggressor. As this was described by Anna Freud, identification with the aggressor is a defensive maneuver that protects the ego against real or feared aggression by allowing the individual to share in the power of the feared one.

2. The interdependence of the two partners is extreme; the identification is carried out in order to avoid a separation, which would be unendurable.
3. Heredity may be a predisposing factor.
4. Both persons usually have a long history of poor adjustment.
5. There is close physical association between the two, who have usually lived in relative isolation and often in poverty.
6. The dominant partner is usually brighter.
7. In the prepsychotic relationship, the dominant partner is strongly dependent on the secondary partner and has few outside sources of gratification.
8. The dominant (primary) partner in the relationship is usually the one who has the primary psychotic disorder. The recipient (the secondary partner) of the induced delusions is often submissive, seclusive, and suspicious (i.e., schizoid), but develops these symptoms secondarily.
9. Since the disorder is usually characterized by delusions, the mechanism of projection is also operating. Because the primary partner is afraid of giving up the relationship, emerging hostility toward the secondary partner cannot be expressed directly. The defense used is the projection of the hostility onto an outsider in the form of paranoid delusions. The result is a paranoid psychosis.

G. Treatment
1. Separation of the two involved individuals.
2. Primary treatment directed at the dominant person (primary partner), who has the primary psychotic symptoms. Treatment modalities should be those recommended for the patient's particular paranoid condition, and may include psychotherapy, neuroleptics, hospitalization, and even electroconvulsive therapy.
3. The disorder of the recipient (secondary partner) may clear up without formal treatment, following separation from the primary psychotic partner.

H. Case example

A. T., a sixty-one-year-old single man, and V. T., his fifty-seven-year-old single sister with whom he had lived for many years, were referred to the court's psychiatric consultant for evaluation after they had both been found guilty of violation of the city fire ordinance on a number of occasions. Their offense consisted of hoarding a number of combustible items and trash in their home and on their premises. Neighbors complained, and the fire-prevention bureau, after repeatedly warning them about the combustible nature of the rubbish and other materials, filed a complaint.

The man, upon examination, showed flattened affect and was silly and inappropriate. He showed signs of schizoid behavior, including introversion, lack of verbal spontaneity and blocking, and was overly sensitive and suspicious. The schizoid and paranoid elements in his personality also became evident in the presentence study, where it was learned that he tended to place much of the blame for the collection of rubbish on his sister. His Minnesota Multiphasic Personality Inventory profile was clearly psychotic, showing elevations of the scales on the right-hand side.

The sister, at the time of the examination, seemed very frightened and kept asking if her brother could be present during the interview so he could "support me." She seemed preoccupied with her fantasy, but denied that she had hallucinations or delusions. She was evasive and defensive and had a number of "reasons" for hoarding trash in their home. From her description, she and her brother would collect a number of items and then spend much time going over them to try sorting out things that might have some value. Whenever she was questioned in detail about what valuable items might be in the trash or why the trash continued to accumulate, she would say, "You are trying to upset me."

Our conclusion was that the brother was the one primarily ill, that he had a paranoid, schizophrenic reaction, and that his sister had the same psychotic illness but, because she was the passive, submissive, suggestible one, she had developed it secondarily, through induction.

## VI. Psychotic disorder not otherwise specified
### A. Definition
*DSM*-III-R lists this classification to include disorders in which there are psychotic symptoms, such as delusions, hallucinations, incoherence, marked loosening of association, catatonic excitement or stupor, or grossly disorganized behavior (that do not meet the criteria for any other nonorganic psychotic disorder).
### B. Example
A postpartum disorder or psychosis that did not meet the criteria for other psychosis listed in *DSM*-III-R; a psychotic episode that met criteria for the diagnosis of schizophrenic disorder but occurred initially after the age of forty-five.

# References

American Psychiatric Association. *Diagnostic and Statistical Manual of Mental Disorders*. 3d ed., rev. Washington, D.C.: APA, 1987.

Goldman, H. H., ed. *Review of General Psychiatry*. 2d ed. Norwalk, Conn.: Appleton & Lange, 1988.

Gralnick, A. "*Folie à Deux*: The Psychosis of Association." *Psychiatric Quarterly* 16 (1942): 230.

Kaplan, H. I., and B. J. Sadock, eds. *Comprehensive Textbook of Psychiatry/V*. 5th ed. Baltimore: Williams & Wilkins, 1989.

# 27 Organic Mental Syndromes and Disorders

Now the time has fled—the world is strange,
Something there is of pain and change;
My books lie closed upon the shelf;
I miss the old heart in myself.

**A student: Adelaide Proctor (nineteenth century)**

## I. Definition
*DSM*-III-R makes a distinction between organic mental syndromes and organic mental disorders.
  - A. *Organic mental syndrome* refers to a constellation of psychological or behavioral signs and symptoms without reference to etiology (e.g., organic anxiety syndrome, dementia).
  - B. *Organic mental disorder* designates a particular organic mental syndrome in which the etiology is known or presumed (e.g., alcohol withdrawal delirium, multi-infarct dementia).

    In the *DSM*-III-R classification the term *disorder* is used when an organic mental syndrome is associated with an Axis III physical disorder or condition, as in organic delusional disorder due to a brain tumor.
  - C. The essential feature of all these disorders is a psychological or behavioral abnormality associated with transient or permanent dysfunction of the brain.
  - D. Organic mental disorders are distinguished from functional mental disorders, such as mood disorders and schizophrenic disorders, in that they have known biologic causes and pathophysiologic mechanisms, whereas functional disorders do not.

## II. Characteristics
  - A. Organic mental disorders are a heterogeneous group; therefore, no single description can characterize them all. The differences in clinical presentation reflect differences in the localization, mode of onset, progression, duration, and nature of the underlying pathophysiologic process.

B. The fundamental process is the (presumed) destruction or damage of neurons (nerve cells).

C. It is this damage, rather than the quality of the destructive process, that is responsible for the typical clinical picture.

D. Although physical damage to the brain is necessary for the production of organic mental disorders, the degree of organic insult, and the rate at which cerebral involvement occurs, strictly speaking, the cerebral damage does not fully account for the occurrence of abnormal behavior. Psychological and sociocultural factors also play a role.

1. Psychological factors
   These include: a) intelligence and education; b) previous personality; c) the manner in which the person previously coped with environmental stresses and internal conflicts; d) the manner of dealing with the organic deficit, which is determined by the person's adjustive patterns and coping mechanisms; and e) current conflicts and psychological stresses.

2. Sociocultural factors
   These include: a) the demands of the environment; b) the psychosocial setting in which the illness develops; c) the person's cultural background; d) the degree of social isolation versus support; and e) the excessiveness or insufficiency of sensory impact.

E. The reactions in organic mental disorders might be regarded as being released by the brain damage and superimposed upon it.

F. The most common organic mental syndromes are delirium, dementia, intoxication, and withdrawal.

III. **Symptomatology**

A. There is usually some evidence of an organic factor from the history, physical, neurological, or laboratory examinations. For example, cerebral concussion or contusion in patients with skull fractures; paralysis, paresis, reflex or sensory changes in patients with brain tumors; urinary or blood chemistry changes in people who have had heavy metal poisoning; spinal fluid changes in patients with deliria caused by infectious illnesses; evidence of cerebral atrophy on computerized cranial tomography (CT scan) in patients with degenerative diseases such as Alzheimer's, Pick's, or senile dementia; history of excessive alcoholic intake in persons with dementia associated with chronic alcoholism; history of exposure to some industrial toxin in a person with toxic delirium.

B. Common signs and symptoms of organic mental disorders. Certain signs and symptoms suggest organicity:

1. Memory impairment

2. Disorientation
3. Cognitive impairment (for example, reduced fund of information or dyscalculia—inability to perform arithmetic operations)
4. Visual hallucinations or illusions
5. Formication (subjective sensation of insects creeping in or under the skin)
6. Floccillation (aimless picking or plucking—usually at nightclothes or bed covers)
7. Fluctuating performance on serial mental status examinations
8. Presence of (or history of) prior physical illness or physical symptoms
9. History of recent medication or drug intake
10. Autonomic symptoms (such as fever, sweating, tachycardia, hypertension)
11. Sudden onset of symptoms without any history of previous psychiatric illness
12. Lack of response to traditional treatment
   (All of the preceding are suggestive of organically caused mental disorder but may at times be present in functional disorders.)
C. The symptomatology associated with the various organic mental syndromes (modified from *DSM*-III-R)
   1. Delirium (acute brain syndrome)
      All the symptoms listed next develop over a short period of time, fluctuate rapidly, and are evidenced by physical, neurological, or laboratory examinations, or by a history of specific organic factors.
      a) Reduced ability to maintain attention to external stimuli
      b) Disorganized thinking, as indicated by rambling, irrelevant, or incoherent speech
      c) At least two of the following:
         (1) Reduced level of consciousness (e.g., difficulty keeping awake during examination)
         (2) Perceptual disturbances: misinterpretations, illusions, or hallucinations
         (3) Disturbances of sleep-wake cycle with insomnia or daytime sleepiness
         (4) Increased or decreased psychomotor activity
         (5) Disorientation to time, place, or person
         (6) Memory impairment
   2. Dementia (may be reversible, e.g., normotensive hydrocephalus)

a) Demonstrable evidence of impairment in short- and long-term memory
b) At least one of the following:
   (1) Impairment in abstract thinking, as indicated by inability to find similarities and differences between related words and concepts, and other similar tasks
   (2) Impaired judgment, as indicated by inability to make reasonable plans to deal with interpersonal, family, and job-related problems and issues
   (3) Other disturbances of higher cortical function, such as aphasia (disorder of language), apraxia (inability to carry out motor activities despite intact comprehension and motor function), agnosia (failure to recognize or identify objects despite intact sensory function), and "constructional difficulty" (e.g., inability to copy three-dimensional figures, assemble blocks, or arrange sticks in specific designs)
   (4) Personality change, that is, alteration or accentuation of premorbid traits
c) The disturbance in *a* and *b* significantly interferes with work or usual social activities or relationships with others.
d) Not occurring exclusively during the course of delirium
e) Either (1) or (2):
   (1) There is evidence from the history, physical examination, or laboratory tests of a specific organic factor (or factors) judged to be etiologically related to the disturbance.
   (2) In the absence of such evidence, an etiologic organic factor can be presumed if the disturbance cannot be accounted for by any nonorganic mental disorder (e.g., major depression accounting for cognitive impairment).

3. Amnestic syndrome
   a) Demonstrable evidence of impairment in both short- and long-term memory disturbance, in the absence of dementia or delirium.
   b) Not occurring exclusively during the course of delirium, and does not meet the criteria for dementia (i.e., no impairment in abstract thinking or judgment, no other disturbances of higher cortical function, and no personality change).
   c) There is evidence from the history, physical examination, or laboratory tests of a specific organic factor (or factors) judged to be etiologically related to the disturbance.

4. Organic delusional syndrome (delusions predominate)
   a) Prominent delusions
   b) Evidence from physical examination, laboratory tests, or history of a specific organic factor
5. Organic hallucinosis (hallucinations predominate)
   a) Persistent or recurrent hallucinations in a state of full wakefulness and alertness.
   b) There is evidence from the history, physical examination, or laboratory tests of a specific organic factor (or factors) judged to be etiologically related to the disturbance.
6. Organic mood syndrome
   a) Prominent and persistent depressed, elevated, or expansive mood.
   b) There is evidence from the history, physical examination, or laboratory tests of a specific organic factor (or factors) judged to be etiologically related to the disturbance.
7. Organic anxiety syndrome
   a) Prominent, recurrent panic attacks or generalized anxiety.
   b) There is evidence from the history, physical examination, or laboratory tests of a specific organic factor (or factors) judged to be etiologically related to the disturbance.
8. Organic personality syndrome
   a) A persistent personality disturbance, either lifelong or representing a change or accentuation of a previously characteristic trait, involving at least one of the following:
      (1) Affective instability (e.g., marked shifts from normal mood to depression, irritability, or anxiety)
      (2) Recurrent outbursts of aggression or rage that are grossly out of proportion to any precipitating psychosocial stressors
      (3) Markedly impaired social judgment (e.g., sexual indiscretions)
      (4) Marked apathy and indifference
      (5) Suspiciousness or paranoid ideation
   b) There is evidence from the history, physical examination, or laboratory tests of a specific organic factor (or factors) judged to be etiologically related to the disturbance.
   c) This diagnosis is not given to a child or adolescent if the clinical picture is limited to the features that characterize attention-deficit hyperactivity disorder.
9. Intoxication

a) Development of a substance-specific syndrome due to recent ingestion of a psychoactive substance. (*Note:* More than one substance may produce similar or identical syndromes.)

b) Maladaptive behavior during the waking state due to the effect of the substance on the central nervous system (e.g., belligerence, impaired judgment, impaired social or occupational functioning).

c) The clinical picture does not correspond to any of the other specific organic mental syndromes, such as delirium, organic delusional syndrome, organic hallucinosis, organic mood syndrome, or organic anxiety syndrome.

10. Withdrawal

a) Development of a substance-specific syndrome that follows the cessation of, or reduction in, intake of a psychoactive substance that the person previously used regularly.

b) The clinical picture does not correspond to any of the other specific organic mental syndromes, such as delirium, organic delusional syndrome, organic hallucinosis, organic mood syndrome, or organic anxiety syndrome.

11. Organic mental syndromes not otherwise specified (NOS) are syndromes that do not meet the criteria for any of the other organic mental syndromes and in which there are maladaptive changes during the waking state, with evidence, from either physical examination, laboratory tests, or history, of a specific organic factor that is judged to be etiologically related to the disturbance. Examples include the "neurasthenic" picture associated with early Addison's disease and unusual disturbances of consciousness or behavior occurring during seizures.

D. Organic mental disorders

1. Organic mental disorders may be grouped into three categories:

a) Disorders related to aging of the brain

b) Disorders due to an ingestion of a substance

c) Organic mental disorders whose etiology or pathophysiologic process is an Axis III physical disorder or condition, or is unknown

2. Among the dementias arising in the senium and presenium is primary degenerative dementia of the Alzheimer type. (It should be remembered that the definitive diagnosis of this condition is dependent on histopathologic findings.) The

second type of dementia due to aging is multi-infarct dementia.

a) In Alzheimer disease the dementia is of insidious onset with a generally progressive deteriorating course, whereas with the multi-infarct dementia, the dementia has a course characterized by stepwise deterioration with "patchy" distribution of deficit.

b) Evidence from history, physical examination, or laboratory tests of significant cerebrovascular disease (recorded on Axis III) and has focal neurologic signs and symptoms.

3. Psychoactive substance-induced organic mental disorder can be produced by any of the psychoactive substances listed in chapter 19, which include alcohol, amphetamines, caffeine, cannabis, cocaine, hallucinogens, inhalants, nicotine, opioids, phencyclidine (PCP) or similarly acting arylcyclohexylamines, and various sedatives, hypnotics, or anxiolytics.

## IV. Etiology

A. Any condition that causes cerebral tissue impairment may lead to organic mental disorder.

B. Among the potential causes of organic mental disorder are[1]

1. Endocrine dysfunction
   a) Thyroid disease
   b) Parathyroid disease
   c) Adrenal dysfunction
   d) Hypoglycemia

2. Metabolic and electrolytic abnormalities
   a) Liver disease
   b) Kidney disease
   c) Lung disease
   d) SIADA acidosis, alkalosis
   e) Wilson's disease
   f) Porphyria

3. Nutritional and deficiency states
   a) Vitamin deficiencies such as thiamin, niacin, and vitamin B-12
   b) Iron deficiency
   c) Pernicious anemia

4. Drugs and medications
   a) Alcohol
   b) Various sedatives
   c) Anticholinergic drugs

1. G. C. Peterson, "Organic Brain Syndrome," *Psychiatric Clinics of North America* 1, no. 1 (April 1978): 21.

d) Steroids

e) Amphetamines

f) Antihypertensive drugs

5. Toxic conditions

a) Heavy metal such as lead, mercury, arsenic, thalium

b) Solvents

c) Organophosphates

6. Infections

a) Brain abscess

b) CNS syphilis

c) Meningoencephalitis

d) Pneumonia

e) Septicemia

7. Post-traumatic reactions

a) Subdural hematoma

b) Normotensive hydrocephalus

c) Contusion

8. Degenerative and "slow viral" diseases

a) Alzheimer's disease

b) Pick's disease

c) Amyotropic lateral sclerosis

d) Huntington's disease

9. Vascular disorders

a) Hypertension

b) Cerebral embolism and thrombosis

c) Cerebral atherosclerosis

d) Congestive heart failure

10. Neoplastic disorders

a) Primary brain tumor

b) Metastic cancer

11. Other causes

a) Intractible seizures

b) Status petit mal

c) Remote effects of carcinoma

d) AIDS

C. The most common organic brain disorders seen in clinical practice are the dementias, occurring in the geriatric population.

## V. Prevalence

A. Organic mental disorders are common and may occur at any age.

1. Some, such as primary degenerative dementia of the Alzheimer type, are found in late life.

2. Others, such as Pick's disease (a presenile focal degenerative disease of the brain affecting the cerebral cortex, particularly the frontal lobes), are found in late middle life.

3. Others, resulting from head injuries, are more commonly found in early life.
4. Organic brain syndromes associated with infectious diseases, psychoactive substance abuse, or alcohol abuse may occur at almost any age.

B. Variable incidence
1. Some organic mental disorders seem to be increasing in frequency, as, for example, primary degenerative dementia of the Alzheimer's type and normotensive hydrocephalus (a nonabsorptive communicating type of hydrocephalus that develops in the absence of a demonstrable lesion). These are increasing because of the aging of the population.
2. Others are decreasing in frequency as, for example, the organic mental brain disorder associated with syphilis of the central nervous system (general paresis).

## VI. Treatment

A. Treatment depends upon the underlying etiology. Treatment is directed at the underlying mental, medical, or neurological disorder.
B. Certain medications are prescribed. For example, neuroleptics are sometimes cautiously prescribed for agitation accompanying senile behavior; benzodiazepines may be used for restlessness or during the withdrawal periods from various substances. In many of these cases, only the smallest dose should be used, since patients with brain syndromes are frequently quite sensitive to these drugs.
C. Management of the patient's behavior frequently involves repeating simple explanations and giving help with orientation, as well as frequently adopting a reassuring attitude.
D. Patients who have deliria do better with constant light. Shadows and darkness increase their illusions and frighten them.
E. Some patients need protection from harming themselves or others.

## VII. Case examples

A. Case example, alcohol withdrawal

A thirty-five-year-old man was admitted to the hospital for a leg injury. He gave a history of alcoholism dating back to age eighteen and said that he had been drinking at least one pint of whiskey daily for several months prior to admission.

The morning following admission, the nurses noted that he seemed confused and could not give the correct date or the name of the hospital. By late afternoon he appeared anxious, and swept his hand along his torso and extremities as if brushing something off. On inquiry, he admitted to "seeing" tiny green animals crawling over his body. By late evening he was very excited and fearful, especially if left by himself in the darkened room. He was transferred to the psychiatric ward, where he recovered from the acute psychotic episode after two days.

In this case, note the history of substance use disorder (chronic alcoholism), the sudden onset of disorientation, mood change, and the vivid, visual hallucinations. Note also the rapid recovery from the acute episode.

(The previous case antedates the present-day period of heightened awareness of substance use disorders.)

### B. Case example, delirium

A seventy-four-year-old man developed symptoms of enlarged prostate, or benign prostatic hypertrophy (frequent urination, nocturia, dysuria, and urinary retention). The urinary retention became so severe that he had to be hospitalized.

Two days after admission, he became confused, disoriented, and unruly. He had visual hallucinations (e.g., he saw his son outside his hospital room) and was delusional (he was paranoid about some of the nurses and at times thought he was God). Examination revealed a markedly enlarged prostate gland and an elevated blood urea nitrogen (indicative of uremia). Following surgical resection of the enlarged prostate, his uremia cleared up and his mental symptoms disappeared.

Note that his symptoms were produced by uremia and disappeared when this was cleared up by treating the underlying cause of the uremia.

### C. Case example, primary degenerative dementia, presenile onset

A forty-eight-year-old woman was brought to the hospital by her son, who said she was disoriented, showed poor judgment, was difficult to manage, and behaved in a childish manner. The onset of symptoms was noted two years earlier, when she first complained of impaired memory of recent events and forgot some of the routine tasks associated with her job as a receptionist. Very shortly after, she showed poor judgment in dealing with people and made obscene remarks to her colleagues. Because of this behavior, she was fired. At home, she progressively deteriorated: she became slovenly in dress, careless of excreta, and markedly disoriented. At the time of admission, she was incapable of carrying out even simple household tasks.

Examination revealed her to be completely disoriented about time and place. Recent and remote memory were totally defective. She was apathetic, disinterested, and passively cooperative. At times she seemed to be responding to auditory hallucinations. Physical and neurological examinations were essentially negative. A pneumoencephalogram (X-ray examination of the skull after replacing the cerebrospinal fluid with air) revealed findings compatible with generalized cerebral atrophy. She was transferred to a state hospital, where her behavior progressively deteriorated.

Note the typical organic symptoms and their progressive nature, a result of the permanent and progressive cerebral atrophy. This generalized cerebral atrophy, occurring in middle life, is called Alzheimer's disease. The pathological changes in the brain are similar to those found in senile dementia.

(This case antedates computerized tomography.)

## D. Case example, primary degenerative dementia, senile onset

A seventy-six-year-old widow was admitted to the hospital complaining of memory loss and hallucinations. She had been well until about a year earlier, when her family first noticed that she was forgetful and had trouble remembering the date. Shortly, she began complaining about strange noises in her apartment. The family was not especially concerned by this complaint because they knew that one of her neighbors had frequent parties and that another kept a dog and other pets in his apartment. About four months before admission, the patient began complaining that her next-door neighbor was a gangster and accused him of shooting someone in the apartment. One week before admission, she went to the manager of the apartment building and complained about the people who were walking through her closed doors and windows. Her family was summoned, and they brought her to the hospital.

Examination revealed her to be grossly disoriented about time and place. Both recent and remote memory were impaired. She had visual hallucinations (e.g., she saw dogs in her room) and was mildly suspicious of the staff. Physical and neurological studies were negative except for X-ray evidence of mild rheumatoid arthritis. After a few weeks, her hallucinations and delusions cleared up, and she recognized that she had experienced a psychotic episode. At the time of her discharge two months later, she was still disoriented about time and had a fair amount of recent memory impairment. However, she was able to return to her apartment and adjust with only minimal supervision.

This is primary degenerative dementia, senile onset. Note the onset in late life of behavioral changes in the absence of any specific positive physical, neurological, or laboratory findings. The "improvement" following hospitalization is not unusual in this type of reaction, although, as in this case, there is usually some residual permanent brain damage (disorientation and memory loss persisted after discharge).

(This case antedates computerized tomography.)

## References

American Psychiatric Association. *Diagnostic and Statistical Manual of Mental Disorders.* 3d ed., rev. Washington, D.C.: APA, 1987.

Goldman, H. H., ed. *Review of General Psychiatry.* 2d ed. Norwalk, Conn.: Appleton & Lange, 1988.

Goodwin, D. W., and S. B. Guze. *Psychiatric Diagnosis.* 2d ed. New York: Oxford University Press, 1979.

Kaplan, H. I., and B. J. Sadock, eds. *Comprehensive Textbook of Psychiatry/V.* 5th ed. Baltimore: Williams & Wilkins, 1989.

Peterson, G. C. "Organic Brain Syndrome in Symposium on Brain Disorders." *Psychiatric Clinics of North America* 1 (April 1978): 21.

# Appendix Symptomatology of Mental Disorders

The symptoms of disease are marked by purpose, and the purpose
is beneficent.
The processes of disease aim not at the destruction of life,
but at the saving of it.

**Frederick Treves, address to the Edinburgh Philosophical Institution
(October 31, 1905)**

I. **Introduction**
   A. Symptoms of mental disorders are expressions of the whole organism, not just the psyche or soma alone.
   B. The manifestations of mental disorders are the result of multiple forces, some of which are extrapsychic (i.e., from the environment) and some of which are intrapsychic (i.e., from within the personality).
   C. Thus, although symptoms may seem perplexing and unusual, they have cause and meaning.
      1. Symptoms represent the patient's effort to maintain his or her emotional equilibrium.
      2. In order to understand their meaning, one must know the patient's life history, including the psychological, sociocultural, and biological needs and the forces that have been of importance in the person's development.
   D. Symptoms of mental disorders are thus really psychobiological reactions.

II. **Somatic symptoms**
   Physical symptoms of mental disorders are of three types.
   A. Physiological reflections of anxiety
      Such symptoms are either
      1. The predominant manifestation of the disturbance, as in panic disorders and generalized anxiety disorders, or

2. Experienced if the person attempts to control symptoms, as in resisting obsessions or compulsions in an obsessive-compulsive disorder or in confronting the feared situation or object in a phobic disorder.

B. Physical symptoms

These symptoms are found in most somatoform disorders in which physical symptoms suggest physical disorder without demonstrable organic findings, without known physiological mechanisms, and for which there is positive evidence or a strong presumption that the symptoms are linked to psychological factors or conflicts (*DSM*-III-R). Such symptoms are not under voluntary control. Included among these are somatization disorder (Briquet's syndrome), somatoform pain disorder, hypochondriasis, and undifferentiated somatoform disorder.

C. Symbolic expressions of underlying conflicts

1. Found in the conversion disorders (symbolic somatization)
2. Examples are
   a) Hysterical deafness as a defense against hearing something feared or forbidden
   b) Hysterical paralysis as a defense against taking action

## III. Psychological symptoms

Psychological symptoms may be manifested in many ways. They are discussed in each of the sections describing the kinds of mental disorders. In previous editions of this Outline, this chapter was part of the regular text, but in this edition we are placing this information in the Appendix.

A. Disturbances of affect (mood, feeling, or emotion)

1. Anxiety

   *Anxiety* may be defined as a diffuse, unpleasant uneasiness, apprehension, or fearfulness stemming from anticipated danger, the source of which is unidentifiable. It can be divided into degrees.

   a) *Free-floating anxiety* is severe, persistent, generalized, and unattached anxiety. It is typically found in anxiety disorders and is often a precursor of panic.
   b) *Agitation* is a state of mental perturbation and of restlessness and uneasiness often characterized by such muscular manifestations as motor restlessness. (Anxiety overflows into the muscular system.)
   c) *Tension* is tautness, motor and emotional restlessness, dread.
   d) *Panic* is an acute anxiety attack of overwhelming severity that leads to disorganization of ego functions. It produces physiological changes and terror. (The word is derived from Pan, the Greek god who suddenly appeared

to unsuspecting travelers in the woods, causing them to "panic.")

e) *Normal anxiety (stress).* The source of the anxiety is actual and realistic.

2. Depression

*Depression* is a feeling of sadness, loneliness, dejection, or hopelessness, typically found in major depressive disorder and bipolar depressive disorder. It must be differentiated from grief, which is a state of sadness proportionate to a loss. It is extremely common in psychiatric patients.

3. Euphoria

*Euphoria* is an exaggerated sense of well-being not consistent with reality. It is most commonly found in manic disorders and in certain organic mental disorders, including disorders resulting from the use of toxic substances. It may be divided into degrees.

a) *Elation* is marked euphoria accompanied by increased motor activity.

b) *Exaltation* is intense elation accompanied by grandiose feelings.

c) *Ecstasy* is the feeling of intense but tranquil rapture. Religious feelings are often an integral part of this feeling. It is found in dissociative states, depersonalization, convulsive disorders, and schizophrenic disorders.

4. Apathy

*Apathy* is the lack of feeling, emotion, interest, or concern; impassiveness or unfeelingness.

5. Inappropriateness

*Inappropriateness* is an affect opposite to what would be expected. It is observed in schizophrenic disorders—for example, laughter when a sad message is being expressed.

6. Ambivalence

*Ambivalence* is the coexistence of two opposing feelings toward the same individual or object; these feelings may be conscious, unconscious, or both. It is characteristic of the unconscious of children. It is found in many emotional disorders, but especially in depressive and obsessive-compulsive disorders, and is one of the fundamental symptoms of the schizophrenic disorders.

7. Hostility

*Hostility* is anger, antagonism, opposition, or resistance in thought or behavior. It is the affective counterpart of aggression, to which it is closely allied. It is found in an extreme degree in antisocial personalities and in certain other personality disorders. Unexpressed and internalized hostility is important in the psychodynamics of some depressive disorders. (Violence is a behavioral expression of extreme hostility.)

8. Depersonalization

   *Depersonalization* is the pervasive feeling of unreality, strangeness, or altered identity. It is found in depersonalization disorder, schizophrenic disorder, and bipolar affective illness. It may occur in normal persons who have suffered exhaustion or shock.

9. Derealization

   *Derealization* is the feeling that the environment has changed. It is found in depersonalization disorders and is characterized by alternating periods of euphoria or anxiety and depression. It is also found in cyclothymic disorder (cyclothymic personality).

B. Disturbances of memory

1. Definition

   Memory is composed of three processes.

   a) Registration

      The ability to establish a record of an experience in the central nervous system.

   b) Retention

      The persistence or permanence of a registered experience.

   c) Recall

      The ability to recount a registered experience.[1]

2. All of these processes may be disturbed in various ways.

3. Amnesia

   *Amnesia* is a pathological loss of memory. It may be of organic etiology (e.g., head injury) or psychogenic, as in certain dissociative disorders (e.g., psychogenic amnesia).

   a) *Anterograde amnesia* is loss of memory of events that occur after a particular time.

   b) *Retrograde amnesia* is loss of memory of events that occurred before a particular time.

4. Fugue state

   A *fugue state* is dissociation, a flight from the immediate environment, characterized by an inability to remember what is happening. The individual escapes from the environment and, during this state, apparently acts purposefully. However, when the person regains consciousness, he or she cannot recall the episode, or fugue. It is found in psychomotor equivalents of convulsive disorders and also in the dissociative disorder, psychogenic fugue.

---

1. Adapted from *Modern Synopsis of Comprehensive Textbook of Psychiatry,* vol. 2 edited by A. M. Freedman, H. I. Kaplan, and B. J. Sadock (Baltimore: Williams & Wilkins, 1976), p. 392.

5. Hypermnesia

   *Hypermnesia* is abnormally vivid or complete memory, or the reawakening of impressions seemingly long forgotten. It is found both in normal persons and in certain manic and paranoid disorders.

6. Paramnesia

   *Paramnesia* is a distortion or falsification of memory in which the individual confuses reality and fantasy. It includes the illusion of remembering scenes and events not experienced before.

   a) *Confabulation* is a falsification of memory in which gaps in memory are filled in by imaginary (fabricated) experiences that seem plausible and are recounted in detail. Found in certain organic mental disorders, especially alcohol amnestic disorder (Korsakoff's syndrome).

   b) *Retrospective falsification* is the unconscious distortion of past experiences to conform to present emotional needs. It is found in certain paranoid disorders.

   c) *Fausse reconnaissance* is a false recognition of the unfamiliar.

   d) *Déjà vu* is the sensation that an experience that is really happening for the first time has occurred previously. It occurs in normal people and is found in many mental disorders.

   e) *Jamais vu* is a false feeling of unfamiliarity with a real situation that one has experienced before.

C. Disturbances of consciousness

   1. Definition

      a) *Consciousness* is synonymous with awareness, "clear mindedness."

      b) It also means *apperception,* a mental act in which the mind becomes aware or has knowledge of itself as it perceives.

   2. Both of these aspects of consciousness may be distorted.

   3. Confusion

      *Confusion* is disorientation in respect to time, place, or person and is accompanied by perplexity. It is sometimes accompanied by disturbances of consciousness and is commonly associated with organic mental disorders.

   4. Clouding of consciousness

      *Clouding of consciousness* is impairment of retention, perception, and orientation. It is commonly associated with organic mental disorders, both acute and chronic.

5. Dream state
   *Dream state* is also known as twilight state. It is a transient clouding of consciousness of intrapsychic origin, during which the person is unaware of reality and behaves violently or opposite to his or her usual pattern. It is found in dissociative disorders, convulsive disorders, and in association with the use of certain drugs (e.g., scopolamine or atropine-like drugs).

6. Delirium
   *Delirium* is characterized by disturbance in affect, orientation, memory, and consciousness. There are obvious changes in mood, there are illusions, and there are hallucinations. Delirium may be caused by any agent that produces temporary and reversible cerebral metabolic insufficiency, such as alcohol or drugs. It is also seen in delirious disorders from acute infectious diseases.

7. Coma
   *Coma* is stupor, a state of unawareness, nonreactiveness, profound unconsciousness. It is found in certain organic mental disorders and in the stuporous form of catatonic schizophrenia.

8. Deterioration
   *Deterioration,* or dementia, is the progressive loss of intellectual and emotional functions. It is found in degenerative diseases of the brain such as Alzheimer's disease, and in primary degenerative dementia. Reversible deterioration is found in schizophrenic disorders.

D. Disturbances of orientation
   1. Definition
      *Orientation* is awareness of one's relationship to time, surroundings, and other persons.
   2. Disorientation
      *Disorientation* is loss of awareness of one's relationship to time, surroundings, or other persons. It is usually reversible in certain substance-induced disorders (toxic deliria) and irreversible in chronic mental disorders such as senile and presenile dementia.
   3. Disorientation in respect to time is the most common, followed by place and person.

E. Disturbances of perception
   1. Definition
      *Perception* is the awareness and intended integration of sensory impressions of the environment and their interpretation in light of experience.
   2. Perception may be disturbed or heightened in several ways.

3. Illusions

   *Illusions* are misinterpretations of sensory experiences, usually optical or auditory. They are frequently normal.

   a) *Optical illusions* are sometimes called mirages, as, for example, when heat rays shimmering on a road look like pools of water. They are common in acute but reversible substance-induced disorders such as the withdrawal delirium from alcohol, also known as delirium tremens.

   b) *Auditory illusions* are mistaken interpretations of sounds, as, for example, the roaring of the wind heard as the moaning of a human voice.

4. Hallucinations

   *Hallucinations* are false sensory perceptions that are not caused by external stimuli.

   a) They may be auditory, visual, olfactory, gustatory, tactile (haptic), or kinesthetic (phantom limb is a kinesthetic hallucination).

   b) Hallucinations occur in substance use disorders (caused by alcohol, cocaine, or hallucinogenic drugs such as LSD, peyote, or mescaline). They may also be found in certain other psychotic conditions such as schizophrenic and manic disorders. Different types of disorders tend to produce different types of hallucinations.

   (1) Colorful or vivid *visual hallucinations* are most typically found in the deliria from acute infectious diseases or in the substance-induced delirious disorders.

   (2) *Auditory hallucinations* are commonly found in schizophrenic disorders.

   (3) *Olfactory hallucinations* occur in schizophrenic disorders and in lesions of the temporal lobe of the brain.

   (4) *Tactile hallucinations* (hallucinations of touch) are found in cocaine intoxication and alcohol withdrawal delirium (delirium tremens).

   (5) *Kinesthetic hallucinations* are found in phantom limb syndrome.

   c) An exception to these generalizations about hallucinations is amphetamine-induced organic mental disorder, which commonly produces auditory hallucinations, and sometimes tactile and olfactory ones as well.

   d) *Hypnagogic hallucinations* (hypnagogic imagery) are mental images that sometimes occur just before sleep. Images seen in dreams that persist after awakening are called *hypnopompic*. Both types are normal and are familiar to healthy individuals. Hypnagogic states in particular are sometimes experienced by persons who are very tired but unable to find the time or place to sleep. Some believe that hypnagogic and hypnopompic hallucinations are found more frequently in persons who ultimately develop hypersomnolence or narcolepsy.

In *Oliver Twist,* Charles Dickens writes: "There is a drowsy state between sleeping and waking when you dream more in five minutes with your eyes half-open and yourself half-conscious of everything that is passing around you, than you would in five nights with your eyes fast closed, and your senses wrapped in perfect consciousness. At such times, a mortal knows just enough of what his mind is doing to form some glimmering conceptions of its mighty powers, its bounding from earth and spurning time and space, when freed from the restraint of its corporeal associate."

Edgar Allan Poe was concerned with such sleepless dreams. In *Marginalia* he writes that "these 'fancies' have in them a pleasurable ecstasy as far beyond the most pleasurable of the world of wakefulness or of dreams, as the Heaven of the Northman theology is beyond its Hell. I regard the visions, even as they arise, with an awe which in some measure moderates or tranquilizes the ecstasy."

e) Both hallucinations and illusions may occur in normal people during prolonged periods of isolation.

f) Pseudohallucinations are transient visual perceptual distortions that may be associated with anxiety or fear.

g) Night terrors (pavor nocturnus) are nightmares occurring in children in which they awaken screaming with fright, the alarm persisting for a time during a state of semi-consciousness. They remain in a twilight state and cannot be awakened. They then fall into a deep, peaceful sleep. There is complete amnesia for the attack as well as the dream content (Campbell 1981).

5. Eidetic imagery
*Eidetic imagery* consists of vivid, accurate, and detailed visual afterimages sometimes called photographic memory. Such experiences are normal and are to be distinguished from hallucinations. "Perhaps the artists have a greater eidetic power than most adults," wrote Franz Boaz. It is found frequently in young children, much less frequently in adults.

6. Misperceptions

*Misperceptions* are associated with conversion disorders (hysterical misperceptions).

a) Perceptual distortions may occur in any of the sensory areas.

b) Sensation may be exaggerated or, more commonly, reduced. For example, *hyperesthesia* and *hyperalgesia* or, conversely, *hypesthesia* and *hypalgesia* may occur in conversion disorder.

c) *Macropsia* is visualization of objects as larger than they really are; conversely, *micropsia* is visualization of objects as smaller than they really are.

F. Disturbances of thinking

1. Definition

*Thinking* is the exercise of powers of judgment, conception, or inference, as distinguished from simple sensory perception. It is prey to many disorders.

2. Fantasy

*Fantasy,* or phantasy, is a fabricated series of mental pictures or sequences of events; daydreaming.

a) Fantasy may express unconscious conflict, gratify otherwise unobtainable wishes, or provide an escape from reality.

b) It may serve as the springboard for creative activities.

c) It may lead to a harmful distortion of reality.

3. Phobias

*Phobias* are persistent, irrational fears of specific objects, activities, or situations. Examples include fear of height, closed spaces, open spaces, strangers, animals, dirt, or school. Certain fears, as of harmless bugs and snakes, are extremely common and not considered pathological, but phobias are typically found in phobic disorders.

4. Obsessions

*Obsessions,* also called ruminations, are recurrent, persistent ideas, thoughts, images, or impulses that remain conscious despite their irrationality. They are typically found in obsessive-compulsive disorders.

5. Preoccupations

*Preoccupations* are excessive concerns with one's own thoughts; engrossment.

6. Delusions

*Delusions* are fixed, false beliefs that are not in keeping with the individual's cultural or intellectual level. They are found in various types of psychotic disorders—organic mental disorders, schizophrenic disorders, and certain of the affective disorders. They may be

    a) *Persecutory,* a belief that one is singled out for oppression, attack, or harassment.

    b) *Grandiose,* an exaggerated belief in one's own importance.

    c) *Somatic,* a deluded interpretation of physical symptoms.

    d) *Referential,* a belief that the irrelevant remarks or acts of others refer to oneself.

    e) *Influential,* a belief that one can control or be controlled by another's behavior or thoughts; most commonly observed in paranoid or schizophrenic disorders.

        (1) Ideas of *active influence,* the psychotic belief that one controls others.

        (2) Ideas of *passive influence,* the psychotic belief that one is being controlled by others.

    f) *Nihilistic,* the belief that oneself, the environment, or the world does not exist.

    g) *Self-accusatory,* the belief that one is responsible for harm.

    h) Other types of delusions include sin, guilt, impoverishment, illness, and infidelity.

7. Blocking

*Blocking* is difficulty in recalling or interpreting a stream of speech or thought because of emotional forces that are usually conscious. It is most often found in schizophrenics who, for example, may stop talking, or block, while listening to an imaginary voice or because of conflicting reactions to the message.

8. Magical thinking

*Magical thinking* is the imputation of reality to a thought. "Wishing will make it so" is a primitive, prelogical idea believed by small children, encountered in dreams, and found in the thinking of obsessive-compulsive patients.

9. Incoherence

*Incoherence* is disorderly, illogical thought, sometimes manifested as garbled speech. It is found in schizophrenic disorders, manic disorders, and certain organic mental disorders.

10. Irrelevance

*Irrelevance* is thinking that is erroneous or irrelevant to the subject at hand.

11. Circumstantiality

*Circumstantiality* is incidental or adventitious thinking. The individual cannot distinguish essentials from nonessentials, although the goal of the thinking is ultimately reached. It is commonly found in manic disorder, in some organic mental disorders, and in the mentally retarded.

12. Tangentiality

   *Tangentiality* is inability to reach the goal of the thinking.

13. Perseveration

   *Perseveration* is a persistent, repetitive expression of a single idea in response to various questions. It is found in some organic mental disorders, aphasia, and in certain types of catatonia.

14. Condensation

   *Condensation* is the coalition of several concepts into one.

15. Psychomotor retardation

   *Psychomotor retardation* is the slowing down of mental and physical activity. It is most commonly observed in depressive disorders, but also in some schizophrenic disorders.

16. Psychomotor excitement

   *Psychomotor excitement* is a mentally and physically hyperactive response to internal or external stimuli. It is found in manic disorders and in some catatonic schizophrenic disorders.

17. Flight of ideas

   The *flight of ideas* is skipping from one idea to another in quick succession, without reaching the goal of the thinking. It is most commonly observed in the manic disorders.

18. Autism

   *Autism,* or dereism, is a persistent overindulgence in fantasy. It is found in child schizophrenics (pervasive developmental disorders).

19. Misidentification

   *Misidentification* is the incorrect identification of other people. It is found in certain psychotic disorders.

20. Intellectualization

   *Intellectualization* is the overuse of intellectual concepts and words to avoid feeling or expressing emotion. It is found in adolescents who want to escape their sexual impulses, borderline personalities, obsessive-compulsive patients, and some schizophrenics.

21. Clang association

   *Clang association* is a disturbance in thinking in which the sound of a word, rather than its meaning, sets off a new train of thought. It occurs most often in manic disorders and may lead to senseless rhyming.

G. Disturbances of speech and verbal behavior

   1. Blocking (see F. Disturbances of thinking)

2. Flight of ideas (see F. Disturbances of thinking)
3. Logorrhea
   *Logorrhea,* or volubility, is uncontrollable, rapid, excessive talking. It is most commonly observed in manic disorders.
4. Pressure of speech
   *Pressure of speech* is rapid, accelerated, voluble speech that is difficult to interrupt. It is sometimes found in manic disorders.
5. Neologism
   A *neologism* is a coined word or a condensation of several words to express a complex idea. Often known simply as jargon, it is also found in certain schizophrenic disorders.
6. Wordsalad
   *Wordsalad* is an incomprehensible and incoherent mixture of words and phrases. It is found in some schizophrenic disorders.
7. Echolalia
   *Echolalia* is the pathological repetition of the phrases or words of another person. It is found in some schizophrenic disorders, certain organic mental disorders, and in mental retardation.
8. Echopraxia
   *Echopraxia* is the pathological repetition or imitation of movements the subject is observing. It is found in catatonic disorders.
9. Verbigeration
   *Verbigeration* is the meaningless repetition of incoherent words or sentences. It is observed in certain psychotic reactions and in certain organic mental disorders.
10. Condensation (see also, Condensation under F. Disturbances of thinking)
    *Condensation* is the contraction of several different ideas into one phrase, forming a collage of thought.
H. Disturbances of motor behavior, or conation
   1. Definition
      *Conation* is the basic striving of an individual as expressed in his or her behavior.
   2. Psychomotor retardation (see F. Disturbances of thinking)
   3. Psychomotor excitement (see F. Disturbances of thinking)
   4. Agitation (see A. Disturbances of affect)
   5. Echopraxia (see G. Disturbances of speech and verbal behavior)

6. Catalepsy

   *Catalepsy* is a generalized diminished responsiveness or immobility characterized by trancelike states. It is found in organic mental disorders and certain psychogenic disorders.

7. Waxy flexibility

   *Waxy flexibility,* or cerea flexibilitas, is a condition in which a patient passively retains the position into which he or she has been placed. It is often present in catatonia.

8. Stereotypy

   *Stereotypy* is the persistent repetition of a motor activity. It is sometimes found in schizophrenic disorders.

9. Posturing

   *Posturing* is the assumption and maintenance of an unusual posture, often an uncomfortable one. It is most commonly observed in catatonics.

10. Mannerisms

    *Mannerisms* are stereotyped movements such as blinking, grimacing, and gesturing. They are found in schizophrenic disorders.

11. Negativism

    *Negativism* is opposition, resistance, or refusal to accept reasonable suggestions or advice; a tendency to be in opposition. It may be passive or active. Its most extreme form is found in catatonic schizophrenic disorders.

12. Mutism

    *Mutism* is a form of negativism characterized by refusal to speak, either for conscious or unconscious reasons. It is observed in catatonic schizophrenic disorders, profound depressive disorders, and stupors of organic or psychogenic origin.

13. Automatism

    *Automatism* is unconsciously directed automatic, repetitious, and symbolic behavior observed in schizophrenic, convulsive, and dissociative disorders.

14. Compulsion

    *Compulsions* are repetitive, compelling acts that develop in an attempt to relieve obsessions or fears. They are most commonly found in obsessive-compulsive disorders and include handwashing rituals and self-mutilation.

I. Disturbances of attention

   1. Definition

      *Attention* is the maintenance of focused consciousness to the salient characteristics of the environment.

2. Decreased attention

   *Decreased attention* may result from a lack of interest in or a deliberate shutting out of impinging stimulation.

3. Preoccupation

   *Preoccupation* is concentration on one's own problems, which may diminish attention.

4. Fluctuation

   *Fluctuation of attention* is a greater than normal variation, sometimes to the point of inability to attend in spite of the attempt to do so.

5. Blunting of attention

   *Blunting of attention* is extreme inattention, so that even noxious stimulation may not elicit a response.

6. Increased attention

   *Increased attention,* or hyperprosexia, is unusual attention, usually to details of personal significance.

7. Distractibility

   *Distractibility* is a heightened, rapid fluctuation of attention, so that every new stimulus, regardless of its significance, is responded to by rapid shifts.

IV. **Usefulness of symptomatology**

   A. Knowledge of the preceding symptoms is of importance in examining the mental status of the psychiatric patient.

   B. The symptomatology helps to establish a working diagnosis and a treatment program.

## References

Campbell, R. J. *Psychiatric Dictionary.* 5th ed. New York: Oxford University Press, 1981.

Henderson, D., and R. D. Gillespie. *Textbook of Psychiatry.* 8th ed. London: Oxford University Press, 1956.

Kaplan, H. I., and B. J. Sadock. *Modern Synopsis of Comprehensive Textbook of Psychiatry/III.* Baltimore: Williams & Wilkins, 1981.

Kolb, L. C., and H. K. H. Brodie. *Modern Clinical Psychiatry.* 10th ed. Philadelphia: Saunders, 1982.

Soloman, P., and V. D. Patch. *Handbook of Psychiatry.* Los Altos, Calif.: Lange Medical Publications, 1971.

# Glossary

**Acting out**    A mechanism in which a person acts without reflection or apparent regard for negative consequences.

**Addiction**    Refers to a compulsive pattern of drug use even at the expense of physical harm and psychosocial deterioration.

**Adjustment disorders**    The essential feature of this disorder is a maladaptive reaction to an identifiable psychosocial stressor, or stressors, that occurs within three months after onset of the stressor, and has persisted for no longer than six months.

**Adult character structure**    Includes the ego's usual mode of dealing with the id, the superego, and the external world.

**Agoraphobia**    The fear of being in places or situations from which escape might be difficult (or embarrassing) or in which help might not be available in the event of suddenly developing a symptom that could be incapacitating or extremely embarrassing.

**AIDS (acquired immune-deficiency syndrome)**    A cluster of opportunistic infections and disorders, such as Kaposi's sarcoma (KS), to which the subject is abnormally vulnerable because of the collapse of his or her immune defense system.

**Alcoholism**    Generally, one can say that persons are alcoholics if their drinking interferes in any way with their lives.

**Alexithymic**    Describes persons who define their emotions only in terms of somatic sensations or in behavioral reactions rather than relating them to accompanying thoughts.

**Altruism**    In this mechanism one deals with emotional conflicts or external or internal stress by dedicating oneself to fulfilling the needs of others instead of one's own.

**Ambivalence**    Coexistence of two opposing feelings toward the same individual or object; very prominent in obsessive-compulsive patients.

**Anankastic personality, or anal character**    An individual who needs to feel in control of him- or herself and of the environment.

**Anorexia nervosa**    The essential features are refusal to maintain body weight over a minimal normal weight for age and height; intense fear of gaining weight or becoming fat, even though underweight; a distorted body image; and amenorrhea in females.

**Antipsychotic agents**   Attributed to the blockade of dopamine receptors.

**Antisocial personality disorder**   The essential feature of this disorder is a pattern of irresponsible and antisocial behavior beginning in childhood or early adolescence and continuing into adulthood. For this diagnosis to be given, the person must be at least eighteen years of age and have a history of conduct disorder before the age of fifteen.

**Anxiety and fear**   *Anxiety* as a symptom can be defined as a diffuse, unpleasant uneasiness, apprehension, or fearfulness stemming from anticipated danger, the source of which is unidentifiable.
*Fear* is a response to a recognized external threat.
Components of anxiety
*Free-floating anxiety*   Severe, persistent, generalized, and unattached anxiety. It is typically found in anxiety disorders and is often a precursor of panic.
*Normal anxiety* (stress)   The source of the anxiety is actual and realistic.
*Tension*   Tautness, motor and emotional restlessness, dread.
*Agitation*   A state of restlessness and uneasiness often characterized by such muscular manifestations as motor restlessness; mental perturbation. (Anxiety overflows into the muscular system.)
*Panic*   An acute anxiety attack of overwhelming severity that leads to disorganization of ego functions.

**Anxiety disorders**   The characteristic features of this group of disorders are symptoms of anxiety and avoidance behavior.

**Autistic fantasy**   A mechanism in which a person substitutes excessive daydreaming for pursuits of human relationships, more direct and effective action, or problem solving.

**Avoidant personality disorder**   The essential feature of this disorder is a pervasive pattern of social discomfort, fear of negative evaluation, and timidity, beginning by early adulthood and present in a variety of contexts.

**Behavior therapy**   Used here as a general term that refers to all therapy that is derived from principles of learning.

**Body dysmorphic disorder (dysmorphophobia)**   The essential feature of this disorder is preoccupation with some imagined defect in appearance in a normal-appearing person.

**Borderline personality disorder**   The essential feature of this disorder is a pervasive pattern of instability of self-image, interpersonal relationships, and mood, beginning by early adulthood and present in a variety of contexts.

**Bulimia nervosa**   The essential features are recurrent episodes of binge eating (rapid consumption of a large amount of food in a discrete period of time); a feeling of lack of control over eating behavior during the eating binges; self-induced vomiting, use of laxatives or diuretics, strict dieting or fasting, or vigorous exercise in order to prevent weight gain; and persistent overconcern with body shape and weight.

**Carbamazepine**   An anticonvulsant, structurally related to tricyclics, which may be used alone or in combination with lithium.

**Clarification**   A process by which the physician helps patients to understand their feelings and behavior and to gain a clearer picture of reality.

**Compensation**    A conscious or unconscious attempt to overcome real or fancied inferiorities.

**Compulsions**    Repetitive, purposeful, and intentional behaviors that are performed in response to an obsession, according to certain rules, or in a stereotyped fashion.

**Computerized axial tomography (CAT)**    Uses a moving X-ray detector system to construct successive cross sections of the brain to reveal differences in tissue density, which may indicate tumors, blockage of blood vessels, and shrinking of tissue.

**Conjoint therapy**    Refers to the practice of both members of a couple seeing the same therapist in the same sessions.

**Conscious**    Composed of ideas, feelings, drives, and urges of which the person is aware.

**Consultation liaison psychiatry**    A discipline that bridges psychiatry/psychology, and general medicine and other medical specialties.

**Continuous amnesia**    Failure to recall events subsequent to a specific time and up to, and including, the present.

**Conversion disorder**    The essential feature of this disorder is an alteration or loss of physical functioning that suggests physical disorder, but that instead is apparently an expression of a psychological conflict or need.

**Coprophilia**    A pathological sexual interest in excretions.

**Cosmic consciousness, or illumination**    A fabulous sense of joy or well-being, sometimes produced by hallucinogenic drugs.

**Counterphobic attitude**    At times persons with a phobia seek out the very situation of which they are afraid.

**Countertransference**    The therapist's unconscious or conscious emotional reaction to the patient.

**Couples therapy**    The emphasis of treatment is on the disturbance of the relationship rather than on the disturbed individual.

**Defense mechanisms**    In psychodynamic usage, defense mechanisms are specific, unconscious, intrapsychic adjustments that represent attempts to resolve emotional conflict and reduce anxiety.

*Déjà vu*    A subjective sensation that an experience that is really happening for the first time occurred on a previous occasion.

**Delusional (paranoid) disorders**    The essential feature of this disorder is the presence of a persistent, nonbizarre delusion that is not due to any other mental disorder.

     Types:

               Erotomanic
               Grandiose
               Jealous
               Persecutory
               Somatic
               Litigious

**Denial**    The unconscious disavowal of a thought, feeling, wish, need, or reality that is consciously unacceptable.

**Dependent personality disorder**    The essential feature of this disorder is a pervasive pattern of dependent and submissive behavior beginning by early adulthood and present in a variety of contexts.

**Depersonalization**    A sense of estrangement from oneself.

**Depersonalization disorder**    The essential feature of this disorder is the occurrence of persistent or recurrent episodes of depersonalization sufficiently severe to cause marked distress.

**Depression**    The emotion of feeling sad, blue or unhappy, typically found in affective disorders.

**Derealization**    A feeling that the environment has changed.

**Devaluation**    In this mechanism one deals with emotional conflicts or external or internal stress by attributing exaggerated negative qualities to self or others.

**Diagnosis**    The procedure by which a patient's presenting clinical picture of complaints, concerns, and disturbances are assessed and compared to those of other patients with similar presentations for the purpose of identifying an underlying disorder or disease.

**Diathesis-stress model**    Views mental disorder as the product of a predisposition toward the development of a particular disorder (diathesis) and conditions operating on a person that require an adjustive response (stress).

**Disorders of impulse control**    Characterized by the irresistible, repetitious expression of a single pleasurable impulse.

**Disorganized schizophrenia (also called hebephrenic)**    The essential features are marked incoherence, marked loosening of associations or grossly disorganized behavior, flat or grossly inappropriate affect, and fragmentary, unsystematized delusions or hallucinations with an incoherent theme.

**Displacement**    The redirection of an emotion from the original object to a more acceptable substitute.

**Dissociation**    The unconscious detachment of certain behavior from the normal or usual conscious behavior patterns of an individual, which then function alone (compartmentalization).

**Dissociative disorders**    The characteristic that is common to all the dissociative disorders is a constellation of recent mental events that is out of the patient's awareness but is capable, under certain conditions, of being brought into consciousness.

**Down's syndrome**    A common form of mental retardation, once called mongolism and caused by an autosomal anomaly.

**Drug tolerance**    Refers to a decreasing responsiveness to a drug with continued use.

**Dysthymia**    A chronic disturbance of mood in which there is a history of depressive mood for more days than not for at least two years and which during the first two years of the disturbance the condition does not meet the criteria for major depressive disorder.

**Eclectic approach**    The use of compatible aspects from diverse systems into an integrated whole.

**Ego**    The part of the personality that meets and interacts with the outside world.

**Electroencephalograph (EEG)**    Used to obtain records of general brain wave activity or responses to some types of stimuli.

**Empathy**    The capacity for participating in, or vicariously experiencing, another's feelings, volitions, or ideas. This ability to feel with another is a form of identification found in mature, well-integrated personalities.

**Environmental modification also called,** *environmental intervention* **or** *environmental manipulation.* Altering the environment so as to relieve the patient's symptoms and distress.

**Epidemiology** The study of the temporal and geographic distribution of a disorder within a specified population.

**Eustress** Positive stress situations that require adaptation but are generally viewed favorably.

**Exaggeration** To protect self-esteem and/or emotional balance, certain meanings can be assigned exaggerated values.

**Exhibitionism** The essential feature of this disorder is recurrent, intense sexual urges and sexually arousing fantasies, of at least six months' duration, involving the exposure of one's genitals to a stranger.

**Factitious disorders** Characterized by physical or psychological symptoms that are intentionally produced or feigned; to assume the patient role.

**Factitious disorder with psychological symptoms** The essential feature of this disorder is intentional production or feigning of psychological (often psychotic) symptoms suggestive of mental disorder. The person's goal is apparently to assume the "patient" role and is not otherwise understandable in light of the person's environmental circumstances.

**Family therapy** A form of group therapy wherein the nuclear family is the unit.

**Fantasy** A fabricated series of mental pictures or sequence of events; daydreaming.

**Fascination, or fixation** A trancelike state induced in individuals (e.g., pilots) who are compelled to focus on a given object for long periods of time.

**Feelings of derealization** Feelings that the environment has changed.

**Feelings of estrangement** A sense of detachment from people, the environment, or concepts.

**Feelings of unreality** Feelings that one is unreal.

**Fetishism** The essential feature of this disorder is recurrent, intense sexual urges and sexually arousing fantasies, of at least six months' duration, involving the use of nonliving objects (fetishes).

**Fixation** The arrest of maturation at an immature level of psychosexual development.

**Free-association** The spontaneous, uncensored verbalizations by the patient of whatever comes to mind.

**Frotteurism** The essential feature of this disorder is recurrent, intense sexual urges and sexually arousing fantasies, of at least six months' duration, involving touching and rubbing against a nonconsenting person.

**Ganser's syndrome** "The syndrome of approximate answers" to questions, commonly-associated with other symptoms such as amnesia, disorientation, perceptual disturbances, fugue, and conversion symptoms. Named for Sigbert J. M. Ganser.

**Gender identity disorder of adolescence or adulthood, nontranssexual type (GIDAANT)** The essential features of this disorder are a persistent or recurrent discomfort and sense of inappropriateness about one's assigned sex, and persistent or recurrent cross-dressing in the role of the other sex, either in fantasy or in actuality, in a person who has reached puberty.

**Gender identity disorders**     The essential feature of the disorders included in this subclass is an incongruence between assigned sex (i.e., the sex that is recorded on the birth certificate) and gender identity.

**Generalized amnesia**     Failure to recall the individual's entire life.

**Generalized anxiety disorder (GAD)**     The essential feature of this disorder is unrealistic or excessive anxiety and worry (apprehensive expectation) about two or more life circumstances—for example, worry about possible misfortune to one's child (who is in no danger) and worry about finances (for no good reason)—for six months or longer, during which the person has been bothered by these concerns more days than not.

**Genital phase**     The final stage of psychosexual development.

**Grief (uncomplicated bereavement)**     Bereavement is a normal, appropriate, affective sadness in response to a recognizable external loss.

**Group psychotherapy**     Application of psychotherapeutic techniques to a group, including utilization of interactions of members of the group.

**Histrionic personality disorder**     The essential feature of this disorder is a pervasive pattern of excessive emotionality and attention seeking, beginning by early adulthood and present in a variety of contexts.

**HIV (human immunodeficiency virus)**     The cause of AIDS, AIDS-related complex (ARC), and AIDS dementia complex.

**Hostile identification**     Internalization of undesirable personality traits of parents or authority figures.

**Humor**     One might deal with external or internal stress by employing humor and emphasizing the ironic or amusing aspects of the stress or conflict.

**Huntington's disease**     A degenerative disorder of the basal ganglia and cortex characterized by progressive intellectual loss and motor dysfunction; related to a dominant gene, but such simple genetic models have not been found in major mental disorders.

**Hypnagogic hallucinations**     The mental images that occur just before sleep.

**Hypnopompic hallucinations**     Images seen in dreams that persist on awakening.

**Hypochondriasis**     The essential feature of this disorder is preoccupation with the fear of having, or the belief that one has, a serious disease, based on the person's interpretation of physical signs or sensations as evidence of physical illness.

**Iatrogenic factors**     Disorders unwittingly precipitated, aggravated, or induced by the physician's attitude, examination comments, or treatment.

**Idealization**     The overestimation of admired qualities of another person or desired object.

**Identification**     The unconscious, wishful adoption, or internalization, of the personality characteristics or identity of another individual, generally one possessing attributes that the subject envies or admires.

**Identification with the aggressor**     Internalization of the characteristics of a frustrated or feared parent or parent substitute.

**Impostership**     Fabrications of attainments, positions, or worldly possessions.

**Incorporation**     A primitive defense mechanism in which the psychic image of another person is wholly or partially assimilated into an individual's personality.

**Induced psychotic disorder**    The essential feature of this disorder is a delusional system that develops in a second person as a result of a close relationship with another person who already has a psychotic disorder with prominent delusions.

**Insight**    The degree to which the patient can appreciate the nature of his or her condition and the need for treatment.

**Intellectualization**    The overuse of intellectual concepts and words to avoid affective experience or expressions of feelings.

**Intermittent explosive disorder**    The essential features of this disorder are discrete episodes of loss of control of aggressive impulses, resulting in serious assaultive acts or destruction of property.

**Interpersonal therapies**    Therapies that have features similar to both psychodynamic and cognitive therapies.

**Introjection**    The symbolic internalization or assimilation (taking into oneself) of a loved or hated person or external object.

**Involutional melancholia**    Once used to describe a depression of initial onset occurring during the involutional years (forty to fifty-five in women and fifty to sixty-five in men).

**Isolation**    The separation of an unacceptable impulse.

**Kleptomania**    The essential feature of this disorder is a recurrent failure to resist impulses to steal objects not needed for personal use or their monetary value.

**Klismaphilia**    The love of enemas and a dependence on their use for sexual arousal.

**Latency**    The stage between the Oedipal period and the adolescent years.

**Localized anmesia**    Failure to recall all events during a circumscribed period of time, usually the first few hours following a profoundly disturbing event.

**Malingering**    Signs and symptoms of illness are consciously produced and consciously motivated.

**Mania**    The essential feature of a manic episode is an elevated euphoric, expansive, or irritable mood.

**Masculine protest**    Adler's term for the individual's (male/female) attempt to escape from the feminine submissive role.

**Melancholia**    A term used since ancient times to refer to a severe form of depression.

**Minimization**    Revaluing a topic as a means of reducing stress—for example, minimizing blame for behavior to avoid shame and guilt.

**Mood disorders (affective disorders)**    The main characteristic is a primary pervasive disturbance in mood.

**Mood episode (major depressive, manic, or hypomanic)**    A mood syndrome that is not due to a known organic factor and is not part of a nonmood psychotic disorder.

**Mood syndrome**    A group of mood and associated symptoms that occur together for a minimal period of time.

**Multiple personality**    The essential feature of this disorder is the existence within the person of two or more distinct personalities or personality states.

**Münchhausen syndrome**    In this chronic form of the disorder, the person's plausible presentation of factitious physical symptoms is associated with multiple hospitalizations.

**Narcissistic personality disorder**    The essential feature of this disorder is a pervasive pattern of grandiosity (in fantasy or behavior), hypersensitivity to the evaluation of others, and lack of empathy that begins by early adulthood and is present in a variety of contexts.

**Necrophilia**    The deriving of sexual gratification from corpses.

**Neuroleptic malignant syndrome (NMS)**    The rare sometimes fatal complication of treatment with high-potency neuroleptics, consisting of hyperthermia, sweating, neuromuscularigidity, abnormal blood pressure, and usually some disturbance of consciousness.

**Neurons**    Consist of a cell body (soma), a set of extending processes that convey information to the cell body (dendrites), and an extended process that carries information away from the cell (axon).

**Nosology**    The technical term used to refer to the science of classification of disorders.

**Nuclear magnetic response imaging (NMR)**    Produces images of the brain that are superior to those obtained by CAT scan and permit the detection of small variations or deviations in brain structure.

**Obsessions**    Persistent ideas, thoughts, impulses, or images that are experienced, at least initially, as intrusive and senseless.

**Obsessive-compulsive disorders**    The essential feature is recurrent obsessions or compulsions that are sufficiently severe to cause marked distress, are time-consuming, or significantly interfere with the person's normal routine, occupational functioning, or usual social activities or relationships.

**Obsessive-compulsive personality disorder**    The essential feature of this disorder is a pervasive pattern of perfectionism and inflexibility, beginning by early adulthood and present in a variety of contexts.

**Organic mental disorder**    Designates a particular organic mental syndrome in which the etiology is known or presumed.

**Organic mental syndrome**    Refers to a constellation of psychological or behavioral signs and symptoms without reference to etiology.

**Organic mood syndrome**    The essential feature is a prominent and persistent depressed, elevated, or expansive mood, resembling either a manic episode or a major depressive episode, which is due to a specific organic factor.

**Overcompensation**    An exaggerated attempt to overcome inferiorities.

**Panic disorder without agoraphobia**    Essential features of these disorders are recurrent panic attacks, that is, discrete periods of intense fear or discomfort, with at least four characteristic associated symptoms: shortness of breath or smothering sensations, dizziness, unsteady feelings, or faintness.

**Paranoid personality disorder**    The essential feature of this disorder is a pervasive and unwarranted tendency, beginning by early adulthood and present in a variety of contexts, to interpret the actions of people as deliberately demeaning or threatening.

**Paranoid schizophrenia**    The essential feature is preoccupation with one or more systematized delusions or with frequent auditory hallucinations related to a single theme.

**Paraphilias**    Characterized by arousal and response to sexual objects or situations that are not part of normative arousal-activity patterns and that in varying degrees may interfere with the capacity for reciprocal, affectionate sexual activity; and sexual dysfunctions, characterized by inhibitions in sexual desire or the psychophysiologic changes that characterize the sexual response cycle.

**Partialism**    Preoccupation with certain parts of the female body.

**Passive aggression**    A mechanism in which a person indirectly and unassertively expresses aggression toward others.

**Passive-aggressive personality disorder**    The essential feature of this disorder is a pervasive pattern of passive resistance to demands for adequate social and occupational performance, beginning by early adulthood and present in a variety of contexts.

**Pathological gambling**    The essential features of this disorder are a chronic and progressive failure to resist impulses to gamble, and gambling behavior that compromises, disrupts, or damages personal, family, or vocational pursuits.

**Patterns of drinking**    Usually of two types:
Spree or periodic drinkers
Continual drinkers

**Pedophilia**    The essential feature of this disorder is recurrent, intense sexual urges and sexually arousing fantasies, of at least six months' duration, involving sexual activity with a prepubescent child.

**Perpetuating factors**    Conditions that maintain, prolong, or exacerbate the symptoms or course of a disorder.

**Personality**    The sum total of the individual's internal and external patterns of adjustment to life.

**Personality disorders needing further study**

<u>Late luteal phase dysphoric disorder</u>    The essential feature is a pattern of clinically significant emotional and behavioral symptoms that occur during the last week of the luteal phase and remit within a few days after the onset of the follicular phase.

<u>Sadistic personality disorder</u>    The essential feature of this disorder is a pervasive pattern of cruel, demeaning, and aggressive behavior directed toward other people, beginning by early adulthood. The sadistic behavior is often evident both in social relationships (particularly with family members) and at work (with subordinates), but seldom is displayed in contacts with people in positions of authority or higher status.

<u>Self-defeating personality disorder</u>    The essential feature of this disorder is a pervasive pattern of self-defeating behavior, beginning by early adulthood and present in a variety of contexts.

**Persuasion**    Direct suggestion, inducement, or entreatment in an effort to influence a patient's behavior.

**Physical dependence**    Physical dependence on a drug is indicated if a person develops dysfunctional physiological symptoms when the drug is reduced or withdrawn (withdrawal effects).

**Placebo effects**    Reactions to pharmacologically inert substances.

**Positron emission tomography (PET)**    Radioactive isotopes are injected into the bloodstream and permit detection of regional differences in the metabolic activity of the brain.

**Post-traumatic stress disorder**    Introduced in *DSM*-III in 1980 and assembled together a seemingly disparate collection of entities including battle fatigue, war neurosis, concentration camp syndrome, post-Vietnam syndrome and post-disaster syndrome, thus emphasizing the ubiquity of the emotional responses manifested by the individuals faced with a psychological trauma of overpowering magnitude.

**Precipitating factors**    Events that precede and contribute to the clinical onset of a disorder.

**Preconscious**    Midway between the conscious and the unconscious.

**Predisposing factors**    Factors that render the personality susceptible or vulnerable and generally are present over a long period of time.

**Projection**    The attributing, to another person or object, the thoughts, feelings, motives, or desires that are really one's own disavowed and unacceptable traits.

**Projective identification**    The association of uncomfortable aspects of one's own personality with their projection onto another person, resulting in identification with the other person.

**Pseudodementia**    Characterized by exaggerated indifference to one's surroundings, without actual mental impairment, and reversible decline of mental functioning, which occurs in depression.

**Psychoactive substance use disorders**    This diagnostic class deals with the symptoms and maladaptive behavioral changes associated with more or less regular use of psychoactive substances that affect the central nervous system.

**Psychoanalysis**    A theory of how the mind works, an investigative or research method, a specific form of therapy.

**Psychobiology**    Studies not only the person as a whole, as a unit, but also the whole person.

**Psychodynamic psychotherapy**    Based on assumptions that are derived from psychoanalytic theory.

**Psychodynamics**    The study, explanation, or interpretation of behavior or mental states in terms of mental or emotional forces or processes.

**Psychogenic amnesia**    The essential feature of this disorder is sudden inability to recall important personal information, an inability not due to an organic mental disorder.

**Psychogenic fugue**    The essential feature of this disorder is sudden, unexpected travel away from home or customary work locale with assumption of a new identity and an inability to recall one's previous identity.

**Psychogenic hypothesis**    Regards mental disorder as the outcome of psychosocial (environmental) factors that influence the development of personality and the adequacy of the individual to manage the satisfaction of personal needs and the requirements of the circumstances of one's life.

**Psychological dependence**    Not a precisely defined term, but usually refers to a degree of loss of control in drug self-administration which does not entail physical dependence.

**Psychosocial stressors**    Etiology of mental disorders should be regarded as a complex interaction of genetic, physical, and psychosocial factors.

**Psychosomatic approach or movement**    Assumes that psychological and social factors are significant predispositions, onsets, and continuations of any illnesses.

**Psychotherapy**    A process in which a person who wishes to relieve *symptoms* or resolve problems in living or is seeking personal growth enters into an implicit or explicit contract to interact in a prescribed way with the psychotherapist.

**Pyromania**    The essential features of this disorder are deliberate and purposeful (rather than accidental) fire setting on more than one occasion; tension or affective arousal prior to setting the fires; and intense pleasure, gratification, or relief when setting the fires or witnessing or participating in their aftermath.

**Rapport**     The feeling of harmonious accord and mutual responsiveness that contributes to the patient's confidence in the therapist and willingness to work cooperatively. It is to be distinguished from *transference,* which is unconscious.

**Rationalization**     The ascribing of acceptable or worthwhile motives to one's own thoughts, feelings, or behavior that really have unrecognized motives.

**Reaction formation**     The direction of overt behavior or attitudes in precisely the opposite direction of the individual's underlying, unacceptable conscious or unconscious impulses.

**Reassurance**     The imparting or restoration of confidence and freeing the patient from fear and anxiety.

**Regression**     The unconscious return to an earlier level of emotional adjustment at which gratification was assured (turning back the maturational clock and going back to earlier modes of dealing with the world).

**Reliability**     The consistency with which a test measures what it proposes to measure.

**Repression**     The involuntary, automatic banishment of unacceptable ideas, impulses, or feelings into the unconscious (motivated unconscious forgetting).

**Residual schizophrenia**     Equivalent of the category, in partial remission.

**Resistance**     Arises from the conscious or unconscious psychological forces in the patient that oppose bringing repressed (unconscious) material into consciousness.

**Restitution**     The supplanting of a highly valued object that has been lost through rejection by, or death or departure of, another object.

**Sado-masochism**     The occurrence of sadism and masochism in the same person.

**Schizoid personality disorder**     The essential feature of this disorder is a pervasive pattern of indifference to social relationships and a restricted range of emotional experience and expression, beginning by early adulthood and present in a variety of contexts.

**Schizophrenia**     A large group of disorders, usually of psychotic proportion, manifested by characteristic disturbances of language and communication, thought, perception, affect, and behavior, which last longer than six months.

**Schizotypal personality disorder**     The essential feature of this disorder is a pervasive pattern of peculiarities of ideation, appearance, and behavior, and deficits in interpersonal relatedness, beginning by early adulthood and present in a variety of contexts.

**Seasonal affective disorder (SAD)**     The diagnostic criteria for this disorder are: a regular temporal relationship between the onset of an episode of bipolar disorder or recurrent major depression and a particular sixty-day period of the year; full remission or change from depression to mania or hypomania also occurred within a particular sixty-day period of the year.

**Selective amnesia**     Failure to recall some, but not all, of the events occurring during a circumscribed period of time.

**Self-help or support groups**     Groups that function without a professional facilitator. The group experience does not uncover basic conflicts but does offer new shared experiences to the patient.

**Sexual deviancy**     Includes any sexual behavior that is at variance with more or less culturally accepted norms.

**Sexual dysfunctions**    The essential feature of this subclass is inhibition in the appetitive or psychophysiologic changes that characterize the complete sexual response cycle.

**Sexual masochism**    The essential feature of this disorder is recurrent, intense sexual urges and sexually arousing fantasies, of at least six months' duration, involving the act (real, not simulated) of being humiliated, beaten, bound, or otherwise made to suffer.

**Sexual sadism**    The essential feature of this disorder is recurrent, intense sexual urges and sexually arousing fantasies, of at least six months' duration, involving acts (real, not simulated) in which the psychological or physical suffering (including humiliation) of the victim is sexually exciting.

**Sexual urethran**    Erotic arousal through stimulation of the urethra (primarily a female paraphilia).

**Simple phobia**    The essential feature of this disorder is a persistent fear of a circumscribed stimulus (object or situation) other than fear of having a panic attack (as in panic disorder) or of humiliation or embarrassment in certain social situations (as in social phobia).

**Simulation**    Role playing.

**Social phobia**    The essential feature of this disorder is a persistent fear of one or more situations (the social phobic situations) in which the person is exposed to possible scrutiny by others and fears that he or she may do something or act in a way that will be humiliating or embarrassing.

**Somatization disorder**    The essential features of this disorder are recurrent and multiple somatic complaints, of several years' duration, for which medical attention has been sought, but that apparently are not due to any physical disorder.

**Somatoform disorders**    The essential features of this group of disorders are physical symptoms suggesting physical disorder (hence, somatoform), for which there are no demonstrable organic findings or known physiologic mechanisms, and for which there is positive evidence, or a strong presumption, that the symptoms are linked to psychological factors or conflicts.

**Somatoform pain disorder**    The essential feature of this disorder is preoccupation with pain in the absence of adequate physical findings to account for the pain or its intensity.

**Somatogenic hypothesis**    Regards mental disorders as resulting from the malfunction of the central nervous system, reflecting physical influences or genetically transmitted conditions, in a way that affects cognitive, emotional, and expressive processes.

**Splitting**    The inability to unite and integrate the hating and loving aspect of both one's self-image and one's image of another person.

**Standardization**    The establishment of responses of reference groups so that individual performance may be compared with the performance of an appropriate group.

**Sublimation**    The diversion of unacceptable, instinctual drives into socially sanctioned channels.

**Substitution**    An unconscious replacement of a highly valued but unattainable or unacceptable emotional goal or object by one that is attainable or acceptable.

**Superego**    The censoring force of the personality.

**Supportive psychotherapy**    Deals predominantly with conscious material and is centered chiefly on bolstering the individual's strength and assets (enhancing self-esteem and ego strength).

**Suppression**    The voluntary, intentional relegation of unacceptable ideas or impulses to the foreconscious (volitional exclusion, or conscious forgetting).

**Symbolization**    The unconscious mechanism by which a neutral idea or object is used to represent another idea or object that has a forbidden aspect.

**Syndrome**    A cluster of symptoms that occur together as part of a recognizable condition.

**Tardive dyskinesia**    Symptoms include choreiform involuntary movements and dyskinesia of the face and mouth, which produce such things as smacking lips, protuberances of the tongues, and grotesque facial grimaces.

**Telencephalon**    Consists of the cerebral hemispheres.

**Telephone scatologia**    Sexual gratification derived usually by men who telephone women, make obscene remarks, and suggest that the women meet them and engage in sexual activity.

**Trance state**    A psychological stupor characterized by immobility and unresponsiveness to the environment.

**Transference**    The patient's unconscious attachment to the therapist (or others involved in the patient's treatment) of feelings and attitudes that were originally related to important figures (e.g., parents, siblings) in early life.

**Transsexualism**    The essential features of this disorder are a persistent discomfort and a sense of inappropriateness about one's assigned sex in a person who has reached puberty.

**Transvestic fetishism**    The essential feature of this disorder is recurrent, intense sexual urges and sexually arousing fantasies, of at least six months' duration, involving cross-dressing.

**Trichotillomania**    The essential feature of this disorder is recurrent failure to resist impulses to pull out one's own hair.

**Turner's syndrome**    A chromosomal defect in women with a karyotype of XO and with forty-five rather than the usual forty-six chromosomes.

**Unburdening**    The therapeutic release of feelings through conscious, free expression.

**Unconscious**    Made up of drives, feelings, ideas, and urges that are outside of the individual's awareness.

**Undifferentiated schizophrenia**    The essential features are:
   1. Permanent psychotic symptoms (delusions, hallucinations, incoherence, or grossly disorganized behavior) that cannot be classified as catatonic, disorganized, or paranoid, or
   2. Meets the criteria for more than one category

**Undoing**    A primitive defense mechanism in which some unacceptable past behavior is symbolically acted out in reverse, usually repetitiously.

**Urophilia**    A pathologic love for, or interest in, urine.

**Validity**    The accuracy with which a test fulfills its purpose of prediction, selection, or classification.

**Vorbeireden**    Giving the approximate answers or talking past the point.

**Voyeurism**    The essential feature of this disorder is recurrent, intense sexual urges and sexually arousing fantasies, of at least six months' duration, involving the act of observing unsuspecting people, usually strangers, who are either naked, in the process of disrobing, or engaging in sexual activity.

**Wernicke's disease**   A rare disorder of central nervous system metabolism, associated with a thiamine deficiency and seen chiefly in chronic alcoholics.

**Working through**   Follows the development of insight and constitutes a major portion of the treatment time. It includes repeated exploration of the insight gained through interpretation.

**Zoophilia**   The essential feature of this disorder is the use of animals as a repeatedly preferred or exclusive method of achieving sexual excitement.

# Index

Monoamines (biogenic amines) 51
Mood
    disorders 96, 341
    episode 342
    modifiers 153
    syndrome 342
More, Thomas 4
Morel, Benedict Augustin 367
Mowrer, O. H. 127
Multiaxial
    classification 95
    system 95
Multiple personality 206
Münchhausen syndrome 315
Muscular-anal stage 25
Musical therapy 144

Narcissistic personality disorder 251
Narcosynthesis 195
Necrophilia 292
Negative
    reinforcement 37
    symptoms (of schiozophrenia) 373
Nerve action potential 46
Nervous system
    central nervous system (CNS) 46, 52
    peripheral nervous system (PNS) 46
Neurasthenic symptoms 348
Neuroactive substances 50
Neurobiological foundations 45
Neurohormones 54
Neuroleptic malignant syndrome (NMS)
    152
Neuromodulators 54
Neuron 49
Neuropeptides 52
Neuropsychological tests 114
Neuroscience 45
Neurotransmission 49
Neurotransmitters 50, 51
Nicotine 312
n-methyl-d-asparatate (NMDA) 51
Norepinephrine 51
Nosology 91
Nuclear magnetic response imaging
    (NMR) 102

Object
    libido 16
    relations theory 24
Objective personality tests 108
Obsessions 178
Obsessive-compulsive disorders 178
Obsessive-compulsive personality disorder
    256
Obsessive-ruminative state 179
Occupational therapy 143
Oedipus complex 18
Operant
    Conditioning 36, 38, 44, 129

Opioid substances 310
Oral character 19
Organ inferiority 19
Organic
    Anxiety syndrome 403
    causes of 405
    Delusional syndrome 403
    Hallucinosis 403
    Mental disorder 92, 399
    Mental syndrome 399, 403
    Mood syndrome 364, 403
    Personality syndrome 403
Orgasm disorders 296
Outcome expectancies 39, 43
Overcompensation 80

Pain, chronic 201, 202
Panic 167
Panic disorder with agoraphobia 169
Panic disorder without agoraphobia 169,
    172
Paranoia 389
Paranoid
    Personality disorder 235
    Schizophrenia 377
Paraphilias 276
Parasympathetic division 47
Parataxic distortions 24
Paresis, general 6
Partialism 292
Passive aggression 86
Passive-aggressive personality disorder 258
Pathological gambling 269
Patterns of drinking 325
Pavlov, Ivan 6, 34, 126, 128
Pedophilia 284
Penis envy 18
Period
    of concrete operational thought 41
    pf formal operational thought 41
    prevalence 57
Periodic catatonic type 92, 375
Peripheral nervous system 46
Perpetuating factors 56
Persona 21
Personality
    development 11, 19, 232
    disorder, characteristics of 233
    disorders, treatment of 236, 263
    disorders, types of 234
    tests 107, 108, 109, 110, 111, 112
Persuasion 125
Phallic character 19
Pharmacological and somatic treatment
    147
Pharmacological principles 148
Phencyclidine (PCP) 311
Phenelzine (Nardil) 154
Phenomenological reality 29
Phenothiazines 150

Urophilia 293

Validity 104
Van Gogh, Vincent 366
Verbal therapies 145
Vocational and educational tests 114
Voltage changes 49
Von Hartman, Eduard 13
von Krafft-Ebing, Richard 6, 275
Vorbeireden 217
Voyeurism 290

Wagner-Jauregg, Julius 6
Wasserman Test 6
Watson, John 9, 35, 126
Wechsler
    Adult Intelligence Scale (WAIS-R) 107
    Intelligence Scale for Children
        (WISC-R) 107

Preschool Primary Scale of
    Intelligence (WPPSI-R) 107
Weiss, Jay 43
Wernicke's disease 328
Western history
    eras in 2
Weyer, Johann 4
Winnicot, Donald 25
Withdrawal 404
Wolpe, Joseph 127
Working through 121, 122
Wundt, Wilhelm 6

Young adulthood 26

Zoophilia 292